PROGRESS IN CLINICAL AND BIOLOGICAL RESEARCH

RECENT TITLES

See pages 351–352 for previous titles in this series.

THE PROSTATIC CELL: STRUCTURE AND FUNCTION

PART B

PROLACTIN, CARCINOGENESIS, AND CLINICAL ASPECTS

THE PROSTATIC CELL: STRUCTURE AND FUNCTION

PART B

PROLACTIN, CARCINOGENESIS, AND CLINICAL ASPECTS

Editors

GERALD P. MURPHY, MD, DSc
Director, Roswell Park Memorial Institute
Director, National Prostatic Cancer Project
Buffalo, New York

AVERY A. SANDBERG, MD
Department of Genetics and Endocrinology
Roswell Park Memorial Institute
Buffalo, New York

JAMES P. KARR, PhD
Deputy Director for Scientific Affairs
National Prostatic Cancer Project
Buffalo, New York

ALAN R. LISS, INC. • NEW YORK

Address all Inquiries to the Publisher
Alan R. Liss, Inc., 150 Fifth Avenue, New York, NY 10011

Printed in the United States of America.

Library of Congress Cataloging in Publication Data

Main entry under title:

The Prostatic cell.

(Progress in clinical and biological research; 75A-75B)
Proceedings of a workshop conducted by the National Prostatic Cancer Project and held at Roswell Park Memorial Institute, Buffalo, N.Y., Mar. 5–7, 1981.
Includes bibliographical references and index.
Contents: pt. A. Morphologic, secretory, and biochemical aspects — pt. B. Prolactin, carcinogenesis, and clinical aspects.
1. Prostate gland — Cancer — Congresses. 2. Cancer cells — Congresses. 3. Prostate gland — Congresses. I. Murphy, Gerald Patrick. II. Sandberg, Avery A. III. Karr, James P. IV. National Prostatic Cancer Project. V. Series. [DNLM: 1. Prostate — Cytology — Congresses. WI PR668E v. 75 / WJ 750 P965 1981]
RC280.P7P78   616.99'463   81-17146
ISBN 0-8451-0075-0 (set)   AACR2
ISBN 0-8451-0161-7 (pt. A)
ISBN 0-8451-0162-5 (pt. B)

THE PROSTATIC CELL: STRUCTURE AND FUNCTION

A Workshop Organized by the National Prostatic Cancer Project Buffalo, New York, March 5-7, 1981

Chairmen, Organizing Committee

James P. Karr, PhD
Avery A. Sandberg, MD
Gerald P. Murphy, MD, DSc

Host

Roswell Park Memorial Institute

Contents of Part B

CLINICAL STUDIES

Contributors to Part B

John A. Arcadi, Department of Biology, Whittier College Cancer Research Laboratory, Whittier College, Whittier, California 90608 **[329]**

Frederick H. Batzold, Department of Biochemistry, Albany Medical College, Albany, New York 12208 **[269]**

E. Borgström, Department of Urology, Karolinska Institutet, Stockholm, Sweden **[299]**

David Brandes, Department of Pathology, The Johns Hopkins School of Medicine and Baltimore City Hospitals, Baltimore, Maryland 21224 **[207]**

Leif Busk, Department of Toxicology, Swedish Food Administration, S-751 26 Uppsala, Sweden **[191]**

Sham-Yuen Chan, Department of Microbiology, Lobund Laboratory, University of Notre Dame, Notre Dame, Indiana 46556 **[249]**

Andrew Chiarodo, National Organ Site Programs Branch, Division of Resources, Centers and Community Activities, National Cancer Institute, Bethesda, Maryland 20205

Hans Deutsch, Department of Toxicology and Experimental Pathology, c/o Dr. Karl Thomae GmbH, Biberach/Riss, West Germany **[231]**

D.R. Fahmy, Tenovus Institute for Cancer Research, Welsh National School of Medicine, Heath, Cardiff, United Kingdom, CF4 4XX **[31]**

Isaiah J. Fidler, Cancer Metastasis and Treatment Laboratory, National Cancer Institute, Frederick Cancer Research Center, P.O. Box B, Frederick, Maryland 21701 **[257]**

Hans Glaumann, Department of Pathology, Huddinge Hospital, S-141 86, Huddinge, Sweden **[191]**

K. Griffiths, Tenovus Institute for Cancer Research, Welsh National School of Medicine, Heath, Cardiff, United Kingdom, CF4 4XX **[31, 115]**

Jan-Åke Gustafsson, Department of Medical Nutrition, Karolinska Institutet, Box 60400, S-104 01 Stockholm, Sweden **[191, 299]**

Tapio Haaparanta, Department of Pathology, Huddinge Hospital, S-141 86, Huddinge, Sweden **[191]**

Miasnig Hagopian, Section on Chemical Carcinogenesis, Mason Research Institute, Worcester, Massachusetts 01605 **[131]**

M.E. Harper, Tenovus Institute for Cancer Research, Welsh National School of Medicine, Heath, Cardiff, United Kingdom, CF4 4XX **[31, 115]**

Bertil Högberg, Department of Pharmacology, Karolinska Institutet, Box 60400, S-104 01 Stockholm, Sweden **[191, 299]**

Christoph Hohbach, Department of Toxicology and Experimental Pathology, c/o Dr. Karl Thomae GmbH, Biberach/Riss, West Germany **[231]**

Myong Won Kahng, Department of Pathology, University of Maryland School of Medicine, 10 South Pine Street, Baltimore, Maryland 21201 **[183]**

James P. Karr, National Prostatic Cancer Project, 666 Elm Street, Buffalo, New York 14263 **[xxv]**

John A. Katzenellenbogen, Department of Chemistry, University of Illinois School of Chemical Sciences, 461 Roger Adams Laboratory, Box 37, 1209 West California, Urbana, Illinois 61801 **[313]**

Edward J. Keenan, Departments of Surgery and Pharmacology, Hormone Receptor Laboratory, University of Oregon Health Sciences Center School of Medicine, 3181 Southwest Sam Jackson Park Road, Portland, Oregon 97201 **[9]**

Elaine D. Kemp, Departments of Surgery and Pharmacology, University of Oregon Health Sciences Center School of Medicine, 3181 Southwest Sam Jackson Park Road, Portland, Oregon 97201 **[9]**

Leon Lack, Department of Pharmacology, Duke Medical Center, Box 3185, Durham, North Carolina 27710 **[283]**

Joseph Meites, Department of Physiology, Neuroendocrine Research Laboratory, Michigan State University, East Lansing, Michigan 48824 **[1]**

Gerald P. Murphy, National Prostatic Cancer Project and Roswell Park Memorial Institute, 666 Elm Street, Buffalo, New York 14263 **[xxv, 341]**

W.B. Peeling, Department of Urology, St. Woolos' Hospital, Newport, Gwent, United Kingdom **[31, 115]**

Vladimir Petrow, Department of Pharmacology, Duke Medical Center, Box 3185, Durham, North Carolina 27710 **[283]**

C.G. Pierrepoint, Tenovus Institute for Cancer Research, Welsh National School of Medicine, Heath, Cardiff, United Kingdom, CF4 4XX **[31]**

Morris Pollard, Department of Microbiology, Lobund Laboratory, University of Notre Dame, Notre Dame, Indiana 46556 **[249]**

S. Poolsawat, Department of Biology, Whittier College Cancer Research Laboratory, Whittier College, Whittier, California 90608 **[329]**

George Poste, Smith Kline and French Laboratories, Philadelphia, Pennsylvania 19101 **[257]**

Åke Pousette, Department of Medical Nutrition, Karolinska Institutet, Box 60400, S-104 01 Stockholm, Sweden **[191, 299]**

Elizabeth E. Ramsey, Departments of Surgery and Pharmacology, University of Oregon Health Sciences Center School of Medicine, 3181 Southwest Sam Jackson Park Road, Portland, Oregon 97201 **[9]**

Avery A. Sandberg, Department of Genetics and Endocrinology, Roswell Park Memorial Institute, 666 Elm Street, Buffalo, New York 14263 **[xxv, 55]**

P.E.C. Sibley, Tenovus Institute for Cancer Research, Welsh National School of Medicine, Heath, Cardiff, United Kingdom, CF4 4XX **[115]**

Nelson H. Slack, National Prostatic Cancer Project, Roswell Park Memorial Institute, 666 Elm Street, Buffalo, New York 14263 **[341]**

W. Roy Slaunwhite, Jr., Department of Biochemistry, State University of New York at Buffalo Schools of Medicine and Dentistry, Buffalo, New York 14214 **[19]**

Emil R. Smith, Department of Pharmacology, University of Massachusetts Medical School, 55 Lake Avenue North, Worchester, Massachusetts 01605 **[131]**

Mary W. Smith, Department of Pathology, University of Maryland School of Medicine, 10 South Pine Street, Baltimore, Maryland 21201 **[183]**

Peter Söderkvist, Departments of Medical Nutrition and Pharmacology, Karolinska Institutet, Box 60400, S-104 01 Stockholm, Sweden **[191]**

Rune Toftgård, Departments of Medical Nutrition and Pharmacology, Karolinska Institutet, Box 60400, S-104 01 Stockholm, Sweden **[191]**

Frank M. Torti, Division of Oncology, Stanford University School of Medicine, Stanford, California 94305 **[335]**

Benjamin F. Trump, Department of Pathology, University of Maryland School of Medicine, 10 South Pine Street, Baltimore, Maryland 21201 **[183]**

Heinz Ueberberg, Department of Toxicology and Experimental Pathology, c/o Dr. Karl Thomae GmbH, Biberach/Riss, West Germany **[231]**

Willard J. Visek, University of Illinois, 190 Medical Sciences Building, 506 South Matthews Avenue, Urbana, Illinois 61801 **[165]**

Mukta M. Webber, Division of Urology, Department of Surgery, University of Colorado Health Sciences Center, Box C-319, 4200 East 9th Avenue, Denver, Colorado 80262 **[63]**

Raphael J. Witorsch, Department of Physiology, Medical College of Virginia School of Basic Sciences, Virginia Commonwealth University, Box 551, Richmond, Virginia 23298 **[89]**

Contents of Part A: Morphologic, Secretory, and Biochemical Aspects

UNIQUE PROSTATIC PROTEINS

TRACE METALS

Contributors to Part A: Morphologic, Secretory, and Biochemical Aspects

Khalil Ahmed, Department of Laboratory Medicine and Pathology, University of Minnesota; Veterans Administration Medical Center, Toxicology Research Laboratory, 4801 East 54th Street, Minneapolis, Minnesota 55417

Neil G. Anderson, Department of Pharmacology, University of Colorado School of Pharmacy, Campus Box 297, Boulder, Colorado 80309

Gerhard Aumüller, Department of Anatomy and Cell Biology, Philipps-Universität at Marburg, Robert-Koch-Strasse 6, 3550 Marburg, West Germany

Evelyn R. Barrack, Department of Urology and Oncology Center, The James Buchanan Brady Urological Institute, The Johns Hopkins University School of Medicine, Baltimore, Maryland 21205

Richard J. Bartlett, Department of Pediatrics and Cancer Research Center, University of North Carolina, Chapel Hill, North Carolina 27514

S. Battersby, Tenovus Institute for Cancer Research, Welsh National School of Medicine, Heath, Cardiff, United Kingdom, CF4 4XX

Per Björk, AB Leo Research Laboratories, Box 941, S-251 Helsingborg, Sweden

D. Bossyns, Laboratorium voor Experimentele Geneeskunde en Laboratorium voor Biochemie, Faculteit Geneeskunde, Katholieke Universiteit Leuven, Rega Instituut, Minderbroedersstraat 10, B-3000, Leuven, Belgium

N. Bruchovsky, Department of Cancer Endocrinology, Cancer Control Agency of British Columbia, 2656 Heather Street, Vancouver, British Columbia, Canada, V5Z 3J3

M.E. Burns, Department of Biochemistry, Boston University School of Medicine, Boston, Massachusetts 02118

Kjell Carlström, Hormone Laboratory, Sabbatsberg Hospital, Box 6401, S-113 82 Stockholm, Sweden

J.A. Chandler, Tenovus Institute for Cancer Research, Welsh National School of Medicine, Heath, Cardiff, United Kingdom, CF4 4XX

Chawnshang Chang, Department of Biochemistry, The Ben May Laboratory for Cancer Research, The University of Chicago, 950 East 59th Street, Chicago, Illinois 60637

Andrew Chiarodo, National Organ Site Programs Branch, Division of Resources, Centers and Community Activities, National Cancer Institute, Bethesda, Maryland 20205

T. Ming Chu, Department of Diagnostic Immunology Research and Biochemistry, Roswell Park Memorial Institute, 666 Elm Street, Buffalo, New York 14263

Leland W.K. Chung, Department of Pharmacology, University of Colorado School of Pharmacy, Boulder, Colorado 80309

Donald S. Coffey, Department of Urology and Oncology Center, The James Buchanan Brady Urological Institute, The Johns Hopkins University School of Medicine, Baltimore, Maryland 21205

Gary A. Croghan, Department of Diagnostic Immunology Research and Biochemistry, Roswell Park Memorial Institute, 666 Elm Street, Buffalo, New York 14263

Gerald R. Cunha, Department of Anatomy, University of Colorado Health Sciences Center School of Medicine, Denver, Colorado 80262

Karen A. Curto, Department of Pharmacology and Toxicology, West Virginia University Medical Center, Morgantown, West Virginia 26506

P. De Moor, Laboratorium voor Experimentele Geneeskunde en Laboratorium voor Biochemie, Faculteit Geneeskunde, Katholieke Universiteit Leuven, Rega Instituut, Minderbroedersstraat 10, B-3000, Leuven, Belgium

Michael P. Donovan, Department of Pharmacology and Toxicology, West Virginia University Medical Center, Morgantown, West Virginia 26506

William R. Fair, Division of Urology, Washington University School of Medicine, 4960 Audubon Avenue, St. Louis, Missouri 63110

Wells E. Farnsworth, Department of Biochemistry, Chicago College of Osteopathic Medicine, 1122 East 53rd Street, Chicago, Illinois 60615

Björn Forsgren, AB Leo Research Laboratories, Box 941, S-251 09 Helsingborg, Sweden

Frank S. French, Department of Pediatrics, University of North Carolina, Chapel Hill, North Carolina 27514

D.K. Fujii, Departments of Medicine and Ophthalmology, Cancer Research Institute and University of California Medical Center, San Francisco, California 94143

L. Giguere, Department of Medicine and Ophthalmology, Cancer Research Institute and University of California Medical Center, San Francisco, California 94143

D. Gospodarowicz, Departments of Medicine and Ophthalmology, Cancer Research Institute and University of California Medical Center, San Francisco, California 94143

Said A. Goueli, Department of Laboratory Medicine and Pathology, Toxicology Research Laboratory, University of Minnesota, Veterans Administration Medical Center, Minneapolis, Minnesota 55417

John T. Grayhack, Department of Urology, Northwestern University Medical School, 303 East Chicago Avenue, Chicago, Illinois 60611

Jan-Åke Gustafsson, Department of Medical Nutrition, Karolinska Institutet, Box 60400, S-104 01 Stockholm, Sweden [391]

Ferenc Gyorkey, Departments of Pathology, Pharmacology, and Virology, Baylor College of Medicine and Veterans Administration Medical Center, 2002 Holcombe Boulevard, Houston, Texas 77211

Barry M. Heatfield, Department of Pathology, University of Maryland School of Medicine, 10 South Pine Street, Baltimore, Maryland 21201

Walter Heyns, Laboratorium voor Experimentele Geneeskunde, Rega Instituut, Leuven, Belgium

Richard A. Hiipakka, Department of Biochemistry, The Ben May Laboratory for Cancer Research, The University of Chicago, 950 East 59th Street, Chicago, Illinois 60637

Bertil Högberg, Department of Pharmacology, Karolinska Institutet, Box 60400, S-104 01 Stockholm, Sweden

Julius S. Horoszewicz, Department of Viral Oncology, Roswell Park Memorial Institute, 666 Elm Street, Buffalo, New York 14263

John T. Isaacs, Department of Urology and Oncology Center, The James Buchanan Brady Urological Institute, The Johns Hopkins University School of Medicine, Baltimore, Maryland 21205

William B. Isaacs, Department of Urology and Oncology Center, The James Buchanan Brady Urological Institute, The Johns Hopkins University School of Medicine, Baltimore, Maryland 21205

Stephen C. Jacobs, Department of Urology, The Medical College of Wisconsin, 9200 West Wisconsin Avenue, Milwaukee, Wisconsin 53226

Sheila M. Judge, Department of Biochemistry, The Ben May Laboratory for Cancer Research, The University of Chicago, 950 East 59th Street, Chicago, Illinois 60637

James P. Karr, National Prostatic Cancer Project, 666 Elm Street, Buffalo, New York 14263

Manabu Kuriyama, Department of Diagnostic Immunology Research and Biochemistry, Roswell Park Memorial Institute, 666 Elm Street, Buffalo, New York 14263

Russell K. Lawson, Department of Urology, The Medical College of Wisconsin, 9200 West Wisconsin Avenue, Milwaukee, Wisconsin 53226

Oscar A. Lea, Department of Pharmacology, University of Bergen, Bergen, Norway

Chung Lee, Department of Urology, Northwestern University Medical School, 303 East Chicago Avenue, Chicago, Illinois 60611

Susan S. Leong, Department of Viral Oncology, Roswell Park Memorial Institute, 666 Elm Street, Buffalo, New York 14263

Shutsung Liao, Department of Biochemistry, The Ben May Laboratory for Cancer Research, The University of Chicago, 950 East 59th Street, Chicago, Illinois 60637

A. Mariotti, Departments of Urology and Pharmacology, West Virginia University Medical Center, Morgantown, West Virginia 26506

M. Mawhinney, Department of Pharmacology, West Virginia University Medical Center, Morgantown, West Virginia 26506

M.G. McLoughlin, Division of Urology, Department of Surgery, University of British Columbia, Vancouver, British Columbia, Canada, V5Z 1L7

J. Mous, Laboratorium voor Experimentele Geneeskunde en Laboratorium voor Biochemie, Faculteit Geneeskunde, Katholieke Universiteit Leuven, Rega Instituut, Minderbroedersstraat 10, B-3000, Leuven, Belgium

R.E. Muller, Department of Biochemistry, Boston University School of Medicine, Boston, Massachusetts 02118

J. Müntzing, AB Leo, Research Laboratories, Box 941, S-251 09 Helsingborg, Sweden

Gerald P. Murphy, National Prostatic Cancer Project and Roswell Park Memorial Institute, 666 Elm Street, Buffalo, New York 14263

Blake Lee Neubauer, Lilly Research Laboratories, Eli Lilly and Company, Indianapolis, Indiana 46285

Claudia M. Noyes, Department of Medicine, University of North Carolina, Chapel Hill, North Carolina 27514

Amy K. Oberhauser, Department of Biochemistry, The Ben May Laboratory for Cancer Research and the University of Chicago, 950 East 59th Street, Chicago, Illinois 60637

Lawrence D. Papsidero, Department of Diagnostic Immunology Research and Biochemistry, Roswell Park Memorial Institute, 666 Elm Street, Buffalo, New York 14263

Richard Parrish, Washington University School of Medicine, 4960 Audubon Avenue, St. Louis, Missouri 63110

B. Peeters, Laboratorium voor Experimentele Geneeskunde en Laboratorium voor Biochemie, Faculteit Geneeskunde, Katholieke Universiteit Leuven, Rega Instituut, Minderbroedersstraat 10, B-3000, Leuven, Belgium

Peter Petrusz, Department of Anatomy, University of North Carolina, Chapel Hill, North Carolina 27514

Patricia C. Phelps, Department of Pathology, University of Maryland School of Medicine, 10 South Pine Street, Baltimore, Maryland 21201

Å. Pousette, Department of Medical Nutrition, Karolinska Institutet, Box 60400, S-104 01 Stockholm, Sweden

P.S. Rennie, Department of Cancer Endocrinology, Cancer Control Agency of British Columbia, 2656 Heather Street, Vancouver, British Columbia, Canada, V5Z 3J3

Audrey K. Rocco, Department of Pharmacology, University of Colorado School of Pharmacy, Boulder, Colorado 80309

W. Rombauts, Laboratorium voor Experimentele Geneeskunde en Laboratorium voor Biochemie, Faculteit Geneeskunde, Katholieke Universiteit Leuven, Rega Instituut, Minderbroedersstraat 10, B-3000, Leuven, Belgium

Betty Rosoff, Department of Biology, Stern College, Yeshiva University, 245 Lexington Avenue, New York, New York 10016

Diane Haddock Russell, Department of Pharmacology, University of

Arizona Health Sciences Center, Tucson, Arizona 85724

Avery A. Sandberg, Department of Genetics and Endocrinology, Roswell Park Memorial Institute, 666 Elm Street, Buffalo, New York 14263

N. Savion, Departments of Medicine and Ophthalmology, Cancer Research Institute and University of California Medical Center, San Francisco, California 94143

Carl P. Schaffner, Waksman Institute of Microbiology, Rutgers —The State University of New Jersey, P.O. Box 759, Piscataway, New Jersey 08854

Karen Schilling, Department of Biochemistry, The Ben May Laboratory for Cancer Research, The University of Chicago, 950 East 59th Street, Chicago, Illinois 60637

Darrel W. Stafford, Department of Zoology, University of North Carolina, Chapel Hill, North Carolina 27514

Michael T. Story, Department of Urology, The Medical College of Wisconsin, 9200 West Wisconsin Avenue, Milwaukee, Wisconin 53226

J.-P. Tauber, Departments of Medicine and Ophthalmology, Cancer Research Institute and University of California Medical Center, San Francisco, California 94143

Peter F. Tauber, Department of Obstetrics and Gynecology, University of Essen, Essen, West Germany

John A. Thomas, Department of Pharmacology and Toxicology, West Virginia Medical Center, Morgantown, West Virginia 26506

Timothy C. Thompson, Department of Pharmacology, University of Colorado School of Pharmacy, Boulder, Colorado 80309

B.G. Timms, Tenovus Institute for Cancer Research, Welsh National School of Medicine, Heath, Cardiff, United Kingdom CF4 4XX

M.P. To, Department of Cancer Endocrinology, Cancer Control Agency of British Columbia, 2656 Heather Street, Vancouver, British Columbia, Canada, V5Z 3J3

A.M. Traish, Department of Biochemistry, Boston University School of Medicine, Boston, Massachusetts 02118

Benjamin F. Trump, Department of Pathology, University of Maryland School of Medicine, 10 South Pine Street, Baltimore, Maryland 21201

Luis A. Valenzuela, Department of Pathology, St. Joseph's Intercommunity Hospital, 2605 Harlem Road, Buffalo, New York 14225

David H. Viskochil, Departments of Pediatrics and Biochemistry, University of North Carolina, Chapel Hill, North Carolina 27514

I. Vlodavsky, Departments of Medicine and Ophthalmology, Cancer Research Institute and University of California Medical Center, San Francisco, California 94143

Michael P. Waalkes, Department of Pharmacology and Toxicology, West Virginia University Medical Center, Morgantown, West Virginia 26506

Ming C. Wang, Department of Diagnostic Immunology Research and Biochemistry, Roswell Park Memorial Institute, 666 Elm Street, Buffalo, New York 14263

Elizabeth M. Wilson, Departments of Pediatrics and Biochemistry,

University of North Carolina, Chapel Hill, North Carolina 27514
Michael J. Wilson, Department of Laboratory Medicine and Pathology, Toxicology Research Laboratory, University of Minnesota, Veterans Administration Medical Center, Minneapolis, Minnesota 55417
H.H. Wotiz, Departments of Biochemistry and Urology, Boston University School of Medicine, Boston, Massachusetts 02118
Lourens J.D. Zaneveld, Departments of Physiology and Biophysics, and Obstetrics and Gynecology, University of Illinois at the Medical Center, P.O. Box 6998, Chicago, Illinois 60680

Foreword: Organ Site Programs Overview

The National Organ Site Programs of the National Cancer Institute consist of grant-suppported National Projects of targeted cancer research. The program was established to stimulate research on important but neglected cancer problems that had not attracted a level of effort commensurate with the research leads available or with the mortality and morbidity associated with them. Currently there are four National Organ Site Projects concerned with cancer of the urinary bladder, large bowel, pancreas, and prostate. The overall strategy of each Project has been to share major responsibility between the National Cancer Institute and scientists throughout the nation for planning and coordinating a multidisciplinary research program aimed at prevention as well as decreased morbidity and mortality from the disease. Under the leadership of a national project director, this working cadre of laboratory and clinical scientists has developed a national plan of research within which priorities are identified in the areas of Etiology and Epidemiology, Detection and Diagnosis, and Treatment. This forms the basis for soliciting grant applications to help fulfill the aims and objectives of the national plan. Thus, the National Organ Site Programs permit the pursuit of targeted research through investigator-initiated efforts and the application of a spectrum of research disciplines to cancer at specific organ sites. It has involved the biomedical community in a unique scientific and managerial partnership with the National Cancer Institute. The effect has been to create research interest and activities where little existed before.

The National Prostatic Cancer Project, with Gerald P. Murphy as National Project Director, periodically conducts workshops on a timely basis to assess the state of the art in areas deemed ready for immediate implementation. In other instances, workshops are held with the objective of creating an atmosphere in which divergent topics are reviewed and brought into current focus, such that a cross fertilization of disciplines and ideas may stimulate thought for new investigational emphasis and direction. This book is one of two volumes that record the proceedings of such a workshop, entitled *The Prostatic Cell: Structure and Function,* held at Roswell Park Memorial Institute, Buffalo, New York, March 5–7, 1981.

The cordial hospitality and organizational effort mounted by the staff of Roswell Park Memorial Institute contributed to the success of the workshop. Special thanks are also extended to the participants.

June, 1981

Andrew Chiarodo, PhD
Chief, National Organ Site
    Programs Branch
Divison of Resources, Centers
    and Community Activities
National Cancer Institute
Bethesda, Maryland

Preface

The contents of this volume, the second of a two-part series, address the cellular and subcellular mechanisms of the prostate, topics that continue to be the focus of increasingly refined investigation. The common objective of these studies is to broaden the understanding of basic prostatic processes, many of which are specific and unique to the gland, so that new concepts can ultimately be tested in animal models of prostatic disease and applied clinically to human conditions. This volume brings the reader to the forefront of advances in the field.

The first section reflects a renewed interest in the study of prolactin and other polypeptide hormones in relation to the development of prostate tumors. New assays and in vitro and in vivo analyses of the role of prolactin in normal and diseased conditions of the prostate have further advanced our understanding of the hypophyseal hormones and their effects on the functioning and health of the prostate.

The reader will surely be intrigued by the next group of papers, which explores the relatively new field of enzyme induction and carcinogenesis in the prostate. Although these studies have not identified a link between environmental or occupational factors and prostate cancer in humans, the reports describe in detail the mechanisms by which such factors could have a causal effect, assays that may ultimately identify individuals at risk, and agents with potential prophylactic value.

The volume concludes with a number of ongoing investigations of interdisciplinary issues that may some day lead to specific methods of prostate tumor diagnosis and treatment.

The success of the Workshop is evidenced by the new ideas that evolved through the interaction and exchange of views among scientific leaders from diverse disciplines. The mechanisms are clearly in place to advance the concepts developed by the contributors to this volume, and to activate the basic and clinical research projects identified through this common endeavor.

James P. Karr, PhD
Avery A. Sandberg, MD
Gerald P. Murphy, MD, DSc

PROLACTIN

The Prostatic Cell: Structure and Function
Part B, pages 1–8

Relation of Prolactin to Development of Spontaneous Mammary and Pituitary Tumors

Joseph Meites

INTRODUCTION

Spontaneous mammary tumors are the most common type of neoplasm in the female rat, mouse, dog, and human and show the highest incidence with aging [1–4]. In Sprague Dawley rats between two and three years of age, the incidence averages between 50 and 80%. In Long Evans rats of similar age groups, the incidence is 25–40%. Wistar rats also show a high occurrence of mammary tumors. The vast majority of these tumors in rats consists of a single benign fibroadenoma or adenoma, and they usually originate from ductal tissue. In mice the incidence of spontaneous mammary tumors depends on the strain. In the C_3H inbred strain, bred specifically for high mammary tumor occurrence, the incidence reaches more than 90% by 8–10 months of age in both virgins and breeders. Other inbred strains, such as the Balb/c or $C_{57}Bl$ have a low incidence of mammary tumors. The tumors in mice usually are carcinomas, and develop from preneoplastic alveolar nodules. In aging female dogs, about one fourth of spontaneous mammary tumors are adenocarcinomas, and the rest are of a mixed type consisting of epithelial elements, fibrous tissue, bone, and cartilage. Breast cancer in women is believed to be of ductal origin, and is the most common cancer in women between 40 and 60 years of age.

The role of prolactin (PRL) in mammary tumorigenesis depends on the species. In rats and mice, PRL is essential for development of mammary tumors, and also for growth of existing mammary tumors in rats. Established mammary tumors in mice usually are hormone independent. In dogs, there is no evidence that PRL is involved in mammary tumorigenesis. A definite role for PRL in human breast cancer also has not been established. Estrogen is believed to participate in mammary tumorigenesis in the rat, mouse, and women; although, like PRL, its importance varies among the different species. In rats and mice, prolonged estrogen treatment results in a high incidence of mammary cancers, but such cancers do not develop in the absence of the pituitary and appear to be secondary to stimulation of PRL secretion. Estrogen is known to promote PRL secretion by a direct action on the pituitary and also via the hypothalamus.

Both estrogen and PRL receptors have been shown to be present in the mammary tissues of rats, mice, and humans, and both are believed to act synergistically to produce normal and tumorous mammary growth. Other hormones also may have a role in mammary tumorigenesis, but are not believed to rank in importance with PRL and estrogen, except in the dog. In the dog, progesterone and growth hormone appear to be the two most critical hormones for mammary tumorigenesis [1].

Development of spontaneous pituitary tumors also are very common in several strains of old rats of both sexes. It is our impression that most of these are prolactinomas [3]. In contrast to rats, spontaneous pituitary tumors in old mice are less common. In human subjects, large pituitary tumors are relatively rare, but microadenomas are very common in both men and women. Their occurrence increases with age, and most appear to be prolactinomas. The cause for development of spontaneous pituitary tumors in rats and mice appear to be related to the same hypothalamic substances indirectly responsible for development of spontaneous mammary tumors. Little is known about the etiology of human pituitary tumors.

DEVELOPMENT OF SPONTANEOUS MAMMARY TUMORS

Appearance of spontaneous mammary fibroadenomas in aging female Sprague Dawley and Long Evans rats is associated with a significant increase in blood PRL levels, and in the oldest rats, with the presence of PRL-secreting pituitary tumors [1-2]. With cessation of regular estrous cycles at about midlife (10-15 months of age), rats show a reduced capacity to secrete gonadotropins and an increased ability to secrete PRL, as compared with young cycling rats [3-4]. Aging male rats similarly exhibit reduced secretion of gonadotropins (and testosterone), and increased secretion of PRL, as compared with young male rats. Since estrogen secretion by the ovaries and testosterone secretion by the testes are reduced in old rats, the increased PRL secretion cannot be attributed to gonadal steroids and must be caused by other factors.

We have shown that the rise in PRL secretion in aging rats of both sexes is related to changes in hypothalamic regulation of PRL secretion. We found that the concentration and turnover of hypothalamic dopamine and norepinephrine are reduced, whereas serotonin turnover is increased in old as compared to young rats of both sexes [3]. Since hypothalamic dopamine depresses, whereas serotonin stimulates PRL secretion [1,5], the changes that occur in these two neurotransmitters in old rats are believed to be mainly responsible for the increase in PRL secretion. Dopamine has been shown to act directly on the pituitary to inhibit PRL release, whereas serotonin is believed to act via a PRL releasing factor (PRF).

In addition, we have recently found that methionine-enkephalin is increased in the hypothalamus [6] and β-endorphin in the blood (Forman, Sonntag, Van Vugt, and Meites, unpublished) of old male rats. These and other endogenous opiates have been demonstrated to increase PRL secretion [7]. Other hypothalamic neurotransmitters (acetylcholine, GABA, etc) also can influence PRL secretion, and may be altered during aging. Thus the development of spontaneous mammary tumors in aging female rats is believed to be due primarily to the increase in PRL secretion brought about by changes in hypothalamic neurotransmitter function. Why the activity of catecholamines, serotonin, and opiates is altered in the hypothalamus of aging rats is unknown at present, but it could involve changes in enzymes that regulate synthesis and metabolism of neurotransmitters, loss in number of neurotransmitter neurons in the hypothalamus, changes in hypothalamic receptors, and alterations in peptidergic neurons that secrete PRL releasing factor (PRF) or PRL release-inhibiting factor (PIF).

In general, treatments that result in increased PRL secretion have been shown to promote development of spontaneous mammary tumors in rats, whereas treatments that reduce PRL secretion inhibited development of spontaneous mammary tumors. Thus placement of median eminence lesions in ten-month-old intact Sprague Dawley female rats resulted in persistent elevation of blood PRL levels for 25 weeks, and in a significant increase in incidence of mammary tumors, as compared with control sham-operated rats [1,2]. The tumors in the lesioned rats were mainly adenomas, whereas they were mainly fibroadenomas in the controls. When intact two- and eight-month-old Sprague Dawley female rats were grafted with a total of five pituitaries over the inguinal, abdominal, and thoracic regions of the mammary glands, and two underneath the kidney capsule of each rat, a significantly greater number of mammary tumors developed in the pituitary grafted than in control rats nine months later. The number of tumors in rats grafted at eight months of age was much greater than in the rats grafted at two months of age. Almost all of the tumors that developed in the pituitary-grafted rats were adenomas.

Treatment of ten-month-old female Sprague Dawley rats with reserpine for nine months, to promote PRL secretion, increased development of spontaneous mammary tumors; whereas treatment with L-DOPA to depress PRL secretion for a similar period of time inhibited development of mammary tumors (Quadri and Meites, unpublished). Multiparous female rats show a higher incidence of spontaneous mammary tumors than nulliparous female rats, probably reflecting the increase that occurs in placental PRL during each pregnancy [2].

Treatments to increase PRL secretion in mice also have led to development of mammary tumors (carcinomas), even in strains that ordinarily develop few mammary tumors, whereas inhibition of PRL secretion by ergot drug administration inhibited development of mammary cancers in C_3H female mice [2]. Thus, lesions placed in the hypothalamus, pituitary grafts implanted underneath the kidney capsule, or daily injections of PRL greatly increased the incidence of mammary cancers in mice, even in strains in which no mammary cancer inducing viral agent could be found (see [8]). Prolonged administration of reserpine also hastened development of mammary cancers in mice [9]. On the other hand, daily administration of bromocryptine to inhibit PRL secretion almost completely prevented the occurrence of mammary cancers in the C_3H strain [2]. These findings point to the essential role of PRL in mammary cancer development in the mouse. There is no convincing evidence at this time that mouse strains with high mammary cancer incidence have greater blood PRL levels than low-mammary cancer strains.

In the human, no definite role for PRL in breast cancer has yet been demonstrated. Although several retrospective studies in patients with breast cancer reported an association with prolonged usage of reserpine, other retrospective studies failed to confirm these reports (see [2,10]). Prolonged use of other neuroleptic drugs that increase PRL secretion also was not shown to be associated with breast cancer. However, at least one laboratory has reported that in families with a genetic propensity for breast cancer, blood PRL levels in women were higher than in families with a low breast cancer incidence [11]. A complicating factor in assessing the role of PRL in human breast cancer development is that there are actually two sources of PRL in the human pituitary. In addition to PRL itself, growth hormone in humans also has PRL activity, and like PRL, can stimulate growth of the human breast and lactation. Human placental lactogen (HPL, or somatomammotropin), also is secreted in large amounts during pregnancy, in addition to increased release of pituitary PRL. The possible role of growth hormone and HPL in breast cancer development remains to be investigated.

It is of some interest to briefly review the relationship of PRL to *carcinogen*-induced mammary cancers [1–4]. PRL is essential for development of mammary tumors in rats and mice, whether the tumors are spontaneous or carcinogen-induced. Treatments that produce a decrease in PRL secretion, such as administration of L-DOPA or ergot drugs, anti-estrogenic drugs (MER-25 or tamoxifen), or ovariectomy, inhibit development of carcinogen-induced mammary cancers in female rats and mice. However, treatments that promote PRL secretion can either increase or decrease mammary cancer development, depending on whether the treatments are begun *before* or *after* the carcinogen is administered. Thus, if PRL secretion is increased *prior* to carcinogen administration, by placing pituitary grafts underneath the kidney capsule, lesioning appropriate areas of the hypothalamus, inducing pregnancy, or by administering neuroleptic drugs, estrogen, or contraceptive steroids, these result in *suppression* of mammary cancer development. On the other hand, if treatments to *enhance* PRL secretion are begun *after* carcinogen administration, these result in *enhancement* of mammary cancer development. No changes are seen in blood PRL levels or in regularity of estrous cycles during development and growth of carcinogen-induced mammary cancers in rats, indicating that sufficient PRL and estrogen are present under normal conditions to permit cancers to appear and grow.

It is clear that there are some important differences in the relation of PRL to development of spontaneous, as compared to carcinogen-induced mammary cancers in the rat. Spontaneous benign mammary fibroadenomas or adenomas are usually seen only in aging female rats, in the presence of rising blood concentrations of PRL. By contrast, the optimal period for producing mammary adenocarcinomas by carcinogen treatment in female Sprague Dawley rats is between 50–60 days of age, in the presence of normal blood concentrations of PRL.

In C_3H female mice, there also is no evidence for an increase in blood concentrations of PRL during development or growth of mammary adenocarcinomas. In both rats and mice given prolonged estrogen treatment, development of mammary *cancers* is accompanied by and promoted by elevated blood PRL values. Although the role of PRL in women with breast cancer is not clear, no differences in blood PRL values are seen after breast cancers are detected. Thus mammary cancers can develop in rats, mice, and women in the presence of normal blood PRL concentrations.

DEVELOPMENT OF SPONTANEOUS PITUITARY TUMORS

A 10–86% incidence of spontaneous pituitary adenomas was reported in old male and female rats of different strains, and a 0.25–10% incidence in old male and female mice of different strains [8]. Pituitary adenomas are rare before one year of age in these animals, and usually appear between two to three years of age. Most of these tumors are chromophobic, but produce large amounts of PRL [12,13]. Human subjects at autopsy show an incidence of 8–25% of pituitary adenomas, and these increase with age [14]. The majority of these pituitary tumors are chromophobic microadenomas and secrete mainly PRL (prolactinomas).

In mice and rats, most of the evidence points to the hypothalamus rather than to the gonads as the major stimulus for development of pituitary adenomas. Gonadal functions, including secretion of estrogen by the ovaries and testosterone by the testes, are reduced, and there is a corresponding decrease in ability to secrete gonadotropins by the pituitary [3,4]. Regular estrous cycles usually cease in females by midlife. Together with the decline in reproductive functions, there is a significant increase in secretion of PRL in both sexes, and enlargment of the pituitary in females. Serum PRL levels become particularly elevated in rats between 2–3 years of age, and it is at this time that pituitary adenomas are most commonly seen [12,13].

It has been well established that the hypothalamus normally inhibits PRL secretion, and that removal of the pituitary from hypothalamic control results in increased secretion of PRL [5]. Thus, in many mouse strains, transplanting or grafting a pituitary to a site outside of its normal sella turcica location results in development of a chromophobic adenoma that secretes high amounts of PRL. Females are more apt to develop tumors than males. Mammary stimulation and sometimes mammary tumors are seen in mice with pituitary transplants or grafts. Pituitary tumor induction by this method usually takes a year or more to develop.

I believe that occurrence of spontaneous PRL-secreting pituitary adenomas in old mice and rats comes about mainly as a result of a functional disconnection of the pituitary from the hypothalamus. It is well established that dopamine in the hypothalamus is the principal agent responsible for inhibition of PRL secretion, and that it is released into the pituitary portal vessels to directly inhibit the pituitary lactotrophs. Serotonin, on the other hand, can stimulate PRL secretion and apparently acts by promoting release from the hypothalamus into the pituitary portal vessels of a PRL-releasing factor (PRF). We have demonstrated that in old male and female rats, hypothalamic dopamine turnover is significantly reduced, whereas serotonin turnover is significantly increased, as compared with young mature rats of both sexes [3,4]. This could account for the increase in PRL secretion and development of spontaneous pituitary tumors, and also for the large numbers of spontaneous mammary tumors in the old female rats. A similar decrease in dopaminergic activity has been described in old mice [15]. Opiates in the hypothalamus and pituitary of old rats also appear to be increased [6], Forman, Sonntag, Van Vugt, and Meites, unpublished), and opiates are known to increase PRL secretion [7]. Thus development of spontaneous pituitary tumors in old rats and mice probably is due mainly to a decrease in hypothalamic dopamine activity and to an increase in release from the hypothalamus of one or more PRFs.

In rats, pituitaries transplanted to sites removed from the sella turcica do not develop into tumors [8], although PRL secretion is increased. However, such pituitaries can develop into tumors if provided with estrogen stimulation. In a study reported by our laboratory [16], a pituitary was grafted underneath the kidney capsule of intact three-month-old female Sprague Dawley rats. A small tablet containing 12 mg diethylstilbestrol was implanted every three months, and at the end of 16 months the rats were killed and the in situ and grafted pituitaries were excised and weighed. Pituitaries weighing 50 mg or more were arbitrarily designated as tumors. Tumors developed in three of the 17 pituitaries grafted underneath the kidney capsule and the others were enlarged to about three times the original size (average weight, 26.5 mg). By contrast, tumors developed in seven of the 17 in situ pituitaries, and the average weight of the others greatly exceeded that of the grafted pituitaries (average weight, 63.5 mg). It was concluded that estrogen was more effective in evoking tumors in the pituitaries located in the sella turcica because, in addition to its direct stimulating action on the pituitary, it promoted release from the hypothalamus into the pituitary portal vessels of a PRF.

In human subjects, the etiology of spontaneous pituitary prolactinomas is unknown at present. PRL secreting microadenomas are found in young as well as in elderly individuals of both sexes, although they are more common in the latter. A decrease in catecholamines has been reported in the brain, including the hypothalamus, of old human subjects [15], and this may contribute to development of these tumors. There is no clear evidence that prolonged estrogen or steroid-contraceptive treatment can produce pituitary adenomas in human subjects [14], although estrogens can definitely enhance PRL secretion in men and women [17]. During pregnancy, enlargement of the anterior pituitary and high secretion of PRL may be related to the great increase in estrogen secretion that occurs during this period.

Our laboratory reported in 1972 [18] that in rats carrying large transplantable pituitary tumors ($MtT.W_{15}$) which secrete large amounts of PRL and growth hormone, administration of ergot drugs could reduce serum PRL to normal levels and evoke regression of the tumors. Subsequently, treatment with ergot drugs has been shown to decrease PRL secretion and induce regression of human pituitary prolactinomas [14]. This is believed to provide further indirect evidence that a deficiency of hypothalamic dopamine may be partially responsible for development of spontaneous pituitary prolactinomas in rats and human subjects.

ACKNOWLEDGMENTS

Research from our laboratory was supported in part by NIH grants CA10771 from the National Cancer Institute; AM04784 from the National Institute of Arthritis, Metabolism, Diabetes, and Digestive Diseases; AG00416 from the National Institute on Aging; and by the Michigan Agricultural Experiment Station.

REFERENCES

1. Meites J: Relation of the neuroendocrine system to the development and growth of experimental mammary tumors. J. Neural Transmission 48: 25-42, 1980.
2. Welsch CW, Nagasawa H: Prolactin and mammary tumorigenesis: A review. Cancer Res 37: 951-963, 1977.
3. Meites J, Huang HH, Simpkins JW: Recent studies on neuroendocrine control of reproductive senescence in rats. In Schneider EL (ed): "The Aging Reproductive System," Raven Press: New York, 1978, pp 213-235.
4. Meites J, Steger RW, Huang HH: Relation of neuroendocrine system to the reproductive decline in aging rats and human subjects. Fed Proc 39: 3168-3172, 1980.
5. Meites J, Simpkins J, Bruni J, Advis J: Role of biogenic amines in control of anterior pituitary hormones. IRCS J Med Sci 5: 1-7, 1977.
6. Steger RW, Sonntag WE, Van Vugt DA, Forman LJ, Meites J: Reduced ability of naloxone to stimulate LH and testosterone release in aging male rats; possible relation to increase hypothalamic met^5-enkephalin. Life Sci 27: 747-754, 1980.
7. Meites J, Bruni JF, Van Vugt DA, Smith AF: Minireview: Relation of endogenous opioid peptides and morphine to neuroendocrine system. Life Sci. 24: 1325-1336, 1979.
8. Russfield AB: Tumors of Endocrine Glands and Secondary Sex Organs. U.S. Dept. of Health, Education, and Welfare, Public Health Services, Washington, DC: U.S. Government Printing Office, 1966.
9. Lacassagne A, Duplan JF: Le Mecanisme de la cancerisation de la mamelle chez la souris. Considere d'apres le resultats d'experience au moyen de la reserpine. Compt Rend 249: 810-812, 1959.
10. Nagasawa H: Prolactin and human breast cancer: A review. Eur J Cancer 15: 267-279, 1979.
11. Kwa HG, Cleton F, deJong-Barker M, Bulbrook RD, Hayward JL, Wang DY: Plasma prolactin and its relationship to risk factors in human breast cancer. Int J Cancer 17: 441-447, 1976.
12. Ito A, Moy P, Kaunitz H, Kortwright K, Clarke S, Furth J, Meites J: Incidence and character of the spontaneous pituitary tumors in strain CR and W/Fu male rats. J Natl Cancer Inst 49: 701-711, 1972.
13. Huang HH, Meites J: Reproductive capacity of aging female rats. Neuroendocrinology 17: 289-295, 1975.
14. Post KD, Jackson IMD, Reichlin S: The Pituitary Adenoma. New York: Plenum Publishing, 1980.
15. Finch CE: Neuroendocrine and autonomic aspects of aging. In Finch CE Hayflick L (eds): "Handbook of the Biology of Aging," New York: Van Nostrand Reinhold, 1977 pp 262-280.
16. Welsch CW, Jenkins T, Amenomori Y, Meites J: Tumorous development of in situ and grafted anterior pituitaries in female rats treated with diethylstilbestrol. Experientia 27: 1350-1352, 1971.
17. Frantz AG: Rhythms in prolactin secretion. In Krieger DT (ed): "Endocrine Rhythms," New York: Raven Press, 1979, pp 175-186.
18. Quadri SK, Lu KH, Meites J: Ergot-induced inhibition of pituitary tumor growth in rats. Science 176: 417-418, 1972.

The Prostatic Cell: Structure and Function
Part B, pages 9–18
© 1981 Alan R. Liss, Inc., 150 Fifth Avenue, New York, NY 10011

The Role of Prolactin in the Growth of the Prostate Gland

Edward J. Keenan, Elizabeth E. Ramsey, and Elaine D. Kemp

INTRODUCTION

Prolactin is present in the anterior pituitary gland and in the circulation of laboratory animals and man [1–6]. Furthermore, plasma levels of prolactin in male rodents are elevated during puberty suggesting that prolactin may be involved in the development of the testes and/or of the accessory reproductive organs, namely the prostate gland and the seminal vesicles [7–10]. Various aspects of prolactin's role in the function of the male reproductive tract have been outlined in recent reviews [11–13].

The influences of prolactin upon prostate cells may be partially attributed to the hormone's stimulatory effects upon testicular androgen production [14–18]. In addition, it is now well established that prolactin acts directly upon the cells of the prostate gland and/or of the seminal vesicles in several species to augment the effects of androgens [19–25]. Identification of receptors for prolactin in male accessory sex organs lends further support to the concept of a direct role for prolactin in the function of these tissues [26–34].

More recent studies have revealed that prolactin-mediated augmentation of androgen action in male accessory sex organs is related to enhancement of DNA synthesis preceding cell proliferation [35,36]. Consequently, prolactin in association with androgens may be involved in modulating the growth of the prostate gland and seminal vesicles. In view of the role of prolactin in the growth of male accessory sex organs and the importance of prolactin receptors in mediating prolactin's effects, the present studies were conducted to characterize the relationship between alterations in the prolactin receptor content and the rapid development of the rat ventral prostate gland that occurs during sexual maturation.

MATERIALS AND METHODS

Ventral prostate glands from albino rats (Sprague Dawley) of varying ages, as indicated, and the anterior prostate glands (coagulating glands) and seminal vesicles from mice (90–100 days old; Swiss Webster) were obtained following cervical dislocation. These tissues were blotted to remove secretory fluid and trimmed of extraneous connective tissue. Subsequently, the tissues were weighed and were rinsed in 0.9% NaCl prior to freezing in liquid nitrogen and storage at –76°C. Frozen tissues were utilized for the ^{125}I-prolactin binding studies, while fresh tissues were used for evaluation of nuclear dihydrotestosterone receptor content and for the ^{3}H-thymidine incorporation studies.

^{125}I-Prolactin Binding Assay

Specific binding of ^{125}I-prolactin by male accessory sex organs was examined using techniques similar to those described by Shiu and Friesen [37]. Tissues were thawed at 0–4°C, minced with a scissors, resuspended in ice cold 0.3 M sucrose (1:10, weight:volume), and homogenized using a Polytron (Brinkman Instruments, Westbury, NY) homogenizer at a setting of 3.5 (two 10-second bursts with a 30-second cooling interval).

Membrane particles subsequently were obtained by differential centrifugation. A crude particulate fraction was obtained after centrifugation at 1500g for 10 minutes. The resulting supernate was centrifuged at 15,000g for 20 minutes to obtain a crude mitochondrial/Golgi vesicle fraction. A crude plasma membrane/microsomal fraction was prepared by centrifugation of the 15,000g supernate at 100,000g for 90 minutes. After centrifugation the membrane particles were resuspended in 0.05 M tris-hydrochloric acid buffer (pH = 7.6) containing 10 mM calcium chloride and were frozen at –76°C. Prior freezing of the membrane particles in the presence of calcium chloride caused the membranes to aggregate upon thawing, which facilitated isolation of these particles by low speed centrifugation (1500g for 10 minutes).

Aliquots (200 μl) of membrane particles containing 100–300 μg protein, as determined according to the procedure of Lowry and associates [38], were added in triplicate to two sets of plastic tubes (12 × 75 mm) and were maintained in an ice bath. To one set of tubes 200 μl of 0.05 M tris-hydrochloric acid–0.01 M calcium chloride buffer containing bovine serum albumin (0.5% final concentration) were added and to the second set of tubes 200 μl of the same buffer containing in addition 500 ng unlabeled prolactin were added.

The binding reactions were initiated by the addition of 0.1 ml ^{125}I-prolactin (100,000 counts per minute, 60–80 μCi/μg protein). Incubations were conducted at 25°C for 20 hours, since preliminary studies using membrane particles from the lactating rabbit mammary gland and from the rat ventral prostate gland demonstrated that binding equilibrium was established under these conditions. The binding reactions were terminated by the addition of 3 ml ice-cold 0.05 M tris-hydrochloric acid–0.01 M calcium chloride buffer containing 0.5% bovine serum albumin. ^{125}I-prolactin that was bound to the membrane particles was separated from free ^{125}I-prolactin by centrifugation (1500g for 20 minutes). Unbound ^{125}I-prolactin in the supernatant was removed by aspiration.

The amount of ^{125}I-prolactin that was bound to membrane particles was quantitated by gamma counting and was expressed as a percentage of the total ^{125}I-prolactin added to the reaction mixture per 0.1 mg membrane protein. The difference between the amount of ^{125}I-prolactin bound in the absence (total binding) and in the presence of unlabeled prolactin (nonspecific binding) was considered specifically bound ^{125}I-prolactin. Specific ^{125}I-prolactin binding data were expressed as the mean ± standard error of the mean. Approximately 60–80% of the total ^{125}I-prolactin binding in the rat ventral prostate and mouse anterior prostate gland and seminal vesicles was specifically bound. Initial studies showed that the dissociation constant for specific prolactin binding by these tissues was approximately $1-3 \times 10^{-10}$ M as determined by Scatchard analysis [39] and is, thus, reflective of the high-affinity binding characteristic of a prolactin receptor [37].

Ovine prolactin (NIH-P-S10, 25.6 IU/mg) was iodinated using lactoperoxidase according to the method of Frantz and Turkington [40]. After iodination ^{125}I-prolactin was separated from free ^{125}I-prolactin by chromatography on a Sephadex G-75 column (0.9 × 15 cm) equilibrated with 0.05 M tris-hydrochloric acid–0.1% bovine serum albumin buffer. ^{125}I-prolactin was purified further by chromatography using a Sephadex G-100 column (0.9 × 60 cm).

Nuclear Dihydrotestosterone (DHT) Receptor Assay

Ventral prostate tissue (0.5 gm) was homogenized (1:10; wt:vol) as described above in ice-cold, 0.05 M Tris buffer (pH = 7.5) containing 1.5 mM EDTA, 0.5 mM dithiothreitol, and 10% glycerol (w/v). The homogenate was centrifuged (0–4°C) at 800g (10 minutes) to prepare a crude nuclear pellet, which was washed twice with homogenization buffer (10 ml). The final nuclear pellet was resuspended in homogenization buffer (2 ml) containing 0.6 M KCl and was incubated at 0–4°C for 60 minutes. The high-salt extract was subsequently diluted (1:1) with homogenization buffer and centrifuged (100,000g, 30 minutes). The extract was maintained on ice prior to ^{3}H-DHT binding assay. The particulate fraction was resuspended in 2.0 ml of 0.6 N perchloric acid (PCA) and the DNA was extracted by incubation at 85°C for 30 minutes [41]. An aliquot (0.1–0.2 ml) of the PCA extract was analyzed for DNA content by the method of Burton [42].

Aliquots (0.5 ml) of the salt extracts containing nuclear DHT receptors were equilibrated with 0.5–5.0 nM ^{3}H-DHT (specific activity = 131 Ci/mmole, New England Nuclear, Boston, MA) by incubation at 0–4°C for 20 hours. Following equilibration, free ^{3}H-DHT was adsorbed by addition of 0.5 ml of dextran-coated charcoal, suspended in homogenization buffer, and incubated (0–4°C) for 15 minutes with mixing every 5 minutes. Free and bound ^{3}H-DHT were then separated by centrifugation (1500g, 10 minutes). Radioactivity in aliquots (0.5 ml) of the supernates was quantitated by liquid scintillation counting. Specificity of ^{3}H-DHT binding was assessed by incubating in the presence and in the absence of a 100-fold excess of unlabeled DHT. Specific binding of ^{3}H-DHT in the nuclear extracts ranged from 50–60% following incubation with ^{3}H-DHT (5.0 nM) and the equilibrium dissociation constant for specific ^{3}H-DHT binding in the nuclear extracts was 1–2 nM as revealed by Scatchard plot analysis [39]. Specific ^{3}H-DHT binding capacity was expressed in picomoles per mg DNA (pm/mg DNA).

^{3}H-Thymidine Incorporation

Slice preparations (0.5 mm) of ventral prostate tissue were made using a McIlwain tissue chopper (Brinkman Instrument, Westbury, NY). Tissue slices (50–100 mg) were incubated in 1.0 ml of Eagle's minimum essential medium (Grand Island Biological Co., Grand Island, NE) containing ^{3}H-methyl-thymidine (4 μCi/ml, specific activity = 95.4 Ci/mmole, New England Nuclear, Boston, MA). A Dubnoff metabolic incubator was utilized for the incubation procedures, which were carried out at 37°C for 60 minutes under a continuous atmosphere of 95% air and 5% CO_2. Incubations were terminated by the addition of 1.0 ml of ice-cold 1.2 N perchloric acid (PCA), and the incubation tubes were immediately placed in an ice bath. The tissues were subsequently homogenized in 2.0 ml of ice-cold PCA (0.6 N) and centrifuged at 1000g for 5 minutes. After centrifugation the supernatant fluid was discarded and the pellets were washed twice with 3.0 ml of ice-cold PCA (0.6 N). The final pellets were resuspended in 2.0 ml of ice-cold PCA (0.6 N), and the DNA was extracted by incubation at 85°C for 30 minutes [41].

A 0.5-ml aliquot was removed from each extract for quantitation of ^{3}H-thymidine incorporation into DNA by liquid scintillation counting procedures. A 1.0-ml aliquot was also removed for determination of the DNA content of each extract according to the method of Burton [42]. The radioactivity incorporated into accessory sex organ DNA was expressed as dpm/μg DNA and represented mean values of triplicate observations.

Statistical Analysis

Statistical differences among mean values were established by analysis of variance and subsequent application of a multiple-range test.

RESULTS

The specific binding of ^{125}I-prolactin by particulate membranes obtained from the accessory sex organs of adult (90–100 days old), male rats and mice is shown in Table I. In the anterior prostate gland of the mouse, specific ^{125}I-prolactin binding activity was observed in the 15,000g membrane fraction, but was not detectable in the 100,000g membrane component. In contrast, significant binding of ^{125}I-prolactin was localized in both subcellular fractions of the mouse seminal vesicle, although a higher degree of binding activity was observed in the 15,000g as compared to the 100,000g membranes (Table I). Considerable specific binding of ^{125}I-prolactin was localized in both the 15,000g and 100,000g membranes isolated from the rat ventral prostate gland, while only the 15,000g fraction of the seminal vesicles exhibited detectable, although low, specific ^{125}I-prolactin binding activity.

The relationship between development of the rat ventral prostate gland and the subcellular distribution of specific ^{125}I-prolactin binding sites is presented in Table II. In young rats (30–40 days old), specific binding of ^{125}I-prolactin was localized in both the 15,000g and 100,000g particulate fractions with lower binding activity associated with the higher-speed membrane component. Significant increases in specific ^{125}I-prolactin binding occurred in both subcellular fractions by 50 days of age and prior to significant development of the ventral prostate gland as evidenced by increases in organ weights (Table II). The level of specific ^{125}I-prolactin binding activity in the 15,000g fraction remained elevated without significant alterations through 105 days of age. However, the specific ^{125}I-prolactin binding, associated with the 100,000g membranes, decreased between 65 and 80 days of age and subsequently rose again at 95 and 105 days of age to levels similar to those observed in the 15,000g membrane fraction. In older animals (>135

TABLE I. Specific ^{125}I-prolactin binding activity in male accessory sex organs

	Specific ^{125}I-prolactin binding ($\%/0.1$ mg protein)	
Tissue	15,000g	100,000g
Anterior prostate, mouse	2.0 ± 0.2[a]	< 0.1
Seminal vesicles, mouse	2.6 ± 0.1	0.9 ± 0.1
Ventral prostate, rat	5.2 ± 0.5	5.5 ± 0.4
Seminal vesicles, rat	0.4 ± 0.1	< 0.1

[a]Expressed as mean $\pm$ SEM.

TABLE II. Relationship between the subcellular distribution of specific ^{125}I-prolactin binding activity and development of the rat ventral prostate gland

Animal age (days)	Specific ^{125}I-prolactin binding (%/0.1 mg protein)		Organ weight (mg/100 gm body weight)
	15,000g	100,000g	
30	3.3 ± 0.2[a]	1.7 ± 0.1	51 ± 1
40	3.1 ± 0.5	1.0 ± 0.2	47 ± 4
50	5.8 ± 0.5*	2.9 ± 0.5*	42 ± 3
65	5.1 ± 0.4*	3.1 ± 0.5*	85 ± 9*
80	4.4 ± 0.2*	1.9 ± 0.2	96 ± 2*
95	5.7 ± 0.6*	6.0 ± 0.4**	104 ± 7*
105	4.6 ± 0.8*	5.1 ± 0.3**	116 ± 5*
135	1.2 ± 0.1*	2.1 ± 0.2	105 ± 5*
240	0.9 ± 0.3*	1.0 ± 0.1*	104 ± 5*

[a]Expressed as mean ± SEM.
*P ≤ 0.05 vs 30-day-old group.
**P ≤ 0.05 vs 65-day-old group.

TABLE III. Relationship between nuclear dihydrotestosterone (DHT) receptor content and growth of the rat ventral prostate gland

Animal age (days)	Nuclear DHT receptor (pm/mg DNA)	^{3}H-Thymidine incorporation (dpm/µg DNA)	Organ weight (mg/100 gm body weight)
40	1.51 ± 0.07[a]	54 ± 5	60 ± 2
48	1.50 ± 0.09	37 ± 5	65 ± 3
60	2.00 ± 0.06*	50 ± 6	95 ± 4*
80	0.94 ± 0.10*	66 ± 5**	88 ± 3*
100	1.82 ± 0.12*	70 ± 5**	109 ± 6*
125	1.11 ± 0.10*	74 ± 9**	87 ± 7*

[a]Expressed as mean ± SEM.
*P ≤ 0.05 vs 40-day-old group.
**P ≤ 0.05 vs 48-day-old group.

days of age), specific ^{125}I-prolactin binding activity declined in both subcellular membrane fractions and by 240 days of age the specific binding of ^{125}I-prolactin had fallen below the levels that were observed in young animals (30–40 days old). These age-related decreases in prostatic ^{125}I-prolactin binding activity occurred without significant alterations in ventral prostate weights (Table II).

Table III reveals the relationship between nuclear DHT receptor content, ^{3}H-thymidine incorporation, and development of the ventral prostate gland. Prostatic levels of nuclear DHT receptors remained unchanged between 40 and 48 days of age, but were increased by 33% to 2.0 pm/mg DNA at 60 days of age in correspondence with marked increases in organ weights (Table III). Twenty days later significantly lower concentrations of nuclear DHT receptors were observed in the ventral prostate gland in association with significant elevations in ^{3}H-thymidine incorporation into DNA. Levels of nuclear DHT receptors were again elevated at 100 days of age, but declined subsequently at 125 days of age without marked changes in either ³H-thymidine incorporation or in the weights of the ventral prostate gland.

DISCUSSION

The prostate gland and the seminal vesicles of rats and mice have previously been described as responsive to prolactin [11–13, 19–25]. Thus, the demonstration of the presence of prolactin receptors in these organs is consistent with their sensitivity to the direct effects of prolactin [26–32].

Emphasis in these studies on the distribution of prolactin binding sites in the accessory sex organs of male mice revealed that prolactin receptors are apparently localized in different subcellular fractions of the anterior prostate gland and seminal vesicles. Specific ¹²⁵I-prolactin binding activity is found primarily in the crude mitochondrial/Golgi membrane fraction (15,000g) in the anterior prostate gland, but is distributed in the 15,000g and the crude microsomal/plasma membrane fractions (100,000g) of the seminal vesicles. It is interesting that prolactin stimulates cell proliferation in the seminal vesicles, while increasing anterior prostate gland weights without enhancement of DNA synthesis. This suggests that prolactin may exert different roles in these tissues [35,36]. It is presently uncertain if differences in subcellular localization of prolactin receptors are related to variations in the prolactin responsiveness of the accessory sex organs in male mice. Further studies using purified membrane fractions may elucidate the precise cellular location of prolactin binding sites in the accessory sex organs of male mice and the physiological significance of their subcellular distribution.

Development of the prostate gland is seemingly related to the presence of prolactin receptors. Specific ¹²⁵I-prolactin binding activity in the rat ventral prostate gland rises markedly in both subcellular fractions (ie, crude mitochondrial/Golgi and microsomal/plasma membrane) between 40 and 50 days of age. The increases in specific binding of ¹²⁵I-prolactin precede the rapid rise in ventral prostate weight observed between 50 and 60 days of age. Following full development of the ventral prostate gland, the prolactin receptor content falls to basal levels. Similar age-associated decreases in prolactin binding by the rat prostate gland have been reported previously [26,29,32].

The age associated changes in specific ¹²⁵I-prolactin binding activity are apparently independent of alterations in the levels of nuclear DHT receptors. Between 40 and 50 days of age, the concentration of DHT receptors in prostatic nuclei remains unchanged, but does subsequently increase at day 60 of age.

Using ³H-thymidine incorporation into DNA as an index of DNA synthesis [35,36], increases in DNA synthesis occur by 80 days of age and could represent the recruitment of new populations of cells. The presence of new cells may explain the unusual decreases in the prolactin receptor content of the microsomal/plasma membrane fraction, as well as in nuclear levels of DHT receptor that occur at 80 days of age in the rat ventral prostate gland. Replenishment of both prolactin and DHT receptors by 100 days of age might be attributed to maturation of these new cell populations.

Although there appears to be a relationship between the level of prolactin binding activity and development of the prostate gland, the precise nature of prolactin influences upon the prostatic cell remains uncertain. Temporal alterations in the levels of prolactin receptors and nuclear concentrations of DHT receptors suggest a possible sequence of events. Early increases in prolactin receptor content between 40 and 50 days of age may trigger the enhanced localization or prolonged retention of DHT receptors in the nuclei of prolactin-sensitive cell types. These cells may then be stimulated to divide as reflected by the increased incorporation of ^{3}H-thymidine into prostatic DNA. Likewise, low levels of prolactin receptors in the ventral prostate gland of old animals may reflect diminished requirements for cellular proliferation in the fully developed prostate gland.

ACKNOWLEDGMENTS

These studies were supported in part by the Pleasants Foundation for Cancer Research, by grant RR00334 from the General Clinical Research Centers Branch of the Division of Research Resources, National Institutes of Health, and by grant 38.17 from the Medical Research Foundation of Oregon. Ovine prolactin was generously provided by NIAMDD through the Pituitary Hormone Distribution Program. Ms Pamela Fitzgerald is gratefully recognized for her contribution in the preparation of the manuscript.

REFERENCES

1. Riddle 0: Prolactin in vertebrate function and organization. J Natl Cancer Inst 31:1038–1110, 1963.
2. Meites J, Nicoll CS: Adenohypophysis. Ann Rev Physiol 28:57–87, 1966.
3. Bern HA, Nicoll CS: The comparative endocrinology of prolactin. Rec Prog Hormone Res 24:681–720, 1968.
4. Frantz AG, Kleinberg DL, Noel GL: Studies on prolactin in man. Rec Prog Hormone Res 28:527–573, 1972.
5. Nicoll CS, Bern HA: On the actions of prolactin among the vertebrates: Is there a common denominator? In Wolstenholme GEW, Knight J (eds): "Lactogenic Hormones." London: Church Hill Livingstone, 1972, pp 229–324.
6. Nicoll CS: Physiological actions of prolactin. In Knobil E, Sawyer WH (eds): "Handbook of Physiology." Washington, D.C.: American Physiological Society. 1974, pp 253–292.
7. Sinha YN, Selby FW, Lewis VJ, Vanderlaan WP: Studies of prolactin secretion in mice by homologous radioimmunoassay. Endocrinology 91:1045–1053, 1972.
8. Negro-Vilar A, Kruhlich L, McCann SM: Changes in serum prolactin and gonadotropins during sexual development of the male rat. Endocrinology 93:660–664, 1973.

9. Dohler KD, Wuttke W: Serum LH, FSH, prolactin and progesterone from birth to puberty in female and male rats. Endocrinolgy 94:1003–1009, 1974.

10. Barkley MS: Serum prolactin in the male mouse from birth to maturity. J Endocrinology 83:31–33, 1979.

11. Reddi AH: Role of prolactin in the growth and secretory activity of the prostate and other accessory glands of mammals. Gen Comp Endocrinol (suppl) 2:81–86, 1969.

12. Thomas JA Keenan EJ: Prolactin influences upon androgen action in male accessory sex organs. In Singhal RL, Thomas JA (eds): "Advances in Sex Hormone Research." Baltimore: Urban and Schwartzenberg, vol 2, 1976, pp 425–470.

13. Bartke A: Role of prolactin in reproduction in male mammals. Fed Proc 39:2577–2581, 1980.

14. Bartke A, Lloyd CW: The influence of pituitary homografts on the weight of sex accessories in castrated male mice and rats and on mating behavior in male mice. J Endocrinol 46: 313–320, 1970.

15. Hafiez AA, Philpott JE, Bartke A: The role of prolactin in the regulation of testicular function: The effect of prolactin and luteinizing hormone on 3β-hydroxysteroid dehydrogenase activity in the testes of mice and rats. J Endocrinol 50:619–623, 1971.

16. Hafiez AA, Lloyd CW, Bartke A: The role of prolactin in the regulation of testis function: Effects of prolactin and luteinizing hormone on the plasma levels of testosterone and androstenedione in hypophysectomized rats. J Endocrinol 52:327–332, 1972.

17. Musto N, Hafiez AA, Bartke A: Prolactin increases 17β-hydroxysteriod dehydrogenase activity in the testis. Endocrinology 91:1106–1108, 1972.

18. Bartke A: Pituitary-testis relationships: Role of prolactin in the regulation of testicular function. Prog Reprod Biol 1:136–150, 1976.

19. Chase MP, Geschwind II, Bern HA: Synergistic role of prolactin in response of male rat sex accessories to androgen. Proc Soc Exp Biol Med 94:680–683, 1957.

20. Antliff HR, Prasad MRN, Meyer RK: Action of prolactin on the seminal vesicles of guinea pig. Proc Soc Exp Biol Med 103:77–80, 1960.

21. Grayhack JT: Pituitary factors influencing growth of the prostate. Natl Cancer Inst Monog 12:189–199, 1963.

22. Bartke A: Influence of pituitary homografts on the weight of the seminal vesicles in castrated mice. J Endocrinol 38:195–196, 1967.

23. Moger WH, Geschwind II: The action of prolactin on the sex accessory glands of the male rat. Proc Soc Exp Biol Med 141:1017–1021, 1972.

24. Keenan EJ, Thomas JA: Effects of testosterone and prolactin or growth hormone on the accessory sex organs of castrated mice. J Endocrinol 64:111–115, 1975.

25. Negro-Vilar A, Saad WA, McCann SM: Evidence for a role of prolactin in prostate and seminal vesicle growth in immature male rats. Endocrinology 100:729–735, 1977.

26. Aragona C, Friesen HG: Specific prolactin binding sites in the prostate and testis of rats. Endocrinology 97:677–684, 1975.

27. Hanlin ML, Yount AP: Prolactin binding in the rat ventral prostate. Endocrine Res Commun 2:489–502, 1975.

28. Kledzik GS, Marshall S, Campbell GA, Gelato M, Meites J: Effects of castration, testosterone, estradiol and prolactin on specific prolactin-binding activity in ventral prostate of male rats. Endocrinology 98:373–379, 1976.

29. Barkey RJ, Shani J, Amit T, Barzilai D: Specific binding of prolactin to seminal vesicle, prostate and testicular homogenates of immature, mature and aged rats. J Endocrinol 74: 163–173, 1977.

30. Charreau EH, Attramadal A, Torjesen PA, Calandra R, Purvis K, Hansson V: Androgen stimulation of prolactin receptors in rat prostate. Mole Cell Endocrinol 7:1–7, 1977.

31. Barkey RJ, Shani J, Barzilai D: Regulation of prolactin binding sites in the seminal vesicle, prostate gland, testis and liver of intact and castrated adult rats: Effect of administration of testosterone, 2-bromo-α-ergocryptine and fluphenazine. J Endocrinol 81:11–18, 1979.
32. Keenan EJ, Kemp ED, Ramsey EE, Garrison LB, Pearse HD, Hodges CV: Specific binding of prolactin by the prostate gland of the rat and man. J Urol 122:43–46, 1979.
33. Witorsch RJ: Immunohistochemical localization of prolactin binding sites in R 3327 rat prostatic cancer cells. Hormone Res 10:268–281, 1979.
34. Witorsch RJ: The application of immunoperoxidase methodology for the visualization of prolactin sites in human prostate tissue. Hum Pathol 10:521–532, 1979.
35. Keenan EJ, Klase PA, Thomas JA: Interaction between prolactin and androgens in the accessory sex organs of male mice. J Endocrinol 1981 (in press).
36. Keenan EJ, Klase PA, Thomas JA: Effects of prolactin on DNA synthesis and growth of the accessory sex organs in male mice. Endocrinology 109:170–179, 1981.
37. Shiu RP, Friesen HG: Properties of a prolactin receptor from the rabbit mammary gland. Biochem J 140:301–311, 1974.
38. Lowry OH, Rosebrough NJ, Farr AL, Randall RJ: Protein measurement with Folin phenol reagent. J Biol Chem 193:265–275, 1951.
39. Scatchard G: The attraction of proteins for small molecules and ions. Ann NY Acad Sci 51:660–672, 1949.
40. Frantz WL, MacIndoe JH, Turkington RW: Prolactin receptors: characteristics of the particulate fraction binding activity. J Endocrinol 60:485–497, 1974.
41. Schneider WC: Determination of nucleic acids in tissues by pentose analysis. Methods Enzymol 3:680–684, 1951.
42. Burton K: A study of the conditions and mechanism of the diphenylamine reaction for the colorimetric estimation of deoxyribonucleic acid. Biochem J 62:315–323, 1956.

The Prostatic Cell: Structure and Function
Part B, pages 19–29
© 1981 Alan R. Liss, Inc., 150 Fifth Avenue, New York, NY 10011

Inhibitors of Prolactin Secretion: A Mini-Review

W. Roy Slaunwhite, Jr.

This brief review covers only the recent literature, from 1975. Since the emphasis is on mechanisms rather than applications, clinical usage is included only if it illustrates a point. Several recent reviews [1–5] made my task easier.

The title of this review requires further definition. It might better be "Natural Inhibitors of Prolactin Secretion and Their Modifiers," which allows me to include antagonists of inhibitors: these are obviously stimulators but rationally should be included. I shall also include some substances which are "mugwumpers"; that is, they are reported as both inhibitors and stimulants.

For a compound to be judged a *natural* inhibitor of prolactin release from the pituitary, it should meet the following criteria:

a) be present in the hypothalamus;
b) be released by appropriate physiological stimuli;
c) be present in the portal blood serving the adenohypophysis in sufficient concentration to suppress release of prolactin;
d) have receptors in the adenohypophysis which respond specifically to the inhibitor, its agonists, and antagonists;
e) act in vitro on isolated pituitary tissue or cells in a logical, consistent manner.

No substance can meet all these criteria at this time; (b) is especially difficult to define because prolactin release is the *net* resultant of one or more inhibitors plus one or more stimulators of release. Therefore, there is no reason to expect a simple relationship between the concentration of a substance in vivo that modifies release and the release of prolactin in response to a physiological stimulus. It may be some time before one can define "appropriate."

For technical reasons, (d) also presents difficulties. While most biological type experiments are done on rats, most receptor binding studies use pituitaries from the larger domestic animals. Moreover, the values obtained are often critically dependent on the amount of protein assayed and the presence of proteolytic enzymes. Optimum conditions remain to be established.

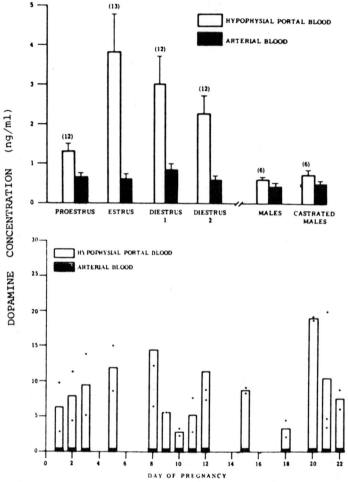

Fig. 1. Dopamine concentration in hypophyseal portal and arterial plasma from rats (from Ben-Jonathan et al [6]).

Dopamine can meet most of the requirements. It is almost certainly a prolactin release-inhibiting hormone (PRIH) and may soon deserve promotion from the status of a PIF. Several critical experiments support this conclusion.

Ben-Jonathan and co-workers [6] were the first to measure dopamine in hypophyseal stalk blood during estrus cycles and during pregnancy (Fig. 1) and later [7] during lactation. This work was soon extended by others (Table I). The values are, on the whole, reasonably consistent except for those of DeGreef and Neill [9] which are perhaps an order of magnitude too great. I reason that values for ovariectomized females should not be much different from males (1–3 nM)

TABLE I. Dopamine concentration in hypophyseal portal blood and prolactin concentration in peripheral blood of rats

Condition		Dopamine		Prolactin ng/ml	Reference
		ng/ml	nM		
Males		0.5	3	—	[6]
Estrous females		1.3–3.8	8–25	—	
Pregnant females		2–18	13–120	—	
Pregnant, 18–21 d		4.9	32	30	[7]
22 d		3.3	22	85	
Lactating		2.7	18	—	
Diestrous, cycling		1.4	9	50	[8]
noncycling		1.2	8	50	
Ectopic pituitary		1.4	9	150	
7315a Tumor		2.0	13	1,600	
Ovariectomized	AM	10	65	3	[9]
	noon	6	39	3	
	PM	7	46	3	
Ovariectomized	AM	6	39	12	
+ cervical	noon	5	33	3	
stimulation	PM	4	26	7	
Males		0.3	2	—	[10]
Males + d-amphetamine (5mg/kg)		1.45	9	—	
Males + d-amphetamine + α-MT		0.4	3	—	
Males + reserpine (2.5 mg/kg)		0.15	1	—	
Males + reserpine + d-amphetamine		0.7	5	—	
Pregnant		2.0	13	—	
Pregnant + α-methyltyr (50 mg/kg)		0.4	3	—	
Males		0.2	1	—	[11]
Males + rPRL (1 μg ivt)		1.1	7	—	
Males + haloperidol (2.5 mg/kg)		1.25	8	—	
Diestrus		3.0	20	6	[21]
Proestrus		1.2	8	16	

Values are minimal values as no correction apparently is applied for loss during collection (0.3%/min for 45–60 minutes [6]) or during analysis. Values are expressed per unit volume of plasma or serum.

and certainly less than those for cycling females (8–25 nM). Values of 39–65 nM appear out of line. A possible reason may be the type of anesthesia used: all [6–8, 10, 11] used pentobarbital except DeGreef and Neill [9] who used urethane anesthesia. Values then fall in the range of 1–30 nM in hypophyseal portal plasma whereas they are less than 1 nM in peripheral plasma.

Are these concentrations sufficiently large to influence prolactin release? Gibbs and Neill [12] attempted to answer this question by infusing dopamine into rats treated with α-methyltyrosine to inhibit synthesis of endogenous dopamine or into rats having lesioned median eminences to prevent release of endogenous dopamine. The arterial concentrations achieved were 8.4–10.7 ng/ml so that the portal concentrations, which were shown to be 70% of arterial, were 5.9–7.5 ng/ml (39–49 nM) by calculation. These concentrations produced no diminution in plasma prolactin of diestrus rats, but a 70% suppression in α-methyltyrosine-treated rats and a 42% suppression in lesioned rats (Fig. 2). It is unfortunate that the α-methyltyrosine experiment was not repeated at lower concentrations of dopamine.

Another approach is the measurement of the dissociation (or association) constant of the dopamine receptor. For the concentrations of dopamine reported in Table I, a K_d of about 10 nM for the dopamine-receptor complex would allow occupancy of the receptor to vary from very low to moderately high. There is still insufficient evidence (Table II) to draw firm conclusions. Note the paucity of data for the combination, dopamine/rat! The single value of 35 nM [14] is based on inhibition of prolactin release from a cell culture of rat anterior pituitary. This value of 35 nM would require operation on the low end of the binding curve, a definite possibility if "spare" receptors were operable. The major difficulty in pursuing this problem is the lack of material and the low concentration of receptors. Agonist/antagonist action on the release of prolactin from isolated rat anterior pituitary cells in culture, however, is closely correlated with binding to bovine anterior pituitary membranes [14].

The pituitary cell line, GH_3, is an interesting variant in that it either has no receptor [17] or it has a defective receptor [18]. Cronin and co-workers [16] compared affinities of a large number of compounds for GH_3 cells (rat) with ovine anterior pituitary membranes (Table III). Certainly there is a weakly binding receptor for dopamine agonists present, but it bears little resemblance to that present in normal tissue. Most striking is the loss of stereoselectivity for d- and l-butaclamol in the GH_3 cells.

Internalization of membrane receptors is currently a very active area of investigation. Nansel and co-workers [19] have found dopamine in apparent association with prolactin secretory granules in the adenohypophysis.

Only in the male or in the ovariectomized female can one sometimes see an inverse correlation of dopamine and prolactin concentrations. If estrogen is present, no correlation can be seen (Fig. 1). Estradiol acts directly on pituitary cells in culture, both canine [20] and rat [5], to increase prolactin release. The latter [5] have concluded "that estrogens have potent antidopaminergic activity on prolactin secretion, not only in anterior pituitary cells in culture but also in vivo, the effect being qualitatively similar in both female and male animals." An example of an in vitro experiment (Fig. 3) shows that preincubation of rat adenohypophyseal cells with 1 nM estradiol-17β reduced the inhibition of prolactin release by bromoergocryptine from 70% to 20% regardless of whether 10 nM TRH was present [5, 22]. Progesterone or 5α-dihydrotestosterone (10 nM)

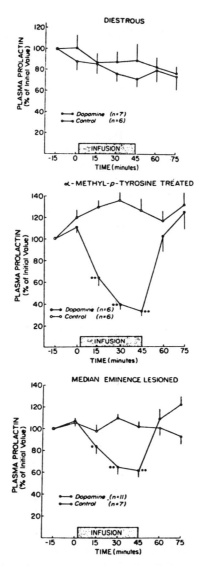

Fig. 2. Effect of dopamine infusion (0.9–1.1 μg/min/kg BW) that mimics hypophyseal stalk plasma dopamine levels on prolactin secretion. Dopamine or distilled water (control) was infused for 45 minutes. Vertical lines indicate SE. *, P<0.05; **, P< 0.01 (from Gibbs and Neill [12]).

TABLE II. Binding to adenohypophyseal dopamine receptors

Substance	Binding sites (fmole/mg protein)	$IC_{50\%}/K_d$ (nM)	Species	Reference
Dopamine	43	—	monkey	[13]
Haloperidol	65	0.7	monkey	
Dopamine	—	35[a] (37°)	rat	[14]
		490 (23°)	cattle	
Dihydroergocryptine	260,208	3.7, 6.0	rat	[15]
	150,373	4.7, 5.2	sheep	
Dopamine	—	776 (K_i)	sheep	
Spiperone	—	0.8	sheep	[16]
Dopamine	—	1,330 (K_i)	sheep	

[a]Value based on PRL release.

TABLE III. Competition for [³H]SPIP binding

Agent	GH_3 (nM)	n	Anterior pituitary (nM)	n
Chlorpromazine	170 ± 70	5	16 ± 6	3
Haloperidol	680 ± 120	3	12 ± 3	4
Pimozide	770 ± 90	4	4 ± 3	3
d-Butaclamol	1,160 ± 240	4	1.6 ± 0.5	5
l-Butaclamol	1,300 ± 250	3	17,000 ± 5,000	3
SPIP	1,490 ± 290	5	0.8 ± 0.4	4
Bromoergocryptine	4,980 ± 470	3	19 ± 15	3
Apomorphine	13,900 ± 2,500	4	220 ± 80	7
l-Sulpiride	>100,000	2	2,200	2
d-Sulpiride	>100,000	2	>40,000	2
DA	>100,000	2	1,330 ± 40	3
Norepinephrine	>100,000	3	18,000 ± 6,000	3
Epinephrine	>100,000	2	22,000 ± 10,000	3
Serotonin	>100,000	2	>40,000	2
Oxymetazoline	>100,000	2	>40,000	2
Histamine	>100,000	2	>40,000	2
TRH	>100,000	2	>40,000	2
Methysergide	>100,000	2		

The K_i values measured in GH_3 cells differ dramatically from those seen in homogenates of sheep anterior pituitaries. GH_3 cells were co-incubated with [³H]SPIP (0.85–1.56 nM) and increasing concentrations of nonradioactive competitor. The K_i was derived from direct measurement of the concentration required to compete for 50% of the [³H]SPIP binding. There was no stereoselectivity for d- and l-butaclamol at these low affinity sites as there is for the high affinity sites in normal anterior pituitary homogenates. We have also observed that d- and l-butaclamol are equipotent in inhibiting PRL secretion at micromolar concentrations in GH_3 cells. n, Number of independent experiments. Values given are the mean ± SEM. From Cronin et al [16] with permission.

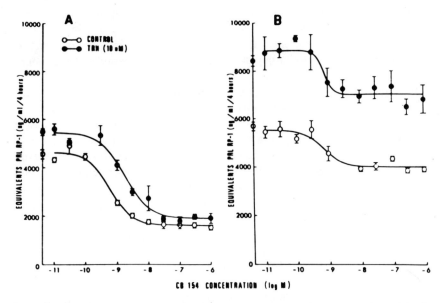

Fig. 3. Effect of estradiol-17β on the prolactin response to increasing concentrations of the dopamine agonist, bromoergocryptine (CB-154) in rat adenohypophyseal cells in culture. The cells were preincubated for 5 days in the presence (B) or absence (A) of 1 nM estradiol before a 4-hour incubation in the presence (●—●) or absence (○—○) of 10 nM TRH and the indicated concentrations of CB-154 (from Ferland et al [5]).

partially reverse the stimulatory action of estradiol [5]. Evidence of a direct action in vivo was also found [23].

Estradiol also stimulates the release of hypothalamic dopamine [5, 24]. Gudelsky et al. [24] directly measured a 2.5-fold increase in dopamine concentration in portal plasma in response to estrogen, but a decreased (60%) internalization of dopamine. Therefore, even though estrogens increase release of dopamine from the hypothalamus, they exert an overbalancing antidopaminergic activity at the pituitary level which leads to increased prolactin secretion.

Suprachiasmatic lesions in ovariectomized rats abolish estrogen-induced surges of prolactin [25]. This observation does not appear compatible with the preceding conclusion.

Prolactin may act in a "short loop" feedback to inhibit its own release. Through the use of the principles of competitive protein binding combined with radioautography, Walsh and co-workers [26] have demonstrated prolactin binding sites in the ependyma of the choroid plexus. Gudelsky and Porter [11] report that 1 μg of rPRL injected intracerebroventricularly raised the dopamine concentration in adenohypophyseal portal plasmas to 1.1 ng/ml (7 nM) compared to 0.2 ng/

ml (1 nM) in controls. Haloperidol (2.5 mg/kg; SC), a dopamine antagonist, gave a similar result, but simultaneous injection of an antiprolactin antiserum largely eliminated the response. Prolactin enhances dopmaine turnover in the median eminence and anterior hypothalamus after a latent period of 10–26 hours [27].

In cell culture, high levels of prolactin can inhibit prolactin release from the pituitary 2B8 cell line [28]. This presumably has no physiological significance.

Ontogeny of prolactin release is interesting. In the female rat [29], plasma prolactin increases gradually to adult levels by day 35. Response to pimozide, a dopamine antagonist, was detectable at day 3 and increased in magnitude up to day 35. The response to estrogen, however, was not present until day 24 and then increased to a maximum at 37 days. In the sheep [30], on the other hand, plasma prolactin rises to high concentrations in the late gestational period (gestation, 147 days) and remains elevated in the early neonatal period. By infusing apomorphine or bromoergocryptine, dopamine agonists, or haloperidol, an antagonist, dopaminergic inhibition of prolactin release was present by the 106th day before the rapid rise in fetal prolactin concentration which occurs between 110–120 days of gestation.

γ-Aminobutyric acid (GABA) is apparently also an inhibitor of prolactin release. Ingestion of enormous amounts (50 or 200 mmoles) [31] or intraventricular injection or infusion of large amounts (2–8 μmoles) of GABA [32, 33], however, may produce anomalous effects, such as no change or a rise in prolactin secretion. Similarly, ingestion of muscimol, a GABA agonist, by human subjects produced a rise in plasma prolactin [34].

The balance of the evidence, however, suggests that GABA is an inhibitor of prolactin release. Schally and co-workers [35] isolated GABA from porcine hypothalami and demonstrated its release-inhibiting activity, both in vitro and in vivo. Grandison and Guidotti [36] firmly established that the rat anterior pituitary has specific high affinity binding sites (K_d, 33 nM) on mitochondrial membranes for GABA. ^{3}H-Muscimol, a specific long-acting GABA agonist when administered intravenously, localized predominantly in the anterior pituitary. Relative to ^{3}H-GABA, muscimol had an IC_{50} of 5 nM, GABA had 50 nM and bicuculline, a specific GABA receptor agonist which does not enter the brain, had an IC_{50} of 50 μM. Muscimol (1 mg/kg; IV) was most potent in vivo in blocking a stimulus for release of prolactin, such as morphine (2–15 mg/kg; SC) or haloperidol (25–500 μg/kg; IV). Muscimol (10–1,000 nM) also reduced the spontaneous release of prolactin from pituitary halves in vitro. Muscimol injected intraventricularly produced a slight stimulation of prolactin release. These results have been confirmed by nearly simultaneous publications [37, 38].

Dopamine and GABA receptors can be distinguished by picrotoxin, which blocks only the GABA receptor, and α-flupenthixol, which blocks only dopamine receptors [37]. Although GABA inhibits prolactin release, its maximal effect in vitro is less than that of dopamine, and, in disagreement with Grandison and

Guidotti [36], the K_d is 1.5 μM [38]. Nevertheless, it is clear that GABA is a second PIF; its physiological significance remains to be established.

Two reports on the effect of pyridoxine have appeared [39, 40]. This vitamin is converted to a co-factor which is required for the decarboxylation of Dopa to dopamine. In female rats [39], pyridoxine (50 mg; IP) prevented the increase in prolactin secretion normally seen at 1300 hours. This effect was also seen after treatment with α-methyltyrosine, an inhibitor of dopamine synthesis! A 300-mg intravenous injection of pyridoxine had no effect on plasma prolactin in nine hyperprolactinemic subjects [40].

Recently several neuropeptides have been tested. Centrally administered bombesin-like peptide (5 μg) had a very potent and long acting inhibitory effect on stress-induced prolactin release [41]. Neurotensin produced equivocal results [42]. Centrally administered at two amounts (0.5 or 2 μg), it decreased prolactin secretion while an intermediate dose (1 μg) increased secretion. Large amounts (>50 ng/ml) added to incubation media containing hemipituitaries promoted prolactin release.

REFERENCES

1. Creese I, Sibley DR, Leff S, Hamblin M: Dopamine receptors: subtypes, localization and regulation. Fed Proc 40: 147–152, 1981.
2. Shaar CJ, Clemens JA: The effects of opiate agonists on growth hormone and prolactin release in rats. Fed Proc 39: 2539–2543, 1980.
3. Clemens JA, Shaar CJ: Control of prolactin secretion in mammals, Fed Proc 39: 2588–2592, 1980.
4. Clemens JA, Shaar CJ, Smalstig EB: Dopamine, PIF and other regulators of prolactin secretion. Fed Proc 39: 2907–2911, 1980.
5. Ferland L, Labrie F, Kelly PA, Raymond V: Interactions between hypothalamic and peripheral hormones in the control of prolactin secretion. Fed Proc 39: 2917–2922, 1980.
6. Ben-Jonathan N, Oliver C, Weiner HJ, Mical RS, Porter JC: Dopamine in hypophysial portal plasma of the rat during the estrous cycle and throughout pregnancy. Endocrinology 100: 452–458, 1977.
7. Ben-Jonathan N, Neill MA, Arbogast LA, Peters LL, Hoefer MT: Dopamine in hypophysial portal blood: relationship to circulating prolactin in pregnant and lactating rats. Endocrinology 106: 690–696, 1980.
8. Cramer OM, Parker CR Jr, Porter JC: Secretion of dopamine into hypophysial portal blood by rats bearing prolactin-secreting tumors or ectopic glands. Endocrinology 105: 636–640, 1979.
9. DeGreef WJ, Neill JD: Dopamine levels in hypophysial stalk plasma of the rat during surges of prolactin secretion induced by cervical stimulation. Endocrinology 105: 1093–1099, 1979.
10. Gudelsky GA, Porter JC: Release of newly synthesized dopamine into the hypophysial portal vasculature of the rat. Endocrinology 104: 583–587, 1979.
11. Gudelsky GA, Porter JC: Release of dopamine from tuberoinfundibular neurons into pituitary stalk blood after prolactin or haloperidol administration. Endocrinology 106: 526–529, 1980.
12. Gibbs M, Neill JD: Dopamine levels in hypophysial stalk blood in the rat are sufficient to inhibit prolaction secretion in vitro. Endocrinology 102: 1895–1900, 1978.
13. Brown GM, Seeman P, Lee T: Dopamine/neuroleptic receptors in basal hypothalamus and pituitary. Endocrinology 99: 1407–1410, 1976.

14. Caron MG, Beaulieu M, Raymond V, Gagne B, Drouin J, Lefkowitz RJ, Labrie F: Dopaminergic receptors in the anterior pitutiary gland. Correlation of ^{3}H-dihydroergocryptine binding in the dopaminergic control of prolactin release. J Biol Chem 253: 2244–2253, 1978.

15. Cronin MJ, Roberts JM, Weiner RI: Dopamine and dihydroergocryptine binding to the anterior pituitary and other brain areas of the rat and sheep. Endocrinology 103: 302–309, 1978.

16. Cronin MJ, Faure N, Martial JA, Weiner RI: Absence of high affinity dopamine receptors in GH_3 cells: A prolactin-secreting clone resistant to the inhibitory action of dopamine. Endocrinology 106: 718–723, 1980.

17. West B, Dannies PS: Antipsychotic drugs inhibit prolactin release from rat anterior pituitary cells in culture by a mechanism not involving the dopamine receptor. Endocrinology 104: 877–880, 1979.

18. Faure N, Cronin MJ, Martial JA, Weiner RI: Decreased responsiveness of GH_3 cells to the dopaminergic inhibition of prolactin. Endocrinology 107: 1022–1026, 1980.

19. Nansel DD, Gudelsky GA, Porter JC: Subcellular localization of dopamine in the anterior pituitary gland of the rat: Apparent association of dopamine with prolactin secretory granules. Endocrinology 105: 1073–1077, 1979.

20. Jones GE, Boyns AR: Oestradiol stimulation of prolactin release from canine pituitary in culture. Acta Endocrinol 82: 706–709, 1976.

21. Plotsky PM, Gibbs DM, Neill JD: Liquid chromatographic-electrochemical measurement of dopamine in hypophyseal stalk blood of rats. Endocrinology 102: 1887–1900, 1978.

22. Raymond V, Beaulieu M, Labrie F: Potent antidopaminergic activity of estradiol at the pituitary level on prolactin release. Science 200: 1173–1175, 1978.

23. Ferland L, Labrie F, Euvrard C, Raynaud J-P: Antidopaminergic activity of estrogens on prolactin release at the pituitary level in vivo. Mol Cell Endocrinol 14: 199–204, 1979.

24. Gudelsky GA, Nansel DD, Porter JC: Role of estrogen in the dopaminergic control of prolactin secretion. Endocrinology 108: 440–444, 1981.

25. Kawakami M, Arita J, Yoshioka E: Loss of estrogen-induced daily surges of prolactin and gonadotropins by suprachiasmatic nucleus lesions in ovariectomized rats. Endocrinology 106: 1087–1092, 1980.

26. Walsh RJ, Posner BI, Kopriwa BM, Brawer JR: Prolactin binding sites in the rat brain. Science 201: 1041–1043, 1978.

27. Gudelsky GA, Simkins J, Mueller GP, Meites J, Moore KE: Selective actions of prolactin on catecholamine turnover in the hypothalamus and on serum LH and FSH. Neuroendocrinology 22: 206–215, 1976.

28. Herbert DC, Ishikawa H, Rennels EG: Evidence for the autoregulation of hormone secretion. Endocrinology 104: 97–100, 1979.

29. Ojeda SR, McCann SM: Development of dopaminergic and estrogenic control of prolactin release in the female rat. Endocrinology 95: 1499–1505, 1974.

30. Gluckman PD, Marti-Henneberg C, Thomsett MJ, Kaplan SL, Rudolph AM, Grumbach MM: Hormone ontogeny in the ovine fetus. VI. Dopaminergic regulation of prolactin secretion. Endocrinology 105: 1173–1177, 1979.

31. Cavagnini F, Invitti C, Pinto M, Maraschini C, DiLandro A, Dubini A, Marelli A: Effect of acute and repeated administration of gamma aminobutyric acid (GABA) on growth hormone and prolactin secretion in man. Acta Endocrinol 93: 149–154, 1980.

32. Mioduszewski R, Grandison L, Meites J: Stimulation of prolactin release in rats by GABA. Proc Soc Exp Biol Med 151: 44–46, 1976.

33. Ondo JG, Pass KA: The effects of neurally active amino acids on prolactin secretion. Endocrinology 98: 1248–1252, 1976.

34. Tamminga CA, Neophytides A, Chase TN, Frohman LA: Stimulation of prolactin and growth hormone scretion by muscimol, a γ-aminobutryic acid agonist. J Clin Endocrinol Metab 47: 1348–1351, 1978.

35. Schally AV, Redding TW, Arimura A, Dupont A, Linthicum G: Isolation of gamma-amino-butyric acid from pig hypothalami and demonstration of its prolactin release-inhibiting (PIF) activity in vivo and in vitro. Endocrinology 100: 681–691, 1977.

36. Grandison L, Guidotti A: γ-Aminobutyric acid receptor function in rat anterior pituitary: evidence for control of prolactin release. Endocrinology 105: 754–759, 1979.

37. Locatelli V, Cocchi D, Frigerio C, Betti R, Krogsgaard-Larsen P, Racagni G, Muller EE: Dual γ-aminobutyric acid control of prolactin secretion in the rat. Endocrinology 105: 778–785, 1979.

38. Enjalbert A, Ruberg M, Arancibia S, Fiore L, Priam M, Kordon C: Independent inhibition of prolaction secretion by dopamine and γ-aminobutyric acid in vitro. Endocrinology 105: 823–826, 1979.

39. Harris ARC, Smith MS, Alex S, Salhanick HA, Vagenakis AG, Braverman LE: Pyridoxine (B_6)-induced inhibition of prolaction release in the female rat. Endocrinology 102: 362–366, 1978.

40. Spiegel AM, Rosen SW, Weintraub BD, Marynick SP: Effect of intravenous pyridoxine on plasma prolactin in hyperprolactinemic subjects. J Clin Endocrinol Metab 46: 686–688, 1978.

41. Tache Y, Brown M, Collu R: Effects of neuropeptides on adenohypophyseal hormone response to acute stress in male rats. Endocrinology 105: 220–224, 1979.

42. Vijayan E, McCann SM: In vivo and in vitro effects on substance P and neurotensin on gonadotropin and prolactin release. Endocrinology 105: 64–68, 1979.

The Prostatic Cell: Structure and Function
Part B, pages 31–53
© 1981 Alan R. Liss, Inc., 150 Fifth Avenue, New York, NY 10011

The Pituitary-Testicular Axis in Prostatic Disease: The Potential of Salivary Steroid Assays

K. Griffiths, M.E. Harper, D.R. Fahmy, W.B. Peeling, and C.G. Pierrepoint

Although the biological control of the prostate would seem to be relatively complex (Fig. 1), the basis of most endocrine studies concerning the gland centers around the fact that its growth, maintenance, and functional activity are largely dependent on the androgenic hormones secreted by the testis. Other hormones, particularly of pituitary origin, indirectly affect the prostate, and there is evidence that certain of them may exert a direct effect on the gland. Luteinizing hormone (LH), for example, controls testicular synthesis of testosterone, the principal circulating androgen, approximately 95% of which originates in the testis [1]. Prolactin appears to have a synergistic role with LH in regulating testosterone production by the testis [2–4]. There is also a considerable body of evidence, however, to suggest that prolactin may have a direct influence on prostatic growth and function, and can accentuate the effects of androgens on the gland. Grayhack and Lebowitz [5] also observed an augmented increase in fructose and citric acid content of the prostate of castrated-hypophysectomised rats when testosterone and prolactin were administered together compared with that caused by testosterone alone, and specific binding sites for prolactin have been reported in prostatic tissue membranes [6,7]. Furthermore, Farnsworth has reported [8] that prolactin may, to some extent, increase testosterone uptake by the prostate gland, and others [9,10] suggest that growth hormone (GH) can also increase prostatic weight. Investigations in our laboratories, however, indicated that treatment of rats for 30 days with an inhibitor of prolactin secretion (2-bromo-α-ergo-cryptine; Sandoz Ltd.) failed to affect the weight of the accessory sex glands. Prolactin levels in the plasma were undetectable in these animals. The treatment had no effect on the ventral prostate lobe but did influence the zinc levels and its distribution in the dorsolateral lobes, consistent with earlier

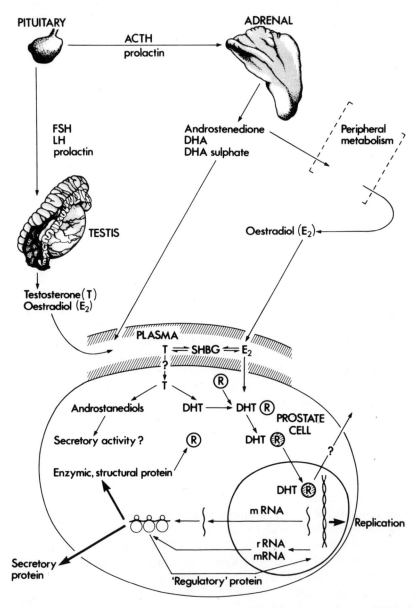

Fig. 1.   Schematic representation of certain aspects of the endocrinology relating to control of the prostate gland. DHA, dehydroepiandrosterone; DHT, 5α-dihydrotestosterone; SHBG, sex hormone binding globulin; R, specific intracellular receptor; DHT-R, steroid receptor complex; mRNA and rRNA, messenger and ribosomal ribonucleic acid respectively. Question marks refer to processes not completely elucidated.

observations [11]. Aragona and Friesen have subsequently reported that prolactin receptors are localized in the dorsolateral lobes of the rat prostate [12].

Follicle stimulating hormone (FSH) or LH may also influence the biochemistry of the prostate gland by controlling oestradiol-17β production by the testis. Receptors for oestradiol-17β have been reported to be present in prostatic tissues, but their precise physiological role has still to be determined. It may be that this role is concerned more with stromal tissue rather than epithelial elements since investigations by ourselves [13] have clearly indicated that the oestradiol-17β receptors of the canine prostate are located mainly in the stroma. ACTH has been reported to stimulate rat prostatic growth [14–17] although its relationship with the prostate must be through the production of adrenal androgens, dehydroepiandrosterone and its sulphate, and androstenedione, which can be metabolized by the prostate [18]. Androstenedione can be peripherally converted to oestrogens [19,20]. The evidence that prolactin is concerned with the production of androgens by the adrenal gland remains equivocal [21]. It must be borne in mind, however, that the adrenal gland is unable to maintain prostatic weight in the castrated man or rat, and adrenal androgens are not sufficient to compensate for the loss of testicular function. The endocrinology of the prostate gland has recently been the subject of at least two major reviews [21,22].

PITUITARY-TESTICULAR AXIS AND PROSTATIC DISEASE

An involvement of pituitary hormones in the development of prostatic neoplasia or benign hyperplasia of the gland has still to be decided. There is, however, little evidence to implicate any hormone in the initiation of prostatic cancer [21]. Clinical data would indicate that carcinoma of the prostate in man is, to some extent, functionally dependent upon androgenic stimulation, yet the role of the various hormones circulating in the blood and synthesized within the prostate, in the aetiology of the disease, remains obscure.

The changes in plasma hormone concentrations associated with ageing in man have been of interest. There are reports that although the ability of the testis to respond to exogenous gonadotrophin is preserved despite ageing and decline in libido [23,24], plasma levels of testosterone decrease after the sixth decade [25]. On the other hand, the plasma oestradiol-17β concentration increases with age in the healthy normal adult man [26], an effect which is probably responsible for the reported increase in sex hormone binding globulin (SHBG) levels in the older man [27]. It is quite possible therefore that changes in the androgen-oestrogen balance in the elderly male and in the proportion of the free nonprotein-bound steroid hormones of plasma which are considered the biologically active moiety of the circulating hormone, could be implicated in the aetiology of prostatic disease.

In the search for the endocrine abnormality that may be implicated in the pathogenesis of prostatic cancer, detailed studies of hormone levels in plasma and tissue from patients with this disease have been undertaken with the view that such data will increase our understanding of its aetiology.

Fundamental to this approach is the possibility that a change in the endocrine status of an individual has activated latent carcinoma or a particular pattern of hormone secretion has promoted early neoplastic growth. Studies from our own laboratories [28] and in association with the British Prostate Study Group [29] have been concerned with the plasma levels of hormones in patients with prostatic disease prior to and during treatment. Patients who presented for treatment in the various urological clinics of the group were assessed and classified in a standardized manner according to their primary tumour grade and metastatic status. Possible differences in the concentration of hormones between the various groups of patients was assessed using a multivariate-statistical analysis technique developed at the Institute [30].

Results obtained from the analysis of plasma obtained from patients with histologically proven prostatic cancer, prior to treatment, were somewhat disappointing, but possibly to be expected from the analysis of a single plasma sample from each patient. When hormone concentrations were classified according to primary tumour staging, using a standard Student t test, no significant differences between the group means were found, with the progression of the disease from stage T0 to T4. Furthermore, there were no significant differences seen in the hormone concentrations of patients with and without metastases. Of interest, however, was the separation found, using canonical variate analysis, between those patients with and without clinically evident metastases. GH levels were higher in those with metastatic disease and together with age, was the principal discriminating component responsible for group separation. High GH levels may be associated with the stress of a more debilitating development of the disease, but such studies indicate that careful assessment of the endocrinology of patients, investigated in depth, many ultimately provide the means to identify factors concerned in the pathogenesis of the disease.

Analysis of these data in relation to patient survival serves to illustrate the point. Patients were separated into groups 1–6 (Table I) depending on the number of years they survived from the time the disease was diagnosed and treatment commenced. Pretreatment hormone results were related to these patient groups (Table II). The analysis clearly indicated that the normality of the pituitary-testicular axis of the patient, on presentation at the clinic, was related to ultimate survival.

The higher the levels of plasma testosterone and oestradiol-17β and the lower those of LH, the longer the patient survived. Those patients with low concentrations of testosterone and oestradiol-17β and high LH levels, died relatively quickly from the disease.

TABLE I. Patient survival groups

		Group	n
Patients who died	< 1 year after initial diagnosis	1	43
" " "	1–2 years " " "	2	32
" " "	2–3 " " " "	3	30
" " "	3–4 " " . " "	4	15
" " "	3–5 " " " "	5	41
Patients alive	4–6 " " " "	6	76

n, Number of patients.

TABLE II. Relationship of survival to hormone concentrations

Survival groups	Plasma hormones (2p values)					
	T	E_2	LH	FSH	GH	Prolactin
1 v 2	NS	NS	NS	NS	NS	NS
1 v 3	NS	0.04	0.04	NS	NS	NS
1 v 4	0.01	NS	0.05	NS	0.01	NS
1 v 5	0.02	0.04	0.02	NS	NS	NS
1 v 6	0.001	0.004	0.02	NS	NS	NS

Mann Whitney U Statistics. NS, not significant; T, testosterone; E_2, oestradiol-17β.

MONITORING HORMONE LEVELS THROUGHOUT TREATMENT

As part of this investigation, plasma hormone levels were measured in patients with prostatic cancer throughout treatment until recurrence and eventual death. The profile of hormone changes seen in Figure 2 was generally found in patients receiving treatment with diethylstilboestrol (DES) diphosphate (Honvan), 100 mg, twice daily. Levels of FSH and LH consistently decreased and subsequently so did the plasma concentration of testosterone. It was interesting that although the testis is generally considered to secrete little oestrogen [20], the levels of oestradiol-17β were always decreased by the order of 50% during treatment (Fig. 3). Prolactin and GH concentration increased under the influence of the high doses of synthetic oestrogen, and in line with the belief that prolactin may exercise some role in either promoting androgen uptake by the prostate or may influence the adrenal in synthesizing androgens, it was obvious that the high dose was contraindicated. Over recent years, a dose of DES of 1 mg t.d.s. has

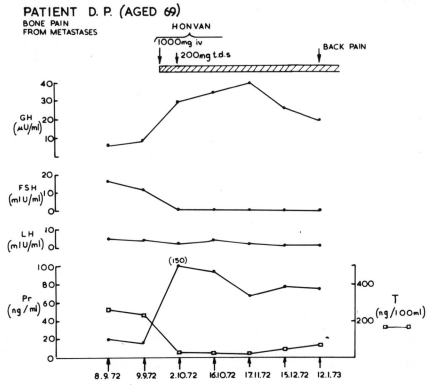

Fig. 2. Patient with prostatic cancer treated with Honvan 100 mg b.d., and the plasma hormones monitored over several months. Pr, prolactin; T, testosterone.

become generally accepted in the United Kingdom as that which provides adequate endocrine control of testicular activity in the patient.

In Figure 2, the increase in testosterone observed in this patient after a year or more of treatment was seen to relate to disease recurrence (Fig. 4), and this rise in testosterone has usually been considered of adrenal origin. In the investigation of more than 300 patients, only rarely did symptoms of disease recurrence relate to an increase in plasma testosterone. The use of adrenal stimulation tests (Synacthen, IM) or dexamethasone suppression tests clearly indicated that the basal 50 ng/100 ml testosterone, with its episodic and circadian rhythm, was of adrenal and not testicular origin, and the clinical value of orchiectomy for treatment of the patient who has relapsed after oestrogen therapy requires reassessment. Although aminoglutethimide, a drug capable of suppressing steroid synthesis, has been used to treat patients with prostatic cancer who have relapsed

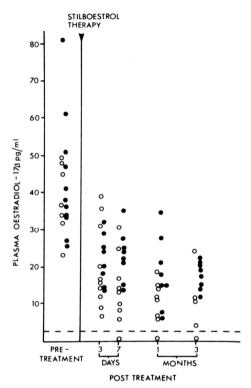

Fig. 3. Changes in plasma oestradiol-17β in patients with prostatic carcinoma before and after treatment with diethylstilboestrol (○) 1 mg t.d.s. or Honvan (●) 100 mg b.d.

after orchiectomy [31], the possibility that it should be used as part of the primary treatment to suppress all testosterone production from all sources must also be considered. Adrenalectomy and hypophysectomy have never been accepted as offering an effective means of controlling recurrent disease, although it has to be accepted that hypophysectomy is of value for the palliation of pain in patients who have failed on endocrine therapy [32]. The possibility that certain hypothalamic-pituitary factors may influence the biochemistry of prostatic cancer cells must also be accepted. It is noteworthy however, that the profiles of hormone changes during various forms of therapy for prostatic cancer are quite different (Fig. 5). The initial clinical response of the patients to treatment can be identical despite vastly different levels of protein hormones in their plasma.

As part of this study throughout treatment, a method for the measurement of DES in plasma was established [33]. This specific radioimmunoassay, developed

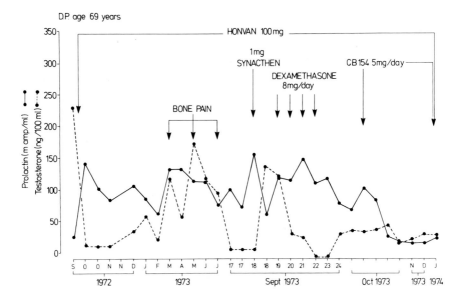

Fig. 4. Changes in plasma prolactin and testosterone in a patient with prostatic carcinoma treated with Honvan. Synacthen test-blood samples taken at 9 AM and 4 PM on control day and at 9 AM followed by Synacthen IM and sample taken at 4 PM on the test day.

using an antiserum raised against DES-carboxymethyl ether and a tritium-labelled radioligand, has a sensitivity of 8.8 pg, corresponding to a plasma level of 132 pg/ml and is adequate for the accurate determination of DES in the plasma of patients with prostatic carcinoma. When validated against gas chromatography-high resolution mass spectrometry, an excellent correlation (r = 0.96) was achieved.

Plasma samples from six patients receiving 1 mg DES t.d.s. were assayed for levels of DES and testosterone. DES was administered at 0630, 1230, and 1700 hours and blood collected via indwelling catheter from 0730–1600 hours on two consecutive days. On the second day, luteinizing hormone-releasing hormone (LH-RH; 100 μg, IV) was administered at 0900 hours.

In Figure 6, the expected marked rise in DES concentration occurred 1.5–2.0 hours after the oral administration of a 1-mg tablet. A less significant rise was observed 4 hours later when DES glucuronides are hydrolyzed in, or reabsorbed from the large intestine. Patients had been on DES for the previous three months.

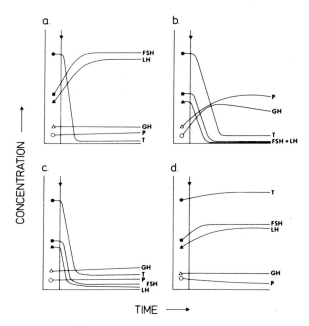

Fig. 5. General hormone profiles with various endocrine therapies. a) Orchidectomy, b) oestrogen therapy, c) antiandrogen therapy, d) antiestrogen therapy. Arrows indicated start of treatment; P, prolactin; T, testosterone.

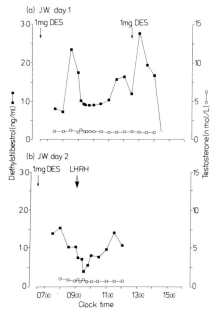

Fig. 6. Plasma testosterone and diethylstilboestrol (DES) concentrations measured at 30-minute intervals. LH-RH (IV 100 μg) administered at 0900 hours on day 2.

Levels of testosterone were low and failed to rise after LH-RH administration (Fig. 6b).

In one of the six patients, however, levels of testosterone were higher than expected after three months of DES treatment (Fig. 7a) and furthermore, were further elevated after LH-RH treatment (Fig. 7b), indicating a responsive pituitary-testicular axis. Although it would seem therefore that 1 mg DES t.d.s. is sufficient to suppress the pituitary-testicular axis in most patients, it can fail occasionally, and the study emphasizes the value of monitoring testosterone levels during treatment.

HORMONAL RHYTHMS

Detailed assessment of the hormone concentrations of patients with prostatic cancer reveals a wide variation in the hormone values found in the differing groups. Concentrations of plasma testosterone in the older patient can be as high as that in 20-year-old men. Such results are probably due to the single sample determination of parameters which exhibit episodic, circadian, and possibly even circatrigintan (monthly) or annual variation. In-depth studies of certain patients with prostatic cancer in whom an indwelling catheter was used to collect blood at 30-minute intervals for periods of 12 or 24 hours illustrated the errors concerned with single sample analysis. This multiple-sampling study clearly indicated the wide differences between patients even within the same age group and disease

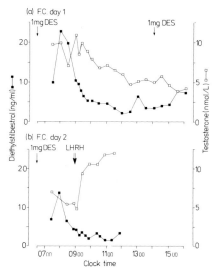

Fig. 7. Plasma testosterone and diethylstilboestrol (DES) concentrations measured at 30-minute intervals. LH-RH (IV 100 μg) administered at 0900 hours on day 2.

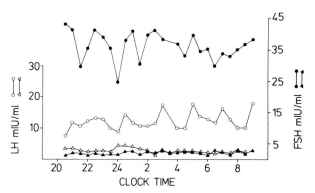

Fig. 8 Plasma gonadotrophin concentrations measured at 30-minute intervals in two patients with BPH: Circles, patient HR, age 71; triangles, patient SB, age 69.

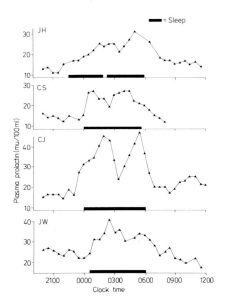

Fig. 9. Plasma prolactin concentrations in 4 BPH patients measured at 30-minute intervals during a 16-hour period.

category. Plasma FSH and LH levels throughout the day and night of two patients with benign prostatic hyperplasia are shown in Figure 8.

Figures 9 and 10 show the concentrations of prolactin and GH in plasma of patients with prostatic cancer from whom blood was collected during their sleep periods. The high prolactin during the early hours of the morning would seem normal, and the elevation of GH immediately on falling asleep would again

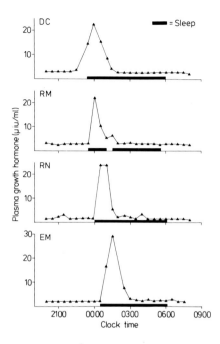

Fig. 10 Plasma growth hormone concentrations in three BPH patients and one prostatic cancer patient (EM) measured at 30-minute intervals during a 12-hour period.

suggest that any differences between patients and clinically normal males may be difficult to identify.

SALIVARY STEROID ANALYSIS

The recognition of the difficulties in assessing the endocrine status of patients by either single sample analysis or use of indwelling catheters stimulated the search for a new approach. The ease with which saliva may be collected and the fact that multiple samples may be taken without detriment to the patient make this an obvious body fluid to revisit; earlier attempts at measuring hormones in this secretion had failed in the fifties and sixties because of the lack of sensitivity of the assays at that time.

Samples of saliva can be collected by patients themselves which is obviously cost effective by saving both clinician-time and the materials required for plasma collection. Equally important is that samples of saliva can be stored at −20°C for 6 months without change in steroid concentrations. The following section serves to illustrate the potential value of salivary steroid analysis in endocrinology.

Steroid concentrations in saliva are low compared to plasma (< 10% plasma value), and their determination requires assays which are sensitive as well as specific. Such radioimmunoassays, and certain enzymeimmunoassays, have now been developed and validated in these laboratories [33–41] and are now in routine use for both natural steroid hormones and also certain synthetic compounds. Table III shows the list of these assays, the volume of saliva required, and the sensitivity of the procedure. All assays have been validated against gas chromatography-high resolution mass spectrometric procedures and excellent correlation achieved. Noteworthy, also, is the fact that the concentration of steroid in whole saliva is the same as that in parotid fluid, collected by fitting a modified

TABLE III. Immunoassays for salivary steroids

Steroid	Sensitivity (pg/tube)	Sample volume[a] (μl)	
Cortisol	4	10	
DHA	7	50	
17α-OH-progesterone	4	200	
Progesterone	7	400	
Testosterone	0.5	200	
Oestriol	12	200	< 36 weeks
	12	100	> 36 weeks
Norethisterone	3	100	

[a]Singlet determination.

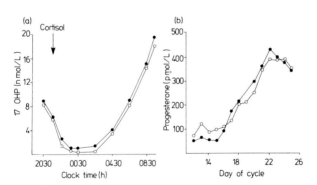

Fig. 11.   a) Concentrations of 17α-hydroxyprogesterone in matched samples of parotid fluid (○), collected under citric acid stimulation, and of mixed saliva (●) collected with no stimulation, from a patient with congenital adrenal hyperplasia. b) Progesterone concentrations in matched samples of parotid fluid (○) collected under citric acid stimulation, and of mixed whole saliva (●) with no stimulation, from a normal woman.

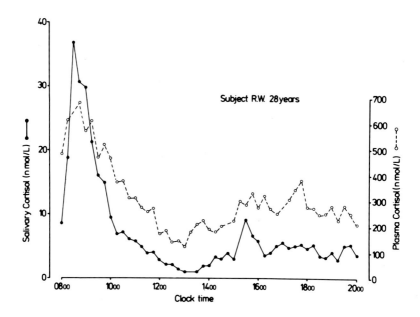

a

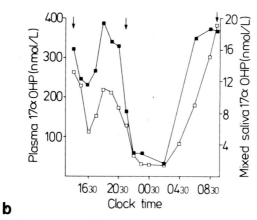

b

Fig. 12. a) Cortisol concentrations in matched plasma and saliva samples collected from a normal male at 15-minute intervals throughout a 12-hour period. b) Concentrations of 17α-hydroxyprogesterone in matched plasma (□) and mixed saliva (■) samples collected from a congenital adrenal hyperplasia patient over a 24-hour period. The arrows indicate the time of cortisol administration.

Carlsen-Crittenden device [42] over the duct of the parotid gland (Fig. 11a). Steroid concentrations in parotid fluid do not change with increasing flow rate, stimulated with citric acid on the tongue. The concentration of 17α-hydroxy-progesterone throughout the day of a patient with congenital adrenal hyperplasia and of progesterone, through the luteal phase of the menstrual cycle, in matched whole-saliva samples and in parotid fluid collected under conditions of maximally stimulated salivary flow rate, showed excellent agreement (Fig. 11).

Concentrations of steroid in whole saliva also adequately reflect the changes occurring in the plasma. Figure 12a illustrates the radioimmunoassay of cortisol in matched samples of saliva and plasma collected at 15-minute intervals through-out the day and Fig. 12b, the concentration of 17α-hydroxyprogesterone in matched saliva and plasma from a patient with congenital adrenal hyperplasia. Figure 13 shows the good correlation for progesterone concentrations between matched samples of blood plasma and saliva taken through one ovulatory cycle and related to basal body temperature. The data indicate the potential value of salivary progesterone in the assessment of ovarian function in cases of subfer-tility. This is further illustrated in Figure 14 which shows salivary progesterone levels in a woman who was seen at an infertility clinic, prior to (a) and after

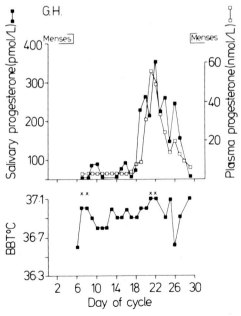

Fig. 13. Plasma and salivary progesterone concentrations throughout the menstrual cycle of a normal female, and the corresponding basal body temperatures (BBT).

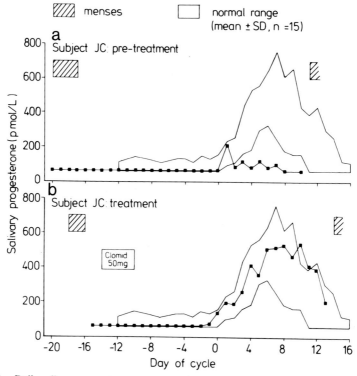

Fig. 14. Daily salivary progesterone concentrations in a female subject with luteal phase insufficiency before and after clomiphene treatment (50 mg/day).

(b) clomiphene treatment. Once therapy has been initiated the levels of progesterone become elevated and are then seen to be in the normal range [43].

Particularly interesting, however, is the fact that the concentration of steroid in saliva closely relates to the level of free non-protein-bound steroid in plasma. The method thus allows the evaluation of the biologically active principle without recourse to the tedious and difficult procedures of separating free and bound steroids in plasma. Table IV shows the levels of free testosterone in blood reported by Vermeulen and his colleagues [27,44] and the close correlation with our saliva data [45]. The two studies indicate that free testosterone declines with increasing age (Fig. 15). Others have also confirmed the close correlation between the concentration of testosterone in saliva and the free nonprotein-bound fraction in plasma [46,47].

The potential value of such assays is obvious. Salivary testosterone levels rise

TABLE IV. Changes in free plasma testosterone[a] and salivary testosterone with age

Age	TBG × 10⁻⁸M (± SE)	% Free T (± SE)	Free T pmole/l	Range pmole/l
20–50	5.2 ± 0.07	2.08 ± 0.08	402.7 ± 24.3	191–694.4
50–70	6.5 ± 0.8	1.72 ± 0.12	298.6 ± 34.7	
70–85	8.9 ± 1.5	1.26 ± 0.14	156.3 ± 27.8	

Age	Saliva/plasma % (± SD)	T In saliva pmole/l (± SD)	Range pmole/l
18–35	1.6 ± 0.42	368 ± 166 (AM)	104–781
		212 ± 131 (PM)	35–538
40–60		158 ± 68 (AM)	51–292
61–80		103 ± 53 (AM)	38–208

[a]Vermeulen, Stoica, and Verdonck, J Clin Endocrinol 33: 759, 1971, with permission.

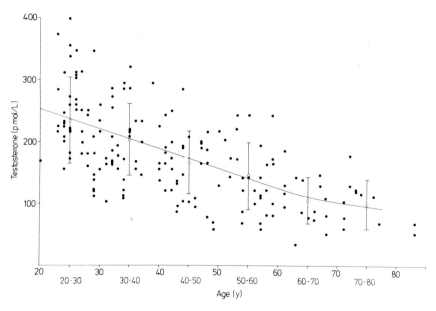

Fig. 15. Salivary testosterone levels in normal men of various ages. The mean (○) and SD for each decade also plotted.

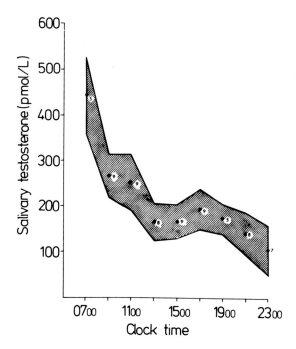

a

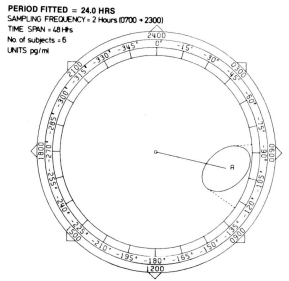

PERISD FITTED = 24.0 HRS
SAMPLING FREQUENCY = 2 Hours (0700 + 2300)
TIME SPAN = 48 Hrs
No. of subjects = 6
UNITS pg/ml

VARIABLE AND ELLIPSE IDENT.	# OF DATA	MESOR	SEM	AMPLITUDE AND (95% LIMITS)	ACROPHASE AND (95% LIMITS)	P VALUE
A NORMAL YOUNG MEN	92	53.09	2.02	21.79 (15.29 , 28.62)	-103 (-85 , -125)	<0.001

b

in parallel with those in plasma in man after HCG stimulation, indicating the value of the assay for assessment of testicular function [39]. The circadian variation in testosterone levels is illustrated in Figure 16a. Cosinar analysis of the data from the subjects studied indicated that a cosine function can be fitted to the results with an acrophase (peak value) at approximately 0700 hours (Fig. 16b).

Obviously, the increase in testosterone production during the night is controlled [48], and it is interesting to speculate on the role of the elevated night prolactin levels. This steady rise in plasma testosterone throughout the night is shown in Figure 17, which illustrates results obtained from patients with prostatic cancer maintained in bed and in whom an indwelling catheter was used to collect blood. Equally interesting in this respect is the comparative rise in prostatic acid

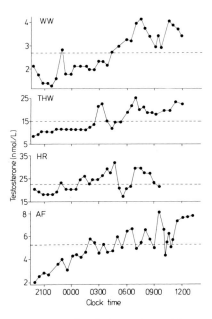

Fig. 17. Plasma testosterone concentrations in four patients with prostatic cancer. Blood samples were collected at 30-minute intervals throughout a 16-hour period. The dotted line represents the mean value of the determinations.

Fig. 16. a) Salivary testosterone was collected from nine normal males at 2-hour intervals throughout a 16-hour period. Shaded area represents mean and standard deviation. The number of samples analyzed at each time point is indicated. b) Cosinor analysis of salivary testosterone showing a significant rhythm.

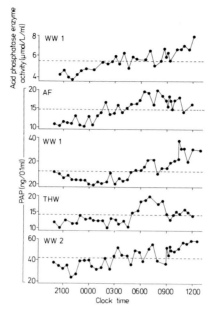

Fig. 18.   Plasma prostatic acid phosphatase (PAP) in three patients with prostatic cancer prior to therapy, and one patient (WW) after cyproterone acetate treatment 200 mg b.d., was measured by RIA. Acid phosphatase enzyme activity was also measured in split plasma samples of patient (WW).

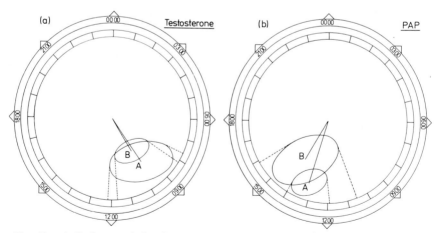

Fig. 19.   a) Cosinor analysis of plasma testosterone concentrations of a prostatic cancer patient. A: pretreatment; B: 6 days post cyproterone acetate therapy 200 mg b.d. A sigificant rhythm seen with peak levels at 0930 hours. b) Cosinor analysis of the same patient's plasma prostatic acid phosphatase (PAP) also revealed a significant rhythm with peak values between 1300–1400 hours.

phosphatase levels (Fig. 18) which appear to display a circadian acrophase, a few hours behind that for testosterone (Fig. 19a, b).

It is clearly obvious that there is still a great deal to be understood about the endocrinology of the prostate and prostatic disease. The use of salivary steroid analysis, a noninvasive multisampling procedure, which can provide information on rhythmic steroid secretion, will do much to increase this understanding. In relation to the use of chronobiological procedures for data analysis and the added potential of assays for protein hormones in saliva, soon to be reported by the Institute [49], these new procedures offer an exciting development in the study of prostatic cancer.

REFERENCES

1. Lipsett MB: Steroid secretion by the human testis. In Rosenberg E, Paulsen CA (eds): "The Human Testis." New York, Plenum Press, 1970, pp 407–421.
2. Hafiez AA, Lloyd CW, Bartke A: The role of prolactin in the regulation of testis function: the effect of prolactin and luteinising hormone on the plasma levels of testosterone and andros-tenedione in hypophysectomised rats. J Endocrinol 52: 327–332, 1972.
3. Hafiez AA, Bartke A, Lloyd CW: The role of prolactin in the regulation of testis function: the synergistic effects of prolactin and luteinising hormone on the incorporation of $|1 - {}^{14}C|$ acetate into testosterone and cholesterol by testes from hypophysectomised rats in vitro. J Endocrinol 53: 223–230, 1972.
4. Ambrosi B, Travaglini P, Beck-Peccoz P, Bara R, Elli R, Paracchi A, Faglia G: Effect of sulpiride-induced hyperprolactinaemia on serum testosterone response to HCG in normal men. J Clin Endocrinol 43: 700–703, 1976.
5. Grayhack JT, Lebowitz JM: Effect of prolactin on citric acid of lateral lobe of prostate of Sprague-Dawley rat. Invest Urol 5: 87–94, 1967.
6. Aragona C, Friesen H: Specific prolactin binding sites in the prostate and testis of rats. Endocrinology 97: 677–684, 1975.
7. Kledzik GS, Marshall S, Campbell GA, Gelato M, Meites J: Effects of castration, testosterone, estradiol and prolactin on specific prolactin-binding activity in ventral prostate of male rats. Endocrinology 98: 373–379, 1976.
8. Farnsworth WE: The normal prostate and its endocrine control. In Griffiths K, Pierrepoint CG (eds): "Some Aspects of the Aetiology and Biochemistry of Prostatic Cancer, 3rd Tenovus Workshop." Cardiff: Alpha Omega Alpha, pp 3–15, 1970.
9. Lostroh AJ, Li CH: Stimulation of sex accessories of hypophysectomised male rat by non-gonadotrophin hormone of the pituitary gland. Acta Endocrinol 25: 1–16, 1957.
10. Chase MD, Geschwind II, Bern HA: Synergistic role of prolactin in response of male rat sex accessories to androgen. Proc Soc Exp Biol Med 94: 680–683, 1957.
11. Gunn SA, Gould TC, Anderson WAD: The effect of growth hormone injections and prolactin preparations on the control of interstitial cell-stimulating hormone uptake. J Endocrinol 32: 205–214, 1965.
12. Aragona C, Friesen HG: Prolactin and aging. Grayhack JT, Wilson JD, Scherbenske MJ (eds): In "Benign Prostatic Hypertrophy." Bethesda: National Institutes of Health, 1975, p 165.
13. Chaisiri N, Pierrepoint CG: Examination of the distribution of oestrogen receptor between the stromal and epithelial compartments of the canine prostate. The Prostate 1: 357–366, 1980.
14. Arvola I: The hormonal control of the amounts of the tissue components of the prostate. Ann Clin Gynaecol Fem 50(Suppl 102): 1–20, 1961.

15. Tisell LE: Effect of cortisone on the growth of the ventral prostate, the dorsolateral prostate, the coagulating glands and the seminal vesicles in castrated, adrenalectomised and castrated non-adrenalectomised rats. Acta Endocrinol 64: 637–675, 1970.
16. Tullner WW: Hormonal factors in the adrenal-dependent growth of the rat ventral prostate. In Vollmer EP (ed): "Biology of the Prostate and Related Tissues." Natl Cancer Inst Monogr 12: 211, 1963.
17. Walsh PC, Gittes RF: Inhibition of extratesticular stimuli to prostatic growth in the castrate rat by antiandrogens. Endocrinology 87: 624–627, 1970.
18. Harper ME, Pike A, Peeling WB, Griffiths K: Steroids of adrenal origin metabolized by human prostatic tissue both in vivo and in vitro. J Endocrinol 60: 117–125, 1974.
19. Longcope C, Kato T, Horton R: Conversion of blood androgens to estrogens in normal adult men and women. J Clin Invest 48: 2191–2195, 1969.
20. MacDonald PC, Grodin JM, Siiteri PK: Dynamics of androgen and estrogen secretion. In Baird DT, Strong JA (eds): "Control of Gonadal Steroid Secretion." Baltimore: Williams & Wilkins, p 157, 1972.
21. Griffiths K, Davies P, Harper ME, Peeling WB, Pierrepoint CG: The etiology and endocrinology of prostatic cancer. In Rose, David P (eds): "Endocrinology of Cancer." Boca Raton: C.R.C. Press, Inc., Vol 2, pp1–55, 1979.
22. Coffey D: Physiological control of the prostatic growth: An overview. In Coffey DS, Isaacs JT (eds): "Prostatic Cancer," UICC Technical Report Series No. 9, Volume 48, Geneva: UICC, pp 4–23, 1979.
23. Kley HK, Nieschlag E, Krüskemper HL: Age dependence of plasma oestrogen response to HCG and ACTH in man. Acta Endocrinol 79: 95–101, 1975.
24. Doerr P, Pirke KM: Regulation of plasma oestrogens in normal adult males. I. Response of oestradiol, oestrone and testosterone to HCG and fluⁿˣymesterone administration. Acta Endocrinol 75: 617–624, 1974.
25. Vermeulen A, Rubens R, Verdonck L: Testosterone ɛ⌣⌣retion and metabolism in male senescence. J Clin Endocrinol 34: 730–735, 1972.
26. Pirke KM, Doerr P: Age related changes in free plasma testosterone, dihydrotestosterone and oestradiol. Acta Endocrinol 193(Suppl): 57–70, 1975.
27. Vermeulen A, Stoica T, Verdonck L: The apparent free testosterone concentration, an index of androgenicity. J Clin Endocrinol 33: 759–767, 1971.
28. Harper ME, Peeling WB, Cowley T, Brownsey BG, Phillips MEA, Groom G, Fahmy DR, Griffiths K: Plasma steroid and protein hormone concentrations in patients with prostatic carcinoma before and during oestrogen therapy. Acta Endocrinol 81: 409–426, 1976.
29. The British Prostate Study Group: Multivariate analysis of plasma hormone concentrations in relation to clinical staging in patients with prostatic cancer. Brit J Urol 51: 382–389, 1979.
30. Wilson DW, Tan SE: In Griffiths K, Pierrepoint CG, Neville AM (eds): "Tumour Markers: Determination and Clinical Significance." Sixth Tenovus Workshop, Cardiff: Alpha Omega Alpha, p 341, 1978.
31. MacDonald PC: Origin of estrogen in men. In Grayhack JT, Wilson JD, Scherbenske MJ (eds): "Benign Prostatic Hyperplasia." Bethesda: National Institute of Health, 1975, pp 191–192.
32. Fitzpatrick JM, Gardiner RA, Williams JP, Riddle PR, O'Donoghue EPN: Pituitary ablation in the relief of pain in advanced prostatic carcinoma. Brit J Urol 52: 301–304, 1980.
33. Kemp HA, Read GF, Riad-Fahmy D, Pike AW, Gaskell SJ, Queen K, Harper ME, Griffiths K: Measurement of diethylstilboestrol in plasma from patients with cancer of the prostate. Cancer Res 1981 (in press).
34. Walker RF, Riad-Fahmy D, Read GF: Adrenal status assessed by direct radioimmunoassay of cortisol in whole saliva or parotid fluid. Clin Chem 24: 1460–1463, 1978.
35. Walker RF, Read GF, Hughes IA, Riad-Fahmy D: Radioimmunoassay of 17α-hydroxyproges-

terone in saliva, parotid fluid, and plasma of congenital adrenal hyperplasia patients. Clin Chem 25: 542–545, 1979.

36. Turkes A, Turkes AO, Joyce BG, Read GF, Riad-Fahmy D: A sensitive solid phase enzymeimmunoassay for testosterone in plasma and saliva. Steroids 33: 347–359, 1979.

37. Walker RF, Hughes IA, Riad-Fahmy D: Salivary 17α-hydroxyprogesterone in congenital adrenal hyperplasia. Clin Endocrinol 11: 631–637, 1979.

38. Walker RF, Read GF, Riad-Fahmy D: Radioimmunoassay of progesterone in saliva: Application to the assessment of ovarian function. Clin Chem 25: 2030–2033, 1979.

39. Walker RF, Wilson DW, Read GF, Riad-Fahmy D: Assessment of testicular function by the radioimmunoassay of testosterone in saliva. Int J Andrology 3: 105–120, 1980.

40. Turkes AO, Turkes A, Joyce BG, Riad-Fahmy D: A sensitive enzymeimmunoassay with a fluorimetric end-point for the determination of testosterone in female plasma and saliva. Steroids 35: 89–101, 1980.

41. Riad-Fahmy D, Walker RF, Read GF: Salivary steroid assays for screening endocrine function. Postgrad Med J 56: 75–78, 1980.

42. Shannon JL, Prigmore JR, Chauncey HH: Modified Carlson-Crittenden device for the collection of parotid fluid. J Dent Res 41: 778–783, 1962.

43. Walker S, Walker RF, Mustafa A, Riad-Fahmy D: "The Role of Salivary Progesterone in Studies of Infertile Women." Brit J Obs Gynaecol, 1981 (in press).

44. Vermeulen A, Verdonck L: Some studies on the biological significance of free testosterone. J Steroid Biochem 3: 421, 1972.

45. Read GF, Harper ME, Peeling WB, Griffiths K: Changes in male salivary testosterone concentrations with age. Int J Andrology, 1981 (in press).

46. Baxendale PM, Reed MJ, James VHT: Testosterone in saliva of normal men and its relationship with unbound and total testosterone levels in plasma. Proc. 160th Meeting Soc. for Endocrinology, J Endocrinol 87: 46P, 1980.

47. Smith RG, Besch PK, Dill B, Buttram VC: Saliva as a matrix for the measurement of free androgens: comparison with serum androgens in polycystic ovarian disease. Fertil Steril 31: 513–517, 1979.

48. Rubin RT, Poland RE, Tower BB: Prolactin-related testosterone secretion in normal adult men. J Clin Endocrinol 42: 112–116, 1976.

49. Groom G, Evans G, Griffiths K: Pituitary hormones in saliva. Submitted for publication.

The Prostatic Cell: Structure and Function
Part B, pages 55–62
© 1981 Alan R. Liss, Inc., 150 Fifth Avenue, New York, NY 10011

Some Experimental Results With Prolactin: An Overview of Effects on the Prostate

Avery A. Sandberg

The physiologic effects of prolactin in some areas (eg, lactogenesis and steroidogenesis) are more evident and distinct than those in the prostate [1–4]. Some of the factors and circumstances which may contribute to the less than clear-cut effect of prolactin on the prostate are listed in Table I. Not only do the results obtained with prolactin vary with the species used, age of the animals, type of experimental design, and origin of the prolactin but also with the prostatic parameter (eg, secretory, weight, androgen metabolism, etc) being followed. Further complicating studies of the influence of prolactin on the prostate is the complexity of cell types existing in the prostate, differences among lobes of the gland in anatomic, functional, and cellular components, and indications that the action of prolactin is dependent on the physiological background or immediate past of the cells being affected and the strong possibility that prolactin is a regulator or modulator of metabolic events rather than a primary controlling factor (eg, it enhances many of the manifestations produced by testosterone but usually cannot initiate these).

Some of the mechanisms of prolactin effects have been delineated or established more rigorously than others. In Table II these mechanisms are listed, though only a few have been investigated in prostatic tissues (Tables III and IV). Thus, receptors for prolactin have been demonstrated in animal and human prostates [21–26], though little is known of how that interaction affects cellular functions of the gland. The high concentrations of prostaglandins and polyamines in the prostate may be related to prolactin effects, though here again definitive data are lacking. It is possible that ion-mediated (through Na^+ and K^+) may be reflected in water imbibition resulting in increased size and weight of the rodent prostate, as has recently been demonstrated in our laboratory [27] (Tables V and VI).

Some of the prostatic effects of prolactin may be mediated through actions on the testes (Table IV). Thus, it has been shown that prolactin increases the binding of LH to the Leydig cells, increasing the effects of LH on steroid hormone synthesis and spermatogenesis. Since prolactin also causes an increased

TABLE I. Some factors related to prolactin studies

1) Prolactin—nearly 100 different actions in diverse biological systems.
2) How any one of the many actions is carried out is not completely understood.
3) Most studied has been the effect on lactogenesis.
4) Effects depend on species (strain), tissue, and experimental design.
5) The action of prolaction is "critically dependent on the background physiological situation" [3].
6) Prolactin is a regulator of fluid and electrolyte metabolism in mammals; it is a *modulator* rather than a primary *controlling factor* [3].

TABLE II. Possible mechanisms of action of prolactin

1) Internalization
   (active hormone? important for action?)
2) Plasma membrane receptors
   (concentration? different types?)
3) Membrane-associated Na^+, K^+
   ATPase (decreases Na^+; increases K^+)
   conflicting data with ovabain, an inhibitor of Na^+, K^+ -ATPase
4) Calcium
   Its absence decreases casein and RNA synthesis in mammary explants stimulated by prolactin
5) Cyclic nucleotides (cGMP vs cAMP)
6) Prostaglandins
   (Indomethacin and prostaglandin synthetase; phospholipase A_2)
7) Polyamines

Based on Rilemma [4].

release of FSH from the pituitary, it is the FSH which may be responsible for the augmented binding of LH to the Leydig cells. It has also been shown that seminal plasma contains concentrations of prolactin exceeding those in the circulation. The function of prolactin in the seminal fluid is unknown, though its concentration correlates with that of zinc.

The effects of prolactin on the prostate are listed in Table III. It is generally agreed that prolactin augments some of the effects of testosterone, though by itself it seems to have a very minor effect on prostatic anatomy or function. Since the binding of prolactin to cellular membranes of the prostate is androgen-dependent, the interdependence of these hormones (androgens and prolactin) is obvious. Furthermore, decreased weight and secretory activity of the prostate can be induced by antiprolactin serum and inhibition of prolactin release. Other effects of prolactin are related to the uptake of testosterone and DHT by the gland, effects on cyclic AMP activity, and DNA synthesis.

TABLE III. Effects of prolactin on prostate

1) Prolactin alone causes a small but detectable increase in weight (not mediated through the pituitary or adrenal) in castrated rats and mice [5,6].
2) Prolactin binding to prostate membranes and cytosol is androgen dependent; possibly accounts for reduced responsiveness of prostate to prolactin in the absence of endogenous or exogenous testosterone [7,8].
3) Decreased weight and secretory activity can be induced by surpression of prolactin levels by:
   a) Antiprolactin serum [9].
   b) Ergocornine or 2-bromo-α-ergocriptine [10,12].
   c) Dopamine.
   d) 2-Hydroxyestrone [13].
4) Substances which increase release of prolactin:
   a) Serotonin may stimulate release of PRF.
   b) Epinephrine and norepinephrine regulate prolactin release at the level of hypothalamus.
5) Prolactin stimulates DNA synthesis, with little effect on RNA; increases adenylate cyclase activity; increases uptake of T and DHT [14–20].
6) No studies available on prolactin effects on androgen receptor levels.

TABLE IV. Actions and characteristics of prolactin related to possible effects on the prostate

1) Increases binding of LH to Leydig cells, leading to increased testicular function (spermatogenesis, testosterone production).
2) Causes release of FSH, which increases LH binding in testes (potentiates LH effect on testosterone production).
3) Presence and function (?) of prolactin in seminal plasma (correlates with levels of Zn, sperm count (?), and motility).

TABLE V. Effects of estradiol (E_2) and a prolactin release inhibitor (I) on prostatic weights and serum prolactin levels in Wistar-Furth rats

Substance administered	VP (mg)	DLP (mg)	Prolactin μg/ml
Control	87 ± 21	141 ± 30	173 ± 99
E_2	112 ± 41	126 ± 44	786 ± 119
E_2 + I	94 ± 21	118 ± 35	312 ± 130
I	75 ± 11	126 ± 21	9 ± 5.3

Taken from Corrales et al [27].
± = SD.

TABLE VI. Control serum prolactin levels and effects of estrogen administration on prostatic weights in Wistar-Furth and Copenhagen rats

Rat strain	Ventral prostate (mg)		Dorsolateral prostate (mg)		Prolactin (μg/ml)
	Control	Estrogen treated	Control	Estrogen treated	
Wistar-Furth	93 ± 16	103 ± 18	132 ± 48	132 ± 23	20.2 ± 6.3
Copenhagen	52 ± 13	111 ± 25	81 ± 41	119 ± 30	75.1 ± 8.8

Taken from Corrales et al [27].
± = SD.

In our laboratory we have addressed ourselves to the effects of prolactin on some parameters of the rat prostate, primarily on 5α-reductase and arginase activities and zinc concentrations [27–29]. These effects have been obtained either through the administration of prolactin to intact, hypophysectomized or castrated animals or following drug induced inhibition of prolactin release with 6-methyl-8-ergolenylacetamide and related compounds.

Prostatic weights, 5α-reductase, and arginase activities were utilized as indexes for the effects of prolactin in short-term experiments in intact, hypophysectomized or castrated rats [29]. Experiments were performed in which a dose-related response in the above parameters was obtained with testosterone administration in castrated mature and immature rats in order to evaluate the effects of simultaneously administered prolactin (Tables VII–IX). This approach was necessitated by the failure of prolactin alone to affect the parameters listed in intact, castrated or hypophysectomized rats. It was shown that ovine prolactin may have an enhancing effect on the prostatic weight, 5α-reductase, and arginase activities, but that this effect is neither consistent nor striking when compared to that of testosterone. Nevertheless, it is still possible that the long-term effects of prolactin, even if they are only of an enhancing quality, may play an important role in normal prostatic physiology and in abnormal states.

The zinc uptake in the dorsolateral prostate of rats was studied after different hormonal manipulations (Table X). Orchiectomy reduced the uptake of ^{65}Zn. Administration of estradiol benzoate to orchiectomized rats doubled the ^{65}Zn uptake, a phenomenon which was not observed in orchiectomized-adrenalectomized rats [29]. Adrenalectomy in orchiectomized rats had no effect on the concentration of radioactivity beyond the castration-induced decrease. A prolactin release inhibitor, 6-methyl-8-ergolenylacetamide, reduced the radioactivity concentration without changing the weight of the gland. Cyproterone acetate reduced the weight but not the radioactivity concentration. The concentration of ^{65}Zn in the ventral prostate was not changed by orchiectomy, adrenalectomy, or the administration of estradiol benzoate, prolactin release inhibitors, or cyproterone acetate. The results suggest an important role for prolactin in the zinc uptake in the dorsolateral prostate but not in the ventral prostate.

TABLE VII. Effects of various doses of bovine prolactin and 50 μg of testosterone on prostatic weights and 5α-reductase and arginase activities in immature rats

Prolactin	Prostate wt (mg) Ventral prostate	Dorsolateral prostate	5α-Reductase activity (nmole DHT/gm/hr) Ventral prostate	Dorsolateral prostate	Arginase activity (μmole urea/gm/min) Ventral prostate	Dorsolateral prostate
None	46.3	37.8	11.0	4.4	1.9	3.5
1 IU	44.2	37.1	8.7	5.0	3.1	4.5
5 IU	47.3	37.6	10.0	5.4	1.6	1.9
15 IU	43.5	38.7	6.8	6.8	1.6	3.4
45 IU	50.0	45.4	8.2	4.9	1.6	3.9
60 IU	47.8	47.8	5.8	4.9	1.8	1.9

Taken from Yamanaka et al [28].

TABLE VIII. Effects of testosterone and prolactin on prostatic weights and 5α-reductase and arginase activities in intact, castrated, and hypophysectomized adult rats

	Prostatic wt (mg) VP	DLP	5α-Reductase activity (μmole DHT/gm/hr) VP	DLP	Arginase activity (μmole urea/gm/min) VP	DLP
Intact						
Control	548.8		19.7		2.4	
Testosterone	600.9		19.3		4.6	
Prolactin	509.5		8.7		3.1	
Testosterone and prolactin	565.2		16.2		4.2	
Castrated						
Control	48.3		1.5		2.2	
Testosterone	147.5		30.1		9.3	
Prolactin	65.2		2.5		2.3	
Testosterone and prolactin	198.3		38.5		10.5	
Control	59.0	96.5	0.46	0.3	2.2	9.0
Testosterone	255.5	273.0	4.4	6.8	3.0	7.5
Prolactin	56.5	100.0	0.68	0.5	3.0	8.0
Testosterone and prolactin	260.0	297.0	7.7	2.9	3.7	8.4
Hypophysectomized						
Control	38.6		4.0		2.3	
Testosterone	173.6		17.6		5.3	
Prolactin	42.1		2.4		3.3	
Testosterone and prolactin	160.7		35.7		4.2	

VP, ventral prostate.
DLP, dorsolateral prostate.
Taken from Yamanaka et al [28].

TABLE IX. Effects of a prolactin inhibitor on prostatic weights and 5α-reductase and arginase activities in mature and immature rats

	Prostatic wt (mg)		5α-Reductase activity (μg DHT/min/gm)		Arginase activity (μmole urea/min/gm)	
	VP	DLP	VP	DLP	VP	DLP
Mature rats						
Control (1 wk)	436.5	263.5	0.73	2.74	2.4	6.5
Inhibitor (1 wk)	415.0	232.0	0.85	2.92	2.2	8.5
Control (2 wk)	467.5	288.3	0.44	0.99	2.3	5.2
Inhibitor (2 wk)	429.5	241.0	0.15	0.29	2.0	8.0
Immature rats						
Control (1 wk)	46.1	21.7	6.8	12.1	4.2	13.1
Inhibitor (1 wk)	45.6	24.2	5.6	7.5	3.7	9.3
Control (2 wk)	58.3	28.3	3.9	7.3	4.2	13.2
Inhibitor (2 wk)	58.3	28.8	2.2	4.0	4.5	12.9

Values are means ± SE. The immature rats were 21 days old and the mature rats were 13–14 weeks. The prolactin inhibitor 2-chloro-6-methylergoline-8β-acetonitrile was given for 1 or 2 weeks intraperitoneally (3 mg/kg) dissolved in water.
VP, ventral prostate; DLP, dorsolateral prostate; DHT, dihydrotestosterone.
Taken from Yamanaka et al [28].

TABLE X. Effects of estradiol benzoate (EB) and prolactin release inhibitor (I) on zinc concentration in the rat prostate

	Prostatic wt (mg)		^{65}Zinc concentration (DPM/min/gm × 10^{-3})	
Treatment	VP	DLP	VP	DLP
Control	131	159	39.0	65.2
EB	155	185	32.6	141.7
I	116	155	31.7	58.2
EB + I	160	188	94.4	81.6

VP, ventral prostate; DLP, dorsolateral prostate.
Taken from Müntzing et al [29].

The mechanism by which estrogens inhibit castration atrophy has been investigated morphologically and biochemically in the ventral prostate of Copenhagen rats [27]. The suppression of weight loss and the gross edematous appearance of the prostate associated with the in vivo effect of 17β-estradiol (E$_2$) could not be accounted for by DNA and protein synthesis. Light microscopy demonstrated that the main effects were on the stroma, characterized by large interglandular areas almost totally devoid of collagen, resulting in an edematous appearance. Electron microscope studies showed an abundance of fluid localized adjacent to the capillary endothelium and some red blood cells, indicating disturbances in capillary permeability. The combination of a prolactin secretion inhibiting agent with E_2 partially prevented the fluid accumulation and weight increase produced by E_2 alone, indicating an involvement of prolactin in the estrogen effect (Table V). Differences in blood prolactin concentration between strains of rats may influence the sensitivity of the prostate to estrogens (Table VI).

A clear view of the effects of prolactin on the prostate is not available at present. Whether prolactin has, in fact, all the effects shown in the tables or whether these reflect events mediated through only a few mechanisms has yet to be settled. The experimental prostatic systems used to date have not been sufficiently sensitive or specific to yield unequivocal evidence of a unique action of prolactin on the prostate. Thus, it is hoped that future studies, utilizing more appropriate test systems, will unravel the enigma of the role of prolactin in normal and abnormal prostatic states.

ACKNOWLEDGMENTS

This study was supported in part by grant CA-15436 from the National Cancer Institute.

REFERENCES

1. Bartke A: Role of prolactin in reproduction in male mammals. Fed Proc 39: 2577–2581, 1980.
2. Clemens JA, Shaar CJ: Control of prolactin secretion in mammals. Fed Proc 39: 2588–2592, 1980.
3. Horrobin DF: Prolactin as a regulator of fluid and electrolyte metabolism in mammals. Fed Proc 39: 2567–2570, 1980.
4. Rillema JA: Mechanism of prolactin action. Fed Proc 39: 2593–2598, 1980.
5. Bartke A, Lloyd CW: The influence of pituitary homografts on the weight of sex accessories in castrated male mice and rats and on mating behavior in male mice. J Endocrinol 46: 313–320, 1970.
6. Negro-Vilar A, Saad WA, McCann SM: Evidence for a role of prolactin in prostate and seminal vesicle growth in immature male rats. Endocrinology 100: 729–737, 1977.
7. Charreau EH, Attramadal A, Torjesen PA, Purvis K, Calandra R, Hansson V: Prolactin binding in rat testis: Specific receptors in interstitial cells. Mol Cell Endocrinol 6: 303–307, 1977.
8. Kledzik GS, Marshall S, Campbell GA, Gelato M, Meites J: Effects of castration, testosterone, estradiol, and prolactin-binding activity in ventral prostate of male rats. Endocrinology 98: 373–379, 1976.
9. Asano M, Kanzaki S, Sekiguchi E: Inhibition of prostatic growth in rabbits with antiovine prolactin serum. J Urol 106: 248–252, 1971.
10. Bartke A: Effects of inhibitors of pituitary prolactin release on testicular cholesterol stores, seminal vesicles weight, fertility and lactation in mice. Biol Reprod 11: 319–325, 1974.
11. Hostetter NW, Piacsek BE: The effect of prolactin deficiency during sexual maturation in the male rat. Biol Reprod 17: 574–577, 1977.

12. Ravault JP, Courot M, Garnier D, Pelletier J, Terqui M: Effect of 2-broma-α-ergocyptine (CB 154) on plasma prolactin, LH and testosterone levels, accessory reproductive glands and spermatogenesis in lambs during puberty, Biol Reprod 17: 192–197, 1977.

13. Fishman J, Tulchinsky D: Suppression of prolactin secretion in normal young women by 2-hydroxyestrone. Science 210: 73–74, 1980.

14. Thomas JA, Keenan EJ: Prolactin influences upon androgen action in male accessory sex organs. In Singhal RL, Thomas JA (eds): "Cellular Mechanisms Modulating Gonadal Hormone Action." Baltimore: University Park Press, 1976, pp 425–470.

15. Golder MP, Boyns AR, Harper ME, Griffiths K: An effect of prolactin on prostatic adenylate cyclase activity. Biochem J 128: 725–727, 1972.

16. Baker HWG, Worgut TJ, Santen RJ, Jefferson LS, Bardin CW: Effect of prolactin on nuclear androgens in perfused male accessory sex organs. In Troen P, Nankin HR (eds): "The Testis in Normal and Infertile Men." New York: Raven Press, 1977, pp 379–385.

17. Farnsworth WE: Prolactin and the prostate. In Boyns AR, Griffiths K, (eds): "Prolactin and Carcinogenesis." Cardiff, Wales: Alpha Omega Alpha, 1972, pp 217–228.

18. Johansson R: Effect of prolactin, growth hormone and insulin on the uptake and binding of dihydrotestosterone to the cultured rat ventral prostate. Acta Endocrinol 81: 854–864, 1976.

19. Johansson R: Effect of prolactin, growth hormone and insulin on the uptake and binding of dihydrotestosterone to the cultured rat ventral prostate. Acta Endocrinol 81: 854–864, 1976.

20. Golder, MP, Boyns AR, Harper ME, Griffiths K: An effect of prolactin on prostatic adenylate cyclase activity. Biochem J 128: 725–727, 1972.

21. Kledzik GS, Marshall S, Campbell GA, Gelato M, Meites J: Effects of castration, testosterone, estradiol, and prolactin on specific prolactin-binding activity in ventral prostate of male rats. Endocrinology 98: 373–379, 1976.

22. Barkey RJ, Shani J, Barzilai D: Regulation of prolactin binding sites in the seminal vesicle, prostate gland, testis and liver of intact and castrated adult rats: Effect of administration of testosterone, 2-bromo-α-ergocryptine and fluphenazine. J Endocrinol 81: 11–18, 1979.

23. Nagasawa H, Sakai S, Banerjee MR: Minireview. Prolactin Receptor. Life Sci 24: 193–208, 1979.

24. Aragona C, Bohnet HG, Friesen HG: Localization of prolactin binding in prostate and testis: The role of serum prolactin concentration on the testicular LH receptor. Acta Endocrinol 81: 402–409, 1977.

25. Keenan EJ, Kemp ED, Ramsey EE, Garrison LB, Pearse HD, Hodges CV: Specific binding of prolactin by the prostate gland of the rat and man. J Urol 122: 43–46, 1979.

26. Edwards WD, Thomas JA: Morphologic and metabolic characteristics of ventral, lateral, dorsal and anterior prostate transplants in rats. Effect of testosterone and/or prolactin. Hormone Res 13: 28–39, 1980.

27. Corrales JJ, Kadohama N, Chai LS, Høisaeter PA, Hampton MT, Murphy GP, Sandberg AA: Fluid imbibition as a factor in estrogen-induced increase of prostatic weight in castrated rats. The Prostate (in press).

28. Yamanaka H, Kirdani RY, Saroff J, Murphy GP, Sandberg AA: Effects of testosterone and prolactin on rat prostatic weight, 5α-reductase, and arginase. Am J Physiol 229: 1102–1109, 1975.

29. Müntzing J, Kirdani R, Murphy GP, and Sandberg AA: Hormonal control of zinc uptake and binding in the rat dorsolateral prostate. Invest Urol 14: 492–495, 1977.

The Prostatic Cell: Structure and Function
Part B, pages 63–88
© 1981 Alan R. Liss, Inc., 150 Fifth Avenue, New York, NY 10011

Polypeptide Hormones and the Prostate

Mukta M. Webber

INTRODUCTION

The development, growth, differentiation, and functions of the prostate are considered to be controlled primarily by androgens. Although the central role of testosterone cannot be questioned, evidence is accumulating to suggest that polypeptide hormones like insulin and prolactin modify the action of testosterone on the prostate and other accessory sex organs. The role of these hormones in prostate physiology, their interactions with androgens, and their mechanism of action are not completely understood. In this author's opinion, prostatic growth and differentiation may be regulated by a complex system involving not only androgens but also a number of other hormones, vitamins, and growth factors. Some evidence will be presented on the role of two protein hormones, namely insulin and prolactin, in prostate physiology.

Most hormones have specific target cells. There is, however, a group of hormones generally known as permissive hormones [1], which have some action on specific target cells but also have ill-defined, less specific effects on a large variety of other cells in the body. This group of hormones includes growth hormone, glucocorticoids, insulin, prolactin, and thyroxine. It is important to note that 75–80% of all known hormones are peptide hormones [1].

My interest in these hormones developed for the following reasons: 1) In order to understand neoplastic transformation, it is important to establish which factors regulate growth and differentiation of human prostatic epithelium. 2) The author is currently developing an in vitro cell model system, which uses human prostatic epithelium, for studies on the etiology of prostatic neoplasia and the mechanisms involved in prostatic carcinogenesis. In order to establish requirements for cell growth, maintenance and differentiation in vitro, it is essential to know which factors regulate them in vivo. 3) It is necessary to develop a chemically defined, serum-free medium for the growth of human prostatic epithelium in vitro so that biochemical studies on cells and media may be performed without any interference from serum. Such a system would be ideal for studying the expression of differentiated function under hormonal control in the form of products secreted into the culture medium, which can then be analyzed.

The development of the cell system used for studies on these hormones has been described earlier [2–4]. In order to develop an in vitro cell model, one must satisfy the following basic requirements: acquisition of viable human tissue, isolation of viable epithelial cells; establishment of in vitro requirements for growth, maintenance, and differentiation and characterization of cells to establish their prostatic epithelial origin. An important point to remember is that different parts of the human prostate respond differently to hormones and other growth stimuli. Hence, it is important that, for studies on benign prostatic hyperplasia (BPH), cells be studied from glands in the periurethral area (Fig. 1), which is the common site of BPH, and for prostatic cancer, cells from the peripheral zone (Fig. 1). In cross sections of the entire prostate removed at the time of total prostatectomy, cystectomy, or autopsy, these zones can be distinguished and separated. Using a collagenase digestion technique, acini from the prostate can be isolated and vigorously growing cultures initiated from them [2]. Elimination of any remaining fibroblasts can be accomplished using the selective toxicity of spermine for fibroblasts in serum containing media [4]. Initially, the cultures consist of a mixture of two types of cells (Fig. 2): the large differentiated postmitotic cells which are lost within the first 10 days in culture, and the small basal cells which multiply and dominate the culture [5]. On the basis of investigations in progress in the author's laboratory on various hormones and growth factors, it is hoped that it would become possible to manipulate these cultures

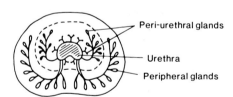

Fig. 1.   A diagram of a cross section of the human prostate showing different regions of the prostate. The periurethral area is the common site of benign prostatic hyperplasia while the peripheral glands are the common site of carcinoma. (After Basmajian, JV: Grant's Method of Anatomy, 10th ed, Baltimore: Williams & Wilkins, 1980.)

Fig. 2.   Cellular composition of the primary cultures of human prostatic epithelium in the early phases of their growth. a) Within 2 days of plating the acini, large epithelial cells form a sheet around the acinus. b) By days 5–7, colonies of small, basal cells (arrows) appear and enlarge. c) By days 10–15, most of the large cells have been lost and the culture primarily consists of actively dividing small cells. Giemsa stain, × 135. (From [5].)

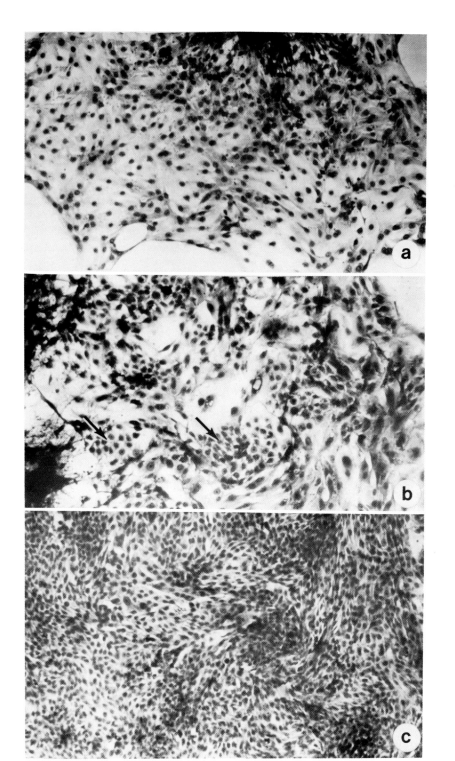

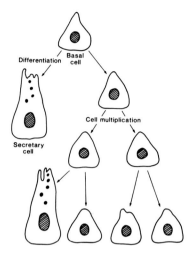

Fig. 3. A diagram to show cell multiplication and cell differentiation, both of which can occur simultaneously in the same culture where different cells may have different fates. Similar phenomena occur in the acinar epithelium in vivo.

in such a way so that they could either be encouraged to multiply and maintain the culture or they could be made to differentiate and express their differentiated functions. Growth and differentiation can occur simultaneously in the same culture where different cells may have different fates (Fig. 3). Generally, under normal conditions, differentiated cells are postmitotic and do not divide. For the in vitro maintenance, growth, and differentiation, a large number of factors are under investigation. This discussion is restricted to insulin and prolactin.

INSULIN

Insulin stimulates cell multiplication in a variety of cells in culture [3,6]. However, little is known about its specific effects on prostatic epithelium in vivo and in vitro. It is appropriate to describe some significant in vivo and in vitro experiments which lead to the present effort to examine the role of insulin in prostate physiology.

Insulin and the Prostate: In Vivo Studies

Rats made diabetic prior to reaching sexual maturity show failure of descent of testes and development of germinal epithelium and have castrate type accessory sex organs. Treatment with insulin corrects all the deleterious effects of diabetes. Testosterone alone does not bring about a complete recovery. Presence of insulin is required for a full restorative effect of testosterone [7].

Insulin and the Prostate: In Vitro Studies

In tissue culture, ventral prostate from adult, orchiectomized mice undergoes castrate type regression. Testosterone has no effect on this fully regressed prostate unless insulin is added to the culture medium. Insulin added alone to the culture medium stimulates extensive repair; however, the response is greater when both insulin and testosterone are present [8]. If the prostate is taken from an orchiectomized donor injected in vivo with testosterone, insulin is not required for the in vitro effect. The marked development of secretory epithelium obtained with testosterone plus insulin surpasses that obtained by insulin alone [8]. In the absence of serum, insulin stimulates RNA, protein, and DNA synthesis in rat ventral prostate explant cultures [9]. The exact mechanism of action of insulin at the subcellular level is not clearly established. However, insulin has been found to stimulate ornithine decarboxylase activity in responsive cells [10,11]. These observations on the effects of insulin on the prostate raise some tantalizing questions about the role of insulin in prostate physiology and about its ability to potentiate the effects of testosterone. A summary of the work done in my laboratory [6,12,13] on the effects of insulin on human prostatic epithelium is given here. The interactions of insulin with a variety of hormones and other factors are discussed in detail elsewhere [5,6,12,13].

Insulin stimulates the growth of human prostatic epithelium in vitro. Figure 4 shows the dose response of epithelial cells from a 21-year-old donor. Cells

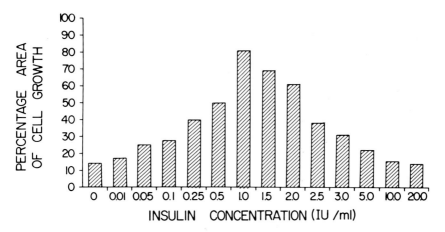

Fig. 4. Effects of insulin on the growth of normal human prostatic epithelium in vitro. These results show a dose-response which fits a bell-shaped curve. The growth of cells increases with the increase in the amount of insulin and reaches a peak at 1.0 IU/ml. Five IU/ml insulin and higher levels were inhibitory. Age of cell donor: 21 years. CMRL-1066 medium containing 10% horse serum and 10% fetal bovine serum was used. (From [6].)

were grown in medium CMRL-1066 containing 10% horse and 10% fetal bovine serum. The response becomes apparent at a low level of 10^{-2} IU/ml. As the dose increases, the response increases and reaches a maximum at 1.0 IU/ml. At concentrations beyond 1.0 IU/ml, growth begins to decline. These results show that insulin has a bell-shaped or a normal dose-response curve (Fig. 5). There is some growth in cultures to which insulin was not added. However, considerable stimulation in cell multiplication is observed in its presence [6]. The growth response of epithelial cells to insulin changes with the age of the donor so that in order to obtain an optimum growth response, higher levels of insulin must be provided. In other words, the cells show decreased sensitivity to insulin with age [6]. Another observation worth noting is that growth in cultures to which insulin was not added showed a rapid decline with time as compared to cultures containing insulin. How does insulin enhance growth? Addition of insulin to responsive cell cultures results in a number of changes in the cell; eg insulin alters the cell membrane permeability, increases pinocytotic activity and the uptake of glucose and amino acids. It also induces an increase in ornithine decarboxylase activity [10,11] and stimulates protein, RNA, and DNA synthesis. Insulin is mitogenic for a variety of cells [3].

Insulin not only stimulates growth but it also alters the spatial distribution of prostatic epithelial cells grown in serum-free media [12]. While cells grow as a monolayer in serum-containing medium, they show a distinct layering similar to the in vivo spatial organization in the presence of insulin in serum-free medium. Cells in the top layer slough off, while cells in contact with the culture dish surface continue to multiply. These cultures, in the presence of transferrin, show blister formation, an indication of the ability of these cells to transport fluids [5,13].

Zinc is considered to have an important role in prostate physiology [13]. It is an essential component of several metalloenzymes in the prostate. Zinc is also an essential component of insulin and at least one atom of zinc is found per three

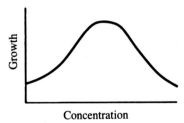

Concentration

Fig. 5. This figure shows a normal, or bell-shaped, dose-response curve. The growth response of prostatic epithelium to insulin or prolactin fits a normal curve. Such a curve indicates that at very low levels, these hormones may have no effect. However, cell growth increases with increase in the concentration of the hormones. It reaches a peak and then begins to decline with further increase in the hormone level. At high levels it may actually become toxic. (From [6].)

molecules of insulin when it is secreted by β-cells of the pancreas [14]. Zinc stabilizes insulin. Prolactin increases zinc uptake by the prostate [15–17], which in turn may enhance insulin stability and thus its effects on prostatic epithelium. On the basis of these observations, zinc may have a greater significance in prostate physiology than has been realized.

Conclusions

Insulin stimulates the growth of prostatic epithelium in vitro and affects its spatial organization. Some of our in vitro studies on the effects of insulin on prostatic epithelium were made in the absence of testosterone where insulin stimulated cell multiplication. These results demonstrate a direct effect of insulin on prostatic epithelium rather than its testosterone potentiating effect.

PROLACTIN

Human prolactin, secreted by the prolactin-secreting cells of the anterior pituitary, was isolated as recently as 1971 [18,19]. The existence of a hormone with the ability to induce lactation was first accidentally recognized in 1928 [20] and experimentally established in 1929 [21]. Since then, prolactin has been identified in a variety of vertebrates from teleosts to mammals. Although the existence of a human prolactin, separate from the growth hormone, was generally accepted 20 years ago, it had not been experimentally demonstrated [22]. The occurrence of prolactin in primates was confirmed only a decade ago. Now, more than 85 different actions have been attributed to prolactin in a number of different biological systems [23]. Its major actions in man, however, are considered to be on the gonads, accessory sex organs, and on the fluid-electrolyte balance [24].

The role of prolactin in the female human physiology is well established [15,25]. In this symposium, the major interest is to examine the role of prolactin in the growth, maintenance, and function of prostatic epithelium; its possible role in the etiology of prostatic neoplasia; and its possible growth enhancing effects on prostatic cancer. In order to develop an understanding of the above roles and to plan critical experiments to investigate these roles, it is necessary first to examine the general properties of this hormone and, more specifically, to evaluate the present knowledge of the actions of prolactin in the human male.

General Properties

Prolactin is a protein which circulates in the plasma in several forms having different molecular size. The human prolactin monomer is a single-chain protein with a molecular weight of about 23,000 [25]. The ovine prolactin, which has generally been used in research, has been shown to be composed of 198 amino acids and has a molecular weight of 22,550 [26]. The half-life of human prolactin in circulation is about 20 minutes [27]. A large number of organs bind prolactin, suggesting a variety of different actions on different organs [15].

Changes in Prolactin Levels With Age in Man

Normal serum prolactin levels in men and women change with age, as shown in Table I. In adult women the serum level falls with age, while in men there is an increase in the prolactin level. In men between the ages of 55–65 years, the mean value of serum prolactin is about 1.5 times higher (13.44 ng/ml) than in men between the ages of 35–45 years (8.82 ng/ml) [28]. In Table I, the age groups used by Vekemans and Robyn [28] are more meaningful in studying changes in prolactin levels with age. However, the purpose of Saroff's [29] studies was to examine differences in prolactin levels between men with normal prostates and those with prostatic neoplasia. Prolactin levels were higher in patients with BPH, prostatic carcinoma, and in patients on estrogen therapy [29]. A recent study by Jacobi et al, [30] did not show increased levels of serum prolactin in aging men.

Species Specificity

Controversy still exists about the species specificity of prolactin. In order to conduct in vivo and in vitro studies, it is essential first to determine the species specificity of the hormone. Because of the recent isolation of human prolactin, most of the experimental work has been done using ovine and bovine prolactin in rats. Both of these prolactins and the human prolactin show activity for rodent tissues [31]. Controversy exists about the effectiveness of prolactins of other than human origin on human cells. Hwang et al [18] have shown that human prolactin shares antigenic determinants with ovine prolactin. Ovine prolactin has

TABLE I. Serum prolactin levels in men and women

Age group	Mean value ng/ml	Reference
Male		
35–45	8.82	[28][a]
45–55	12.20	
55–65	13.44	
23–69	12.2	[29]
Female		
15–25	18.48	[28][a]
45–55	14.70	
55–65	9.24	
22–60	14.9	[29]

[a]Calculated from data provided in mU where 1 mU = 42 ng.

been shown to have mitogenic activity for human mammary epithelial cells of normal [32,33], benign [34], and malignant origin [35] in culture. Others have shown that only human prolactin has growth stimulatory effects on normal human breast tissue in culture and that ovine or bovine prolactin have no effect [36]. It appears that some human mammary tumors respond to ovine prolactin while others do not [37]. This may simply be an indicator of hormone dependence of the tumor rather than an indicator of species specificity.

It is possible that the herbivore prolactin may be less effective in stimulating growth and that maximal response in human cells may only be obtained by human prolactin. In terms of binding specificity, human normal breast and cancer cell lines show binding not only to human prolactin but also to ovine prolactin. Keenan et al [38] have recently shown specific binding of ovine prolactin to a membrane fraction from both benign and malignant human prostatic tissue. In a later section of this paper, new results will be presented which show that ovine prolactin has growth-stimulatory effects on human prostatic epithelial cells [39]. A major problem worth noting is that high levels of prolactin may have been used in studies where no growth response has been reported. The dose-response curve for prolactin is bell-shaped, similar to that for insulin (Fig. 5); hence the true effect of prolactin may be missed if a wide range of concentrations, beginning with the very low physiological levels (1×10^{-4} to 5×10^{-4} IU/ml of serum) to very high levels (eg 10 IU/ml), are not tested.

Effects of Prolactin on Mammary Epithelium

The role of prolactin in normal female reproduction, lactation, and mammary carcinogenesis is now well established [40,41]. The possibility of prolactin as a natural carcinogen has been considered and it does enhance the induction of mammary tumors in rats [41]. The complex interactions of prolactin involved in the induction of neoplasia are demonstrated by the following: Thyrotropin releasing hormone (TRH) stimulates release of thyrotropin, which acts as a prolactin releaser. This explains why goitrous patients with elevated prolactin levels have an increased risk of developing breast cancer. In Japan, where dietary intake of iodine is high, breast cancer incidence is low (see [41]). Thirty-two percent of human breast cancers show prolactin dependence [42]. Suppression of prolactin secretion by bromocriptine inhibits mammary tumorigenesis in carcinogen-treated (7,12 dimethylbenzanthracene) rats [43]. Dexamethasone inhibits mammary tumor growth even in the presence of high serum prolactin [44].

Since mammary epithelial cells have been known for a long time to be target cells for prolactin, most in vitro studies using prolactin have been made on mammary cells. Various effects of prolactin on growth and differentiation and its possible mechanism of action have been elucidated using these cells. A brief examination of the effects of prolactin on mammary epithelium may facilitate our understanding of the role of prolactin in prostate growth and function.

Prolactin appears to have both growth stimulatory and cell differentiation effects on mammary epithelium, depending on the state of differentiation of the cell. Insulin is involved in the maintenance of these cells in vitro, and it also stimulates DNA synthesis and mitosis. Addition of prolactin to insulin-containing media increases DNA synthesis and mitotic activity beyond that induced by insulin or prolactin alone in human, mouse, and rat, normal [32,36], benign [34], and malignant [37] cells in vitro. Prolactin is also able to induce casein and fatty acid synthesis in mammary epithelial cells [31,35,45].

Prolactin, Testes, and the Accessory Sex Organs

Some of the earliest effects of prolactin observed on the accessory sex organs demonstrated its indirect effects on these organs through its influences on the testes. This indirect effect, particularly on the prostate, is clearly demonstrated in Figure 6. Luteinizing hormone (LH) or the interstitial cell stimulating hormone (ICSH) is responsible for stimulating the biosynthesis and secretion of testosterone from Leydig cells in the testes. Leydig cells are the target cells for LH. Prolactin increases the sensitivity of Leydig cells to LH stimulation by increasing the ability of Leydig cells to bind LH [46]. Thus, prolactin is synergistic with LH and indirectly stimulates testosterone production by the testes in adult men [15,46–49]. Increase in testicular weight occurs in hypophysectomized rats given prolactin [50]. This suggests that prolactin may act by increasing testosterone production by the testes. Some prolactin seems to be required for normal testosterone secretion [51]. Prolactin stimulates the release of follicle-stimulating hormone (FSH), which is involved in spermatogenesis. FSH can also increase testicular LH binding to Leydig cells. FSH thus potentiates the effect of LH on testosterone production by Leydig cells [46].

The adrenal cortex has the highest concentration of prolactin receptors in the body. Prolactin stimulates aldosterone production by the adrenals [51]. Aldosterone is the adrenal's contribution to the general pool of androgens. Prolactin potentiates 5α-reductase activity, thus increasing conversion of testosterone to 5α-dihydrotestosterone (5α-DHT) [52,53].

Levels of plasma prolactin in rats increase with sexual maturation [15]. Elevation in plasma testosterone levels in men are preceded by elevation in prolactin levels [54]. Plasma prolactin levels increase sharply before sexual maturation and are higher in adult men than in prepubertal boys [54]. Changes in prolactin levels correlate well with the growth of the accessory sex organs and these organs acquire greater capacity to interact with prolactin at sexual maturity [15]. Inhibition of prolactin during sexual maturation causes inhibition of growth of the accessory sex organs. In mice, serum prolactin levels increase dramatically during pubertal maturation and coincide with rapid growth of the accessory sex organs. This increase precedes the pubertal rise in testosterone levels [55,56].

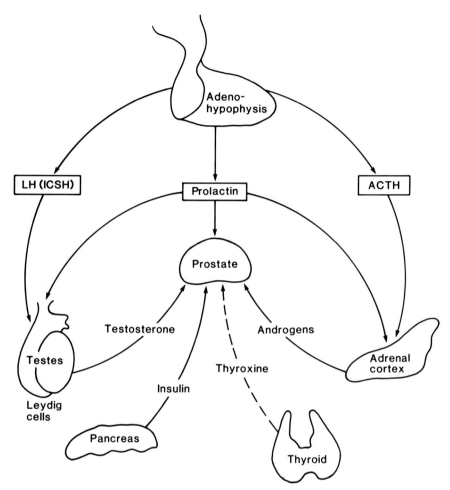

Fig. 6. A picture model to show the direct and indirect effects of prolactin and insulin on the prostate and the effects and interactions of various other hormones which eventually influence prostate growth and function. (From [82].)

Prolactin and the Prostate: In Vivo Studies

The earliest studies which demonstrated synergistic effects of prolactin with testosterone were conducted on the rat ventral prostate using ovine and bovine prolactin. Grayhack [57] did the pioneering experiments which showed the direct effects of prolactin on prostate growth and function. Prostate response to testosterone in both hypophysectomized and castrated rats is not as great as that in castrated rats with pituitary intact. Prolactin administration along with testosterone in hypophysectomized and castrated rats always resulted in an enhancement of the testosterone effect, ie, increase in the weight of the prostate. Thyroxine has a similar but a less striking effect with testosterone [57]. Other investigators some 20 years later [53,58] confirmed Grayhack's findings. In addition, they demonstrated an increase in zinc uptake by the prostate in response to prolactin [15–17,59]. Prolactin acts synergistically with testosterone in promoting citric acid concentration in the prostates of hypophysectomized, castrated rats. A 75% increase over those given testosterone alone occurred [58,60]. Simultaneous injections of 5α-DHT and prolactin to mature castrated rats augment RNA, protein, and DNA synthesis in the prostate [61] and accelerate the uptake of testosterone and formation of 5α-DHT from testosterone [62–64]. The increase in conversion of testosterone to 5α-DHT can be explained on the basis of the fact that prolactin potentiates 5α-reductase activity [52,53].

In 1963 Grayhack [16] proposed certain effects of prolactin on the prostate, independent of testosterone. This idea was based on the following observations: 1) More loss in prostatic weight occurs after hypophysectomy than after castration. 2) Greater decrease in acid and alkaline phosphatase occurs in the prostate after hypophysectomy than after castration. 3) Administration of testosterone after hypophysectomy induces less growth in the prostate than after castration.

Also, inhibition of prolactin during sexual maturation in male rats causes inhibition of prostatic growth [65]. Prolactin increases prostatic weight when injected into castrated, adrenalectomized rats [50]. These results support an independent pituitary effect on the prostate. Evidence for the direct action of prolactin is also supported by the presence of specific prolactin receptors on prostatic epithelial cells [38,46].

In addition to its direct and independent effects, prolactin potentiates the effects of testosterone on the prostate. Uptake of ^{14}C-labelled testosterone is impaired in the rat ventral prostate of hypophysectomized rats [66]. Uptake of testosterone is 25% greater in human prostate minced tissue when incubated with prolactin than with testosterone alone [67]. As stated earlier, prolactin potentiates 5α-reductase activity, thus increasing the converison of testosterone to 5α-DHT [52,53]. Prostates of castrated rats injected with prolactin and testosterone showed 2–2.5 times more RNA and DNA than prostates of rats given testosterone alone [61]. The effects of prolactin on the prostate related to the potentiation of testosterone may be summarized as follows: 1) It increases testosterone binding to prostatic epithelial cells. 2) It increases cytoplasmic and nuclear uptake of testosterone and 5α-dihydrotestosterone. 3) It potentiates the conversion of testosterone to 5α-dihydrotestosterone. 4) It stimulates DNA synthesis in the presence of testosterone.

The synergism between these two hormones works both ways; eg, certain effects of prolactin are androgen-dependent as indicated by the following: 1) the responsiveness of the prostate to prolactin is reduced (but not absent) in the absence of testosterone (see [46]). 2) Prolactin binding to prostate membranes and the cytosol is androgen dependent (see [46]).

Prolactin has been shown to induce cell proliferation in rat ventral prostate [68]. In vitro studies carried out in my laboratory and described in a later section, show that prolactin alone may also have the ability to induce epithelial cell proliferation in the human prostate [39,82]. On the basis of the above data, it may be concluded that prolactin affects the growth and function of the prostate in at least three different ways: 1) It may increase the output of testosterone from the testes and adrenals. 2) It may act synergistically with testosterone by potentiating its effects. 3) It may promote growth and function by acting directly on the prostate.

Prolactin, Estrogens, and the Prostate

It is interesting to note that estrogens have direct effects on the secretion of prolactin from the pituitary and on the response of the prostate to prolactin. Estrogens stimulate prolactin production [24,41,51,69]. Estrogens suppress prolactin-inhibiting factor (PIF) release from the hypothalamus, thus permitting an unlimited secretion of prolactin [70]. Prolactin receptors are increased by estrogens [51]. Estrogens prolong the half-life of testosterone in the serum [71]. Plasma levels of estrogens increase with age in the adult human male [48,72]. A consideration of these results may suggest that since estrogen levels increase with age, this may lead to an increased production of prolactin. Evidence exists to support this suggestion [28]. Estrogens may then increase the sensitivity and response of the prostate to testosterone, even when the levels of testosterone are declining.

Prolactin Receptors in the Prostate

The expression of the biological function of a hormone depends upon the presence of receptors on the target cells. Peptide hormones express their biological function through cell surface receptors. Peptide hormones are hydrophobic, thus they do not easily traverse the lipid bilayer of the cell membrane. In contrast to the cell surface receptors for peptide hormones, steroid hormones are lipid soluble and thus readily cross the cell membrane. Their receptors are in the cytosol and their primary site of action is the nucleus [1].

A variety of different cells have prolactin receptors. Adrenal cortex cells have the highest number of prolactin receptors in the body. Prolactin is involved in the stimulation of androgen synthesis in the adrenals [51]. Prostate is another organ where epithelial cells have specific, high-affinity receptors for prolactin.

Prolactin binding in prostate cells is androgen-dependent. This has been clearly demonstrated by experiments conducted by a number of investigators. Specific binding of ^{125}I-prolactin occurs in rat ventral prostate membrane preparations. However, 90% of this specific binding is lost in castrated rats. Injections of testosterone restore prolactin binding to the normal level [73–78]. Prolactin receptors are further discussed by Witorsch in this volume.

Prolactin and the Prostate in Culture

Little work has been done to date to investigate the effects of prolactin on the growth and differentiation of prostatic epithelium in vitro. The in vitro studies made to date are summarized in Table II. In vitro cell systems are invaluable for studying hormone actions and interactions. In an isolated cell system one is more likely to be able to examine, at the cellular level, the specific effects associated with the hormone without the interference from the complex feedback mechanisms present in vivo.

Lasnitzki [79,80] did her pioneering work during 1970–1972 on the effects of prolactin alone and on its synergism with testosterone using rat ventral and

TABLE II. Effects of prolactin on the prostate in culture

Source of cells	Prolactin used	Effects	Reference
Rat lateral and ventral prostate explants	Ovine and bovine	Low concentrations of P increased epithelial cell number and cell size and enhanced the effect of T.	[79, 80]
Rat ventral prostate explants	Ovine	High concentrations of P stimulated uptake of T.	[95]
Rat ventral prostate explants	Bovine	Stimulated RNA and protein synthesis.	[9]
Rat ventral prostate explants	Bovine	No effect on the conversion of T to DHT; high concentrations stimulated specific uptake of T by nuclei.	[81]
Human prostatic explants and cancer cell lines	Ovine	Stimulation of cell multiplication.	[39, 82]

DHT, 5α-dihydrotestosterone; P, prolactin; T, testosterone.

lateral prostate explants in culture. Her results showed that at low levels (0.01–0.05 IU/ml), prolactin was able to partially maintain prostatic epithelium in the explants. The epithelium was mainly cuboidal and secretory activity was seen in several alveoli. Prolactin also increased the proliferation of epithelial cells in some alveoli. At high concentrations (0.1 IU/.ml), prolactin did not maintain the epithelium. Prolactin (0.05 IU/ml) and testosterone (0.05 μg/ml) combined, however, maintained cell morphology (cuboidal to columnar cells) and partial secretory activity. Laznitzki's more detailed work, published in 1972, is summarized below. Ventral and lateral prostate explants from 8-week-old rats were grown in medium-199 containing horse serum. Explants before culture showed a fully maintained epithelium. After 6 days in culture, in untreated explants, the epithelium lost its folding and was reduced in height. Addition of ovine prolactin (0.01 IU/ml) to the culture medium slightly inhibited this regression. In contrast to the flat cells seen in the control explants, the epithelium was often cuboidal. Low doses of testosterone alone (0.5 μg/ml) were more effective than prolactin alone in maintaining the epithelium and showed some cuboidal and some columnar secretory cells, but it did not induce a full restoration. Prolactin and testosterone in combination were successful in maintaining tall columnar cells and, in addition, induced cell proliferation. This treatment also promoted the formation of new alveoli. The stimulation of testosterone effect by prolactin is dose-dependent and is optimum at a prolactin level of 10^{-2} IU/ml. With increase in the concentration of prolactin, the effect is reversed causing an inhibition in growth.

A number of other important pieces of information emerged from this work: 1) Both ovine and bovine prolactin showed activity for rat cells, and species specificity was not a problem in this case. 2) Ventral prostates from old rats (22 months old) were more responsive to prolactin than prostates from young rats (8 weeks old). Also, they were stimulated by lower concentrations of prolactin (approximately 5×10^{-3} IU/ml) than the young ventral glands (2×10^{-2} IU/ml). 3) The young lateral glands were more sensitive than the ventral glands. 4) Ovine prolactin was more effective than bovine prolactin in inducing growth and function in prostatic epithelium.

The only other in vitro studies on the effects of prolactin on the prostate, except the present work, were made by Johansson [9,81]. Rat ventral prostate explants from 8–12-week-old animals were grown in medium 199 without serum. Bovine prolactin was used. The rationale for using a tissue culture system to elucidate the effects of prolactin on the prostate was as follows: "Because the addition of any hormone in vivo is followed by a series of alterations in the levels of other hormones in the organism, tissue culture is a valuable method for investigating the specific and direct actions of various hormones" [9]. Results showed that prolactin stimulated protein and RNA synthesis when incorporated into the culture medium in the presence of testosterone. Prolactin, insulin, and testosterone together increased RNA and protein synthesis beyond that induced by testosterone plus insulin. It can be concluded that all three hormones are essential for the growth of prostatic epithelium and that prolactin and insulin are synergistic with testosterone [9].

Recent results from studies conducted in my laboratory on the effects of prolactin on human prostate explants in culture show that prolactin has a direct effect on the growth of prostatic epithelium [82]. Explants were maintained suspended in culture medium (RPMI-1640) containing 2% fetal bovine serum for 20 days. As demonstrated earlier [83,84], such explants in culture become encapsulated by epithelial cells migrating from the acini to the surface of the explant. Histological sections of treated and untreated explants were examined [82]. In explants maintained in the basal medium, both the epithelium on the surface and in the acini showed several layers of cells. Addition of 10^{-5} IU/ml ovine prolactin to the culture medium increased the number of cell layers. This effect was more pronounced and the optimum activity was observed at 10^{-4} IU/ml. Several mitotic figures could be seen in the epithelial cell layers. At a concentration of 10^{-3} IU/ml, both the surface and the acinar epithelium showed reduced growth and signs of degeneration. Prolactin at levels of 10^{-2} to 1.0 IU/ml showed toxicity for epithelial cells [82].

Effects of ovine prolactin on the growth of DU-145, a prostatic carcinoma cell line [85,86], were also examined [39]. Preliminary results show that when prolactin levels between 10^{-4} and 10^{-2} IU/ml were tested, 10^{-2} IU/ml induced maximum response in terms of cell multiplication in these cells in vitro (Fig.

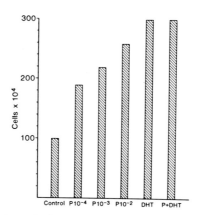

Fig. 7. The effects of ovine prolactin on the growth of a human prostatic carcinoma cell line DU-145. Prolactin induces cell multiplication in these cells at a level of 10^{-4} IU/ml. Maximum response occurred at 10^{-2} IU/ml. 5α-DHT (0.1 μg/ml) alone produced a greater growth response, which was not further enhanced by 10^{-4} IU/ml prolactin. DHT, 5α-dihydrotestosterone; P, prolactin, IU/ml. RPMI-1640 medium + 2% FBS was used. (From [39].)

7). 5α-DHT alone produced a greater response, which was not further enhanced by prolactin at a level of 10^{-4} IU/ml.

Prolactin and Prostate Cancer

The role of prolactin in the enhancement of mammary tumors has already been established [41]. Prolactin enhances DNA synthesis and mitotic activity in rat mammary gland cultures in the presence of insulin [32,26,41].

The basic physiological role of hormones is to regulate cell growth and function. Thus, if the hormonal proliferative stimulus becomes unrestrained, it could lead to excessive, uncontrolled growth and thus to neoplasia. Prolactin is known to enhance cell multiplication not only in mammary epithelial cells but also in 3T3 cells [87] and rat lymphoma cells in culture [88] and in newts [89]. The ability to stimulate growth does not necessarily implicate a hormone in carcinogenesis. However, increasing levels of prolactin, as they occur in the aging human male, in combination with several other physiological and extrinsic factors, may become a contributing factor in the induction of a neoplastic state. The ability of prolactin to stimulate cell multiplication directly in prostatic epithelial cells; its potentiating effects on testosterone and 5α-reductase activity; its enhancing effect on the conversion of testosterone to 5α-dihydrotestosterone; its ability to induce an increase in the uptake of testosterone by prostatic epithelial cells and of 5α-DHT by prostatic epithelial cell nuclei; and its enhancing effect on LH and steroidogenesis in the testes make a case for a serious examination of the possible role of prolactin in the etiology of prostatic neoplasia and in its growth-enhancing effects on prostatic cancer in at least some patients with carcinoma of the prostate.

In patients with metastatic prostatic cancer, inhibitors of prolactin secretion, eg, Levodopa and bromocriptine, relieve bone pain [70,90]. As stated earlier, plasma levels of estrogens increase in the aging human male. Estrogens enhance the secretion of prolactin by inhibiting prolactin-inhibiting factor (PIF). Therefore, in conventional anti-androgen therapy for prostatic cancer which uses estrogens, one may actually be enhancing the growth of certain tumor cell populations rather than suppressing it. Figure 8 shows some possible mechanisms by which changes in prolactin levels may be brought about. This figure further shows how these altered levels may affect the growth of the prostate.

Patients with prostatic cancer secrete more prolactin than age-matched controls, and the levels increase with estrogen administration [29,48,91]. Prostatic carcinoma patients have an increased prolactin pituitary reserve [52]. These patients also have elevated levels of serum 5α-DHT [29]. High prolactin and 5α-DHT levels may be associated with carcinoma [29].

When considering the possible role of prolactin in the growth of the normal prostate and in the etiology of prostatic neoplasia in the aging male, age-associated changes in the levels of several other hormones must also be taken into

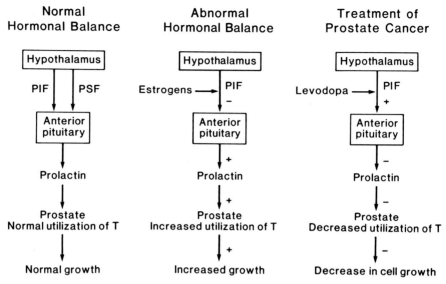

Fig. 8. This figure demonstrates some possible ways in which prolactin levels may affect the growth of prostatic epithelium. Under normal conditions, a balance is maintained between the prolactin-stimulating factor (PSF) and the prolactin-inhibiting factor (PIF) which regulate the secretion of prolactin by the anterior pituitary. This results in the normal growth of prostatic epithelium. Increase in prolactin levels induced by estrogens by inhibition of PIF may disturb the normal balance. The end result of this change may be an increase in prostatic growth as observed in the aging male. Similarly, stimulation of PIF by Levodopa may inhibit prolactin secretion, which may cause a decrease in prostatic growth. This may occur in prostatic cancer patients treated with levodopa. T, testosterone.

TABLE III. Changes in some major hormones in the aging normal human male

Hormone	Basal output	Concentration in blood	Sensitivity of prostate	Sensitivity of other target organs
Testosterone	↓	↓	↑	↓
Estrogen	?	↑	↑	?
Prolactin	↑	↑	↑	?
FSH	↑	↑	—	↓
LH	↑	↑	—	↓
Insulin	↔	↔	↓	↓

Arrow pointing up means increase; arrow pointing down means decrease; horizontal arrow means no appreciable change; ? means results uncertain; horizontal bar means no possible direct effect.
Some information from Goldstein, 1979 [72].

consideration. These changes are shown in Table III. On the basis of the above information, a process-response word model has been constructed (Fig. 9). This model proposes some mechanisms whereby prolactin may be involved in the induction of cell multiplication. This may be a significant factor in neoplastic transformation in the prostate of the aging male [39].

Mechanism of Action of Insulin and Prolactin

Conflicting evidence exists about the mechanism of action of these hormones. Many polypeptide hormones express their biological function by binding with a cell surface membrane receptor and activating adenyl cyclase which initiates a chain of intracellular events leading to the activation of cAMP-dependent protein kinase, transcription, and RNA synthesis [15,27,40]. The end result may be the secretion of a specific cellular protein or DNA synthesis followed by cell division. The immediate events which follow the interaction of prolactin with the cell membrane receptors are not clear. Prolactin and insulin both increase ornithine decarboxylase activity in a number of tissues [23,92,93]. This is followed by polyamine synthesis and macromolecule synthesis resulting in cell division or expression of cell function [23,92,93]. Horrobin's [94] interpretation is that prolactin action on growth and development is dependent on the activation of polyamines and cyclic nucleotide/protein kinase related mechanisms.

Another group of studies has shown that prolactin does increase the adenyl cyclase activity in rat prostate homogenates at low concentrations, but high concentrations have no effect [15,46,95,96]. Testosterone has no effect on the activity of this enzyme [95,96]. It is possible that in cases where activation of adenyl cyclase was not observed, it may have been due to the use of high concentrations of prolactin. The true response may have been missed because low levels were not tested. It should be remembered that a large number of actions of prolactin follow a bell-shaped, dose-response curve, meaning that at very low concentrations it may have no effect. As the concentration increases the effects appear until an optimum is reached beyond which the effects decline. Considerable work still needs to be done to elucidate the mechanisms of action of prolactin and insulin on cells in general and on prostatic epithelium in particular.

Conclusions

Prostatic epithelial cells have cell membrane receptors for prolactin and they appear to be target cells for prolactin. Prolactin maintains cell function and induces cell multiplication in rat lateral and ventral prostate [79,80]. Recent results from the author's laboratory show that ovine prolactin induces cell multiplication in human prostatic epithelium and in a human prostatic carcinoma cell line [39,82]. As shown above, prolactin has direct effects on prostatic epithelium

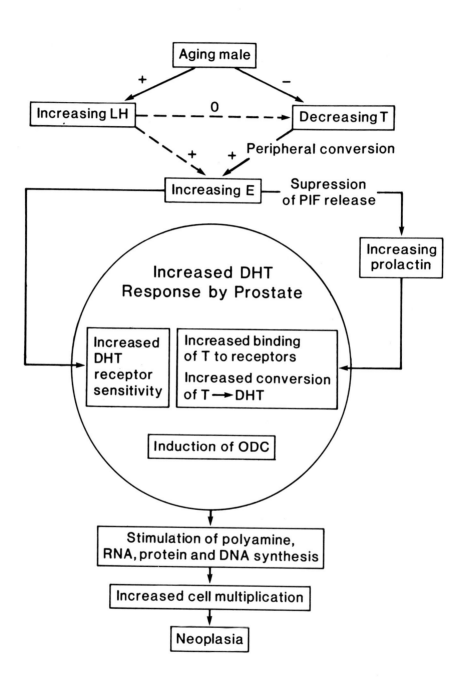

and it also influences these cells indirectly by altering testosterone synthesis and its utilization by these cells. The effects of prolactin on the growth and functions of the prostate can be classified into three groups: 1) It may promote growth and function by acting directly on the prostate. 2) It may increase the output of testosterone from the testes and adrenals. 3) It may act synergistically with testosterone by potentiating its effects.

SUMMARY

Results presented in this paper demonstrate that both insulin and prolactin have direct effects on the growth and functions of prostatic epithelium. They also act on the prostate indirectly by potentiating the effects of testosterone on these cells. Both are capable of inducing cell multiplication and increasing the activity of ornithine decarboxylase in cells. However, the intracellular events which follow the interaction of these hormones with the cell membrane receptors are not clearly understood. Little is known at the present time about the specific effects of insulin and prolactin on prostatic growth regulation and function and about their interactions with other protein and steroid hormones. A considerable amount of further research is needed to establish the basic influences of insulin and prolactin on the prostate. This inquiry is essential before the role of these hormones in normal and abnormal growth of the prostate can be understood.

ACKNOWLEDGMENTS

This work was supported by US Public Health Service Contract NO-1-CP-65849 and grant CA-28279, from the Division of Cancer Cause and Prevention, National Cancer Institute. The author wishes to thank her colleagues who helped in the acquistion of human tissue: Drs. R. Augsberger, R.E. Donohue, G. Miller, S. Mohr, W. Pelander, J. Pitts, R. Pfister, and J.N. Wettlaufer. Technical assistance by Ludmila Jankowsky and Lorna Rolon was invaluable. The author extends special thanks to Susan Gilady for her unfailing dedication to the typing

Fig. 9. A process response word-model to hypothesize the role of prolactin in normal and abnormal growth of the prostate. In the aging male, the following may be observed: decreasing levels of circulating testosterone (T); increasing levels of luteinizing hormone (LH); increasing levels of estrogens (E), primarily derived from the peripheral conversion. It is possible that increasing LH levels may stimulate increased synthesis of estrogens rather than that of testosterone by Leydig cells of the testes. Increased levels of estrogens result in higher prolactin levels. Both estrogens and prolactin increase the utilization and sensitivity of prostatic epithelium to testosterone and 5α-DHT. Prolactin is also capable of enhancing ornithine decarboxylase activity. As a result of the action of 5α-DHT and the direct action of prolactin on cells, stimulation of polyamine, RNA, protein, and DNA synthesis followed by cell multiplication may occur. This may be one of the many contributing factors in the process of neoplastic transformation in prostatic epithelium in the aging male.(From [39].)

and proofreading of this manuscript, to Mel Gabel for drafting the figures, and to Richard Carter and Ralph Black for preparing the photographs. DU-145 cells were provided by Dr. Don Mickey, University of Tennessee.

REFERENCES

1. Roth, J: Receptors for peptide hormones. In Degroot LJ (ed): "Endocrinology." New York: Grune & Stratton, 1979, Vol 3, pp 2037–2054.
2. Webber MM: Normal and benign human prostatic epithelium in culture. I. Isolation. In Vitro 15:967–982, 1979.
3. Webber MM. Growth and maintenance of normal prostatic epithelium in vitro—A human cell model. In Murphy GP (ed): "Models for Prostate Cancer." New York: Alan R. Liss, 1980, pp 181–216.
4. Webber MM, Chaproniere-Rickenberg D: Spermine oxidation products are selectively toxic to fibroblasts in cultures of normal human prostatic epithelium. Cell Biol Int Rep 4:185–193, 1980.
5. Chaproniere-Rickenberg D, Webber MM: A chemically defined medium for the growth of adult human prostatic epithelium in vitro (submitted, Cold Spring Harbor Symposium on Cell Growth in Hormonally Defined Media, 1981).
6. Webber MM: Growth and maintenance of normal human prostatic epithelium in vitro: Effects of insulin (in preparation).
7. Hunt EL, Bailey DW: The effects of Alloxan diabetes on the reproductive system of young male rats. Acta Endocrinologica 38:432–440, 1961.
8. Lostroh AJ: Effect of testosterone and insulin in vitro on maintenance and repair of the secretory epithelium of the mouse prostate. Endocrinology 88:500–502, 1971.
9. Johansson R: RNA, protein and DNA synthesis stimulated by testosterone, insulin and prolactin in the rat ventral prostate cultured in chemically defined medium. Acta Endocrinologica 80:761–774, 1975.
10. Roger LJ, Fellows RE: Stimulation of ornithine decarboxylase activity by insulin in developing rat brain. Endocrinology 106:619–625, 1980.
11. Yamasaki Y, Ichihara A: Induction of ornithine decarboxylase in cultured mouse L cells. I. Effects of cellular growth, hormones and actinomycin D. J Biochem 80:557–562, 1976.
12. Chaproniere-Rickenberg D, Webber MM: The effects of insulin on the spatial distribution of human prostatic epithelium in vitro in serum free media (in preparation).
13. Webber MM, Chaproniere-Rickenberg D: The effects of zinc, insulin and transferrin on the growth of human prostatic epithelium in a defined culture medium (in preparation).
14. Arquilla ER, Packer S, Tarmas W, Miyamoto S: The effect of zinc on insulin metabolism. Endocrinology 103:1440–1449, 1979.
15. Cowie AT, Forsyth IA: Biology of prolactin. Pharmacol Ther B 1:437–457, 1975.
16. Grayhack JT: Pituitary factors influencing growth of the prostate. Natl Cancer Inst Monogr 12:189–199, 1963.
17. Weinstein E, Rosoff B: Effect of prolactin on prostatic weight and zinc-65 uptake in castrated rats. Fed Proc 31:275, 1972.
18. Hwang P, Guyda H, Friesen H: A radioimmunoassay for human prolactin. Proc Natl Acad Sci USA 68:1902–1906, 1971.
19. Lewis UJ, Singh RNP, Seavey BK: Human prolactin: Isolation and some properties. Biochem Biophys Res Commun 44:1169–1176, 1971.
20. Stricker S, Grueter F: Action dc lobe antéreur de l'hypophyse sur la montée laiteuse. C.R. Soc Biol 99:1978–1980, 1928.
21. Evans HM, Simpson ME: Hyperplasia of the mammary apparatus of adult virgin females induced by hypophyseal hormones. Proc Soc Exp Biol Med 26:598, 1929.

22. Pasteels JL: Introduction. In Pasteels JL, Ebling FJG (eds): "Human Prolactin." New York: Elsevier, 1973, pp xi–xiii.

23. Rillema JR: Mechanism of prolactin action. Fed Proc 39:2593–2598, 1980.

24. Horrobin DF: Prolactin: Role in health and disease. Drugs 17:409–417, 1979.

25. Frantz AG: Prolactin. In Degroot LJ (ed): "Endocrinology." New York: Grune & Stratton, 1979, Vol 3, pp 153–168.

26. Li CH: Chemistry of ovine prolactin. In Greep RO, Astwood ER (eds): "Handbook of Physiology, Section 7, Endocrinology, Vol IV. The Pituitary Gland, Part 2." Washington DC: American Physiological Society, 1974, pp 103–110.

27. Turkington RW, Frantz WL, Majumdar GC: Effector-receptor relations in the action of prolactin. In Pasteels JL, Robyn C (eds): "Human Prolactin." New York: Elsevier, 1973, pp 24–34.

28. Vekemans M, Robyn C: Influence of age on serum prolactin levels in women and men. Br Med J 4:738–739, 1975.

29. Saroff J, Kirdani RY, Chu TM, Wajsman Z, Murphy GP: Measurements of prolactin and androgens in patients with prostatic disease. Oncology 37:46–52, 1980.

30. Jacobi GH, Rathgen GH, Altwein JE: Serum prolactin and tumors of the prostate: Unchanged basal levels and lack of correlation to serum testosterone. J Endocrinol Invest 3:14–17, 1980.

31. Bullough WA, Wallis M: An in vitro bioassay for prolactin based on stimulation of casein synthesis by a dispersed cell preparation from mouse mammary gland. J Endocrinol 62:463–472, 1974.

32. Ceriani RL, Contesso GP, Nataf BM: Hormone requirement for growth and differentiation of the human mammary gland in organ culture. Cancer Res 32:2190–2196, 1972.

33. Flaxman BA, Lasfargues EY: Hormone-independent DNA synthesis by epithelial cells of adult human mammary gland in organ culture. Proc Soc Exp Biol Med 143:371–374, 1973.

34. Welsch CW, Dombroske SE, McMantus MJ, Calaf G: Effect of human bovine and ovine prolactin on DNA synthesis by organ cultures of benign human breast tumors. Br J Cancer 40:866–871, 1979.

35. Burke RE, Gaffney EV: Prolactin can stimulate general protein synthesis in human breast cancer cells (MCF-7) in long-term culture. Life Sci 23:901–906, 1978.

36. Dilley WG, Kister SJ: Brief communications: In Vitro stimulation of human breast tissue by human prolactin. J Natl Cancer Inst 55:35–36, 1975.

37. Welsch CW, Delturri GC, Brennan MJ: DNA synthesis of human, mouse, and rat mammary carcinomas in vitro. Influence of insulin and prolactin. Cancer 38:1272–1281, 1976.

38. Keenan EJ, Kemp ED, Ramsey EE, Garrison LB, Pearse HD, Hodges CV: Specific binding of prolactin by the prostate gland of the rat and man. J Urol 122:43–45, 1979.

39. Webber MM, Rolon L: Ovine prolactin stimulates the growth of human prostatic carcinoma cells in culture (in preparation).

40. Aragona C, Friesen HG: Lactation and galactorrhea. In DeGroot LJ (ed): "Endocrinology." New York: Grune & Stratton, 1979, Vol 3, pp 1614–1617.

41. Kim U, Furth J: The role of prolactin in carcinogenesis. Vit Horm 34:107–136, 1976.

42. Salih H, Brander W, Flax H, Hobbs JR: Prolactin dependence in human breast cancer. Lancet 2:1103–1107, 1972.

43. Welsch CW, Brown CK, Goodrich-Smith M, Van J, Denenberg B, Anderson TM, Brooks CL: Inhibition of mammary tumorigenesis in carcinogen-treated Lewis rats by suppression of prolactin secretion. J Natl Cancer Inst 63:1211–1214, 1979.

44. Aylsworth CF, Sylvester PW, Leung FC, Meites J: Inhibition of mammary tumor growth by dexamethasone in rats in the presence of high serum prolactin levels. Cancer Res 40:1863–1866, 1980.

45. Speake BK, Dils R, Mayer RJ: Regulation of enzyme turnover during tissue differentiation. Biochem J 154:359–370, 1976.

46. Bartke A: Role of prolactin in reproduction in male mammals. Fed Proc 39:2577–2581, 1980.
47. Hall P: Testicular hormones: Synthesis and control. In Degroot LJ (ed): "Endocrinology." New York: Grune & Stratton, 1979, Vol 3, pp 1511–1519.
48. Harper ME, Peeling WB, Cowley T, Brownsey BG, Phillips MEA, Groom G, Fahmy DR, Griffiths K: Plasma steroid and protein hormone concentrations in patients with prostatic carcinoma, before and during oestrogen therapy. Acta Endocrinologica 81:409–426, 1976.
49. Rubin RT, Poland RE, Tower BB: Prolactin-related testosterone secretion in normal adult men. J Clin Endocrinol Metab 42:112–116, 1976.
50. Negro-Villare A, Saad WA, McCann SM: Evidence for a role of prolactin in prostate and seminal vesicle growth in immature male rats. Endocrinology 100:729–737, 1977.
51. Horrobin DF: "Prolactin." Montreal: Eden Press, 1976.
52. Giuliani L, Pescatore D, Martorana G, Gilberti C, Barreca T, Rolandi E: Increased serum prolactin pituitary reserve in patients with prostatic neoplasms. Br J Urol 51:390–392, 1979.
53. Yamanaka H, Kirdani RY, Saroff J, Murphy GP, Sandberg AA: Effects of testosterone and prolactin on rat prostatic weight, 5α-reductase and arginase. Am J Physiol 229:1102–1109, 1975.
54. Bartke A: Prolactin and physiological regulation of the mammalian testes. In Troen P, Nankin HR (eds): "The Testis in Normal and Infertile Men." New York: Raven Press, 1977, pp 367–378.
55. Barkley MS: Serum prolactin in the male mouse from birth to maturity. J Endocrinol 83:21–33, 1979.
56. Michael SD, Kaplan SB, Macmillan BT: Peripheral plasma concentrations of LH, FSH, prolactin and GH from birth to puberty in male and female mice. J Reprod Fertil 59:217–222, 1980.
57. Grayhack JT, Bunce PL, Kearns JW, Scott WW: Influence of the pituitary on prostatic response to androgen in the rat. Bull Johns Hopkins Hosp 96:154–163, 1955.
58. Slaunwhite WR, Sharma M: Effects of hypophysectomy and prolactin replacement therapy on prostatic response to androgen in orchiectomized rats. Biol Reprod 17:489–492, 1977.
59. Moger WH, Geschwind II: The action of prolactin on the sex accessory glands of the male rat. Proc Soc Exp Biol 141:1017–1021, 1972.
60. Grayhack JT, Lebowitz JM: Effect of prolactin on citric acid of lateral lobe of prostate of Sprague-Dawley rat. Invest Urol 5:87–94, 1967.
61. Thomas JA, Manandhar M: Effects of prolactin and/or testosterone on nucleic acid levels in prostate glands of normal and castrated rats. J Endocrinol 65:149–150, 1975.
62. Edwards WD, Thomas JA: Effects of androgens and/or prolactin on ventral prostate transplants. Urol Int 32:303–311, 1977.
63. Resnick MI, Walvoord DJ, Grayhack JT: Effect of prolactin on testosterone uptake by the perfused canine prostate. Surg Forum 25:70–72, 1974.
64. Thompson SA, Heidger PM: Synergistic effects of prolactin and testosterone in the restoration of rat prostatic epithelium following castration. Anat Rec 191:31–45, 1978.
65. Hostetter MW, Piacsek BE: The effect of prolactin deficiency during sexual maturation in the male rat. Biol Reprod 17:574–577, 1977.
66. Lawrence AM, Landau RL: Impaired ventral prostate affinity for testosterone in hypophysectomized rats. Endocrinology 77:1119–1125, 1965.
67. Farnsworth WE: Prolactin on androgen mobilization. In Goland M (ed): "Normal and Abnormal Growth of the Prostate." Springfield: Charles C Thomas, 1975, pp 502–508.
68. Baker HWG, Worgul TJ, Santen RJ, Jefferson LS, Bardin CW: Effect of prolactin on nuclear androgens in perfused male accessory sex organs. In Troen P, Nankin HR (eds): "The Testis in Normal and Infertile Men." New York: Raven Press, 1977, pp 379–385.
69. Shin SH: Estradiol generates pulses of prolactin secretion in castrated male rats. Neuroendocrinology 29:270–275. 1979.

70. Farnsworth WE, Gonder MJ: Prolactin and prostate cancer. Urology 10:33–34, 1977.

71. Jacobi GH, Sinterhauf K, Furth KH, Altwein JE: Testosterone metabolism in patients with advanced carcinoma of the prostate: A comparative in vivo study of the effect of oestrogen and anti-prolactin. Urol Res 6:159–165, 1978.

72. Goldstein S: Senescence. In DeGroot LJ (ed): "Endocrinology." New York: Grune & Stratton, 1979, Vol 3, pp 2001–2225.

73. Aragona C, Bohnet HG, Friesen HG: Localization of prolactin binding in prostate and testis: the role of serum prolactin concentration on the testicular LH receptor. Acta Endocrinologica 84:402–409, 1977.

74. Aragona C, Friesen HG: Specific prolactin binding sites in the prostate and testis of rats. Endocrinology 97:677–684, 1975.

75. Barkey RJ, Shani J, Amit T, Barzilai D: Specific binding of prolactin to seminal vesicle, prostate and testicular homogenates of immature, mature and aged rats. J Endocrinol 74:163–173, 1977.

76. Hanlin ML, Yount AP: Prolactin binding in the rat ventral prostate. Endocrine Res Commun 2:489–502, 1975.

77. Kledzik GS, Marshall S, Campbell GA, Gelato M, Meites J: Effects of castration, testosterone, estradiol, and prolactin on specific prolactin-binding activity in ventral prostate of male rats. Endocrinology 98:373–379, 1976.

78. Prasad MSK, Adiga PR: Modulation of prolactin receptors in the male rat. Ind J Exp Biol 17:1166–1170, 1979.

79. Lasnitzki I: The rat prostate gland in organ culture. In Griffiths K, Pierrepoint CG (eds): "Some Aspects of the Aetiology and Biochemistry of Prostatic Cancer." Third Tenovus Workshop. Cardiff, Wales: Alpha Omega Alpha Publishing, 1970, pp 68–73.

80. Lasnitzki I: The effect of prolactin on rat prostate glands in organ culture. In Boyns AR, Griffiths K (eds): "Prolactin and Carcinogenesis." Fourth Tenovus Workshop. Cardiff, Wales: Alpha Omega Alpha Publishing, 1972, pp 200–206.

81. Johansson R: Effect of prolactin, growth hormone and insulin on the uptake and binding of dihydrotestosterone to the cultured rat ventral prostate. Acta Endocrinologica 81:854–864, 1976.

82. Webber MM: Prolactin stimulates the growth of human prostatic epithelium in vitro (in preparation).

83. Webber MM, Stonington OG: Stromal hypocellularity and encapsulation in organ cultures of human prostate: application in epithelial cell isolation. J Urol 114:246–248, 1975.

84. Webber MM, Stonington OG, Poché PA: Epithelial outgrowth from suspension cultures of human prostatic tissue. In Vitro 10:196–205, 1974.

85. Mickey DD, Stone KR, Wunderli H, Mickey GH, Paulson DF: Characterization of a human prostate adenocarcinoma cell line (DU-145) as a monolayer culture and as a solid tumor in athymic mice. In Murphy GP (ed): "Models for Prostate Cancer." New York: Alan R. Liss, 1980, pp 67–84.

86. Webber MM: In vitro models for prostatic cancer: Summary. In Murphy GP (ed): "Models for Prostate Cancer." New York: Alan R. Liss, 1980, pp 133–147.

87. Armelin HA: Pituitary extracts and steroid hormones in the control of 3T3 cell growth. Proc Natl Acad Sci USA 70:2702–2706, 1973.

88. Gout PW, Beer CT, Noble RL: Prolactin-stimulated growth of cell cultures established from malignant Nb rat lymphomas. Cancer Res 40:2433–2436, 1980.

89. Gona O, Gona AG: Thyroid hormone action on the effect of prolactin. J Endocrinol 68:349–350, 1976.

90. Sodoughi N, Razvi M, Bush I, Ablin R, Guinan P: Cancer of the prostate. Relief of bone pain with levodopa. Urology 4:107–108, 1974.

91. Bartsch W, Steins P, Becker H: Hormone blood levels in patients with prostatic carcinoma and

their relation to the type of carcinoma growth differentiation. Eur Urol 3:47–52, 1977.

92. Oka T, Perry JW: Studies on regulatory factors of ornithine decarboxylase activity during development of mouse mammary epithelium in vitro. J Biol Chem 251:1738–1744, 1976.

93. Richards JF: Ornithine decarboxylase activity in tissues of prolactin-treated rats. Biochem Biophys Res Commun 63:292–299, 1975.

94. Horrobin DF: Cellular basis of prolactin in action: involvement of cyclic nucleotides, polyamines prostaglandins, steroids, thyroid hormones, Na/K ATPases and calcium: Relevance to breast cancer and the menstrual cycle. Med Hypoth 5:599–620, 1979.

95. Boyns AR, Cole EN, Golder MP, Danutra MP, Harper ME, Brownsey B, Cowley T, Jones GE, Griffiths K: Prolactin studies with the prostate. In Boyns AR, Griffiths K (eds): "Prolactin and Carcinogenesis." Fourth Tenovus Workshop. Cardiff, Wales: Alpha Omega Alpha Publishing, 1972, pp 207–216.

96. Golder MP, Boyns AR, Harper ME, Griffiths K: An effect of prolactin on prostatic adenylate cyclase activity. Biochem J 128:725–727, 1972

The Prostatic Cell: Structure and Function
Part B, pages 89–113
© 1981 Alan R. Liss, Inc., 150 Fifth Avenue, New York, NY 10011

Visualization of Prolactin Binding Sites in Prostate Tissue

Raphael J. Witorsch

INTRODUCTION

The direct influence of nongonadotrophic pituitary factors on the prostate gland was suggested by the early observations that prostatic atrophy was more marked after hypophysectomy than after orchidectomy and that androgen stimulation of prostatic growth was impaired by pituitary removal [1–3]. Evidence has been accumulating to indicate that prolactin, usually considered the "maternal" hormone, is this hypophyseal prostatotrophic factor. Many studies have shown that prolactin enhances androgen-stimulated prostatic enlargement and this prolactin-androgen interplay on the prostate was also evident when other functional parameters were examined such as zinc uptake, citrate content, nucleic acid content and synthesis, and androgen uptake and metabolism [4].

An additional line of evidence, albeit indirect, that the prostate gland is a prolactin target comes from hormone receptor studies. Sonenberg and Money's report in 1955 that prostate tissue retained radioactivity after ^{131}I-prolactin administration to male rats gave the first suggestion of lactogenic hormone receptors in this tissue [5]. More recently several laboratories have demonstrated specific ^{125}I-prolactin binding (ie, high affinity, saturable, and displaceable) to crude membrane-rich particulate fractions of rat prostate. Prolactin receptor content in prostate appears to be androgen-dependent as it decreases following castration and hypophysectomy and returns in restored prostate glands of castrated or hypophysectomized rats treated with androgen [6–8].

As an alternative to studies using radiolabelled hormone and tissue homogenates (cell-free radioreceptor methods) we attempted to study the prolactin-prostate relationship using an immunohistochemical approach in which we hoped to visualize the loci of prolactin binding in prostate tissue. It was felt that a morphophysiological approach, such as immunohistochemistry, would help define both the mechanism of prolactin action, which was unexplained, and the role of this hormone in normal and abnormal prostate tissue. As an extension of earlier studies in rat lactating mammary gland [9] we initially attempted to localize *endogenous* prolactin bound by prostate in vivo using an immunoperoxidase method. Because of certain methodologic difficulties, which are still under investigation, we were unable to identify immunoreactive endogenous prolactin in prostate tissue. However, in the course of this early immunohistochemical work we found that we could demonstrate intracellular binding sites for exogenous prolactin in rat prostate tissue [10]. This initial observation of intracellular prolactin binding sites in rat prostate tissue served as the basis of our current research program devoted to defining the role of prolactin in normal and abnormal prostate function. In this paper we review our previous immunohistochemical studies of normal and abnormal rat and human prostate and present some recent work in which we characterize prolactin binding sites in human prostate tissue.

MATERIALS AND METHODS

Tissues

Normal ventral and dorsolateral prostate were obtained from adult male Sprague Dawley rats immediately after decapitation. R3327 prostatic cancer tissue was obtained immediately after decapitation from adult male Copenhagen × Fisher F_1 hybrid rats bearing tumor transplants provided by the National Prostatic Cancer Project. Rat tissues were fixed in Bouin's fluid for approximately 18 hours, washed in 70% ethanol, dehydrated in increasing ethanol solutions, and embedded in paraffin. Human prostate tissue specimens were obtained from several sources. Autopsy specimens of normal, hyperplastic, and cancerous prostate tissue previously fixed in formalin and paraffin embedded were provided by the Pathology Department at the Medical College of Virginia. Biopsy specimens of benign prostatic hypertrophy and prostatic cancer, previously formalin fixed and paraffin embedded, were provided by the Pathology Department of the College of Physicians and Surgeons of Columbia University. In more recent studies we received biopsy specimens of benign prostatic hypertrophy and autopsy specimens of normal prostate from the Department of Surgery at the University of Miami. These tissues were placed in nutrient medium and shipped to our laboratory via Federal Express packed in refrigerant. Immediately upon receiving these specimens in our laboratory (24–48 hours following extirpation), specimens were fixed in Bouin's fluid and paraffin embedded as described above for rat tissues. Tissue sections of all specimens were cut serially at 5 μm and mounted on gelatin coated slides, six sections per slide for immunohistochemistry. Additional sections were stained with hematoxylin-Gomori's trichrome for histological observation.

Reagents

NIAMDD was the source of all pituitary hormones and their respective antisera. Highly purified rat prolactin (PRL, lots I-2, I-3 and I-4), human prolactin (lot VLS # 3), and human placental lactogen (HPL) were obtained lyophilized and dissolved in 0.003 N NaOH at a concentration of 0.5 or 1.0 μg/μl and stored as 5–10 μg aliquots at –50°C. Prior to a series of experiments hormone was further diluted in 0.01 M phosphate–0.9% NaCl buffer (phosphate buffered saline, PBS)–0.1% bovine serum albumin (BSA). Hormone solutions (ranging from 6.25 ng/ml to 5 μg/ml) were used over a period of several weeks and stored at 4°C. Rabbit antisera against rat PRL (lots S-2, S-3, S-4, S-6, and S-7), human PRL (lot AFP #1), and HPL (lot CT3399) were received lyophilized and reconstituted in distilled water diluted in PBS-0.05 M EDTA, pH 7.0. Goat antiserum against rabbit γ-globulin (ARγG) was obtained either from Anitbodies Incorporated or Cappel Laboratories and diluted in PBS. Soluble peroxidase-rabbit antiperoxidase (PAP) complex was obtained from Sternberger-Myer, Inc. and diluted in PBS-1% normal goat serum. The immunoperoxidase substrate was a saturated solution of 3,3'diaminobenzidene free base (DAB, Sigma D-8001) + 0.003% H_2O_2 in 0.005 M Tris buffer, pH 7.6. Osmium tetroxide (OsO_4) was obtained from Polysciences, Inc.

Immunoperoxidase Prolactin Binding Protocol

After first exposing prostate tissue sections to exogenous hormone, prolactin binding sites were visualized with an immunoperoxidase staining protocol generally used by others to localize hormones in cells of origin [11]. The basic protocol we use is depicted in Table I. Prior to the assay each slide bearing six serial sections was deparaffinized in xylene and rehydrated in progressively more dilute ethanol solutions (absolute ethanol through 50% ethanol) and finally in PBS. All subsequent reagents were applied as drops to the tissue sections and incubations were carried out at room temperature in a humidified chamber. Between reagent applications, slides were washed thoroughly in PBS to remove unbound reagent. In Step I, section 1 was incubated with hormone vehicle (PBS-BSA) while sections 2–6 were usually incubated with progressively increasing concentrations of hormone. This dose-related design was often modified, depending on the objective of a particular experiment. In studies involving rat tissue we generally used rat PRL, whereas in studies with human specimens we used rat PRL, HPL, and human PRL. After hormone incubation, the tissue sections were exposed to the appropriate primary antiserum (rabbit antisera directed against the hormone used) (Step II). If prolactin binding sites existed in the tissue the hormone would be expected to bind to the tissue and the primary antiserum should then react with the bound hormone. The location of the tissue-bound hormone-antibody complex was then visualized by Steps III through V

TABLE I. Basic protocol for the immunohistochemical localization of prolactin binding sites in prostate tissue

Step	Reagent	Duration
I	Hormone vehicle (PBS-BSA)[a] or hormone[b]	18–24 hr
II	Primary rabbit antiserum against hormone used in step I[c]	18–24 hr
III	Secondary antiserum (goat ARγG)[d], 1:150	30 min
IV	Peroxidase-rabbit antiperoxidase (PAP), 1:80	30 min
V	DAB-H$_2$O$_2$[e]	10 min
VI	0.5% Osmium tetroxide	3 min

[a]Phosphate buffered saline–0.1% bovine serum albumin.
[b]NIAMDD (iodination grade) rat prolactin (PRL), human PRL, human placental lactogen (HPL), concentrations discussed in text.
[c]NIAMDD rabbit anti-rat PRL, rabbit anti-human PRL, rabbit anti-HPL, dilutions presented in text.
[d]Goat antiserum against rabbit γ-globulin.
[e]3,3′Diaminobenzidine + 0.003% H$_2$O$_2$.

of the protocol (ARγG, PAP, DAB-H$_2$O$_2$). The secondary antiserum, goat ARγG, served as a bridge between the two rabbit immunoglobulins used in the procedure, the primary antiserum and antiperoxidase of the PAP complex. In the presence of peroxidase and H$_2$O$_2$, the chromogenic substrate, DAB, was oxidized to a brown precipitate corresponding in location to the initial antigen. Staining was intensified by exposure of tissue sections to OsO$_4$ while unstained areas were unaffected (Step VI). Hormone concentrations and primary antisera dilutions were determined in preliminary experiments to define optimal assay conditions (ie, those producing little or no staining in section 1 and dose-dependent staining in sections 2–6).

Initially we reported in rat sex accessory organs, rat prostate cancer, and human prostate specimens that hormone binding sites could be visualized after exposure of tissue sections to hormone concentrations in the range of 200 ng/ml to 5 μg/ml [12–14]. Most of the tissue sections studied were those exposed to the higher hormone concentrations (1 μg/ml or 5 μg/ml). In later studies with rat tissue, hormone binding sites could be visualized after exposing tissue sections to rat PRL concentrations as low as 25 ng/ml [15] and very recently we have been able to detect binding sites in ventral prostate tissue sections exposed to rat PRL concentrations of 6.25 ng/ml [16], concentrations which are within the physiological range of serum prolactin for the male rat. In the current procedure, rat PRL concentrations range from 6.25–250 ng/ml. Enhancement of the sensitivity of the immunohistochemical binding protocol was brought about by introducing several modifications. The area of the tissue section has been reduced because staining intensity increases as smaller reagent bubbles are added to tissue sections. We currently mount tissue sections on slides within an etched circle 6.5 mm in diameter. Etched circles not only confine the size of the section but also introduce consistency into the method. The circle serves as a guide in order to add the same volume of reagent to each section (approximately 20 μl). Recent batches of NIAMDD antisera to rat PRL (S6 and S7) are used which produce more intense immunostaining reactions than previous batches (S3 and S4). Tissue sections are now osmicated which intensifies staining of reaction product. With information obtained working with rat tissues, we have been able to implement improvements which enhance the sensitivity of the immunohistochemical method when applied to human tissues. These improvements and related developments as applied to human tissue are discussed in the Results and Discussion section.

In order to minimize nonspecific staining reactions and assure immunological specificity of our binding procedure, hormones of the highest purity available were used (iodination grade reagents from NIAMDD radioimmunoassay kits) as well as highly specific primary antisera as determined by radioimmunoassay (also from NIAMDD radioimmunoassay kits). In addition, primary antisera were characterized for specificity using the standard Sternberger immunoperoxidase method (Steps II–VI, Table I) on rat pituitary sections [11]. With this procedure NIAMDD anti-rat PRL revealed only prolactin cells in rat pituitary and staining intensity decreased as antiserum dilution increased. Neutralization (or immunoabsorption) of the antiserum by admixture with highly purified rat PRL (iodination grade) blocked prolactin cell staining in rat pituitary. Admixture of anti-PRL with other hormones including prolactins from other species did not block prolactin cell staining indicating that the antisera against rat PRL were highly specific for this hormone [10,12,13]. We have also reported a similar high degree of specificity for HPL antiserum by immunohistochemistry [17] and the specificity of human PRL antiserum is currently under investigation. In all binding studies in prostate tissue we included pituitary tissue to serve as immunostaining standards and methodologic controls. In addition to demonstrating a dose-related staining reaction for each hormone applied to prostate tissue we have verified that hormone-dependent staining in prostate was immunospecific by showing that the bound hormone was *not* detected by the appropriate specifically absorbed primary antiserum [10,12–14].

RESULTS AND DISCUSSION

Intracellular Prolactin Binding in Normal and Neoplastic Rat Prostate Tissue

Our initial studies in rat ventral prostate showed that when tissue sections were incubated with rat prolactin followed by anti-rat prolactin, an immunoperoxidase reaction sequence produced an immunospecific, hormone dose-related staining reaction in epithelial cells [10]. This staining, indicative of prolactin binding loci, occurred in a supranuclear location corresponding to the area of the ventral prostate epithelial cell designated by Moore et al as the Golgi region [18] (Fig. 1). We further showed that this intracellular prolactin binding was androgen dependent. Golgi region prolactin binding was absent in ventral prostates from long-term (3-month) castrated rats and returned when ventral prostates from castrated rats were restored by androgen replacement [10]. This demonstration of testicular dependence of prostatic prolactin binding, which is consistent with the concept of a prolactin-androgen interplay in this organ, confirmed the observations of other workers cited above using radioreceptor methods to estimate prostatic prolactin binding [6–8]. The Golgi zone has been recognized for some time as a sensitive indicator of the physiological status of ventral prostate epithelial cells [19]. Interestingly, prolactin has been shown by Lasnitski

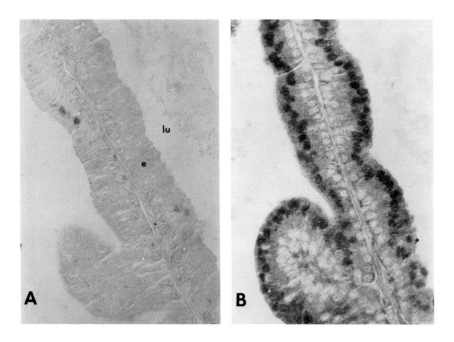

Fig. 1.   Rat ventral prostate showing prolactin binding in the Golgi region of epithelial cells. A) Section exposed to the hormone vehicle, PBS-BSA followed by anti-rat PRL S6(1:200) and the immunoperoxidase staining sequence. Section is unstained although diffraction patterns reveal epithelial cell outlines, basal nuclei, and intraluminal contents. B) Same field of cells from another section exposed to rat PRL (500 ng/ml) followed by anti-rat PRL S6(1:200) and the immunoperoxidase staining sequence. Staining occurs primarily in the Golgi region of the cells indicative of intracellular prolactin binding sites. Epithelial cells, e; lumen, lu. × 570.

to enlarge ventral prostate epithelial cells in organ culture in the vicinity of the Golgi region [20]. Since the Golgi region of ventral prostate epithelial cells contains several organelles [21], the precise location(s) of prolactin binding sites will have to await the results of ultrastructural immunohistochemical studies.

In subsequent studies we examined the patterns of prolactin binding by immunohistochemistry in several other sex accessory organs of the male rat (epididymides, vas deferens, seminal vesicle, and dorsolateral prostate) and observed that prolactin binding activity was ubiquitously found in epithelial cells throughout the male reproductive tract, although the pattern of hormone binding varied from organ to organ [12]. Unlike the stereotyped pattern of Golgi-localized prolactin binding of ventral prostate epithelial cells, hormone binding patterns were quite heterogeneous in epithelial cells of dorsolateral prostate [12]. In these early studies we made no attempt to differentiate between lateral and dorsal regions of the dorsolateral complex because the prevailing literature, with some exception, regards this structure as a unit [4,22]. Because of heterogeneity in prolactin binding patterns in dorsolateral prostate we reexamined this structure in order to compare prolactin binding patterns in the lateral and dorsal regions. Significant differences were found between these zones [15]. In lateral prostate epithelial cells both discrete Golgi-localized and diffuse cytoplasmic prolactin binding were observed. In addition, we frequently found cells devoid of prolactin binding activity interspersed among intensely stained cells (Fig. 2). Dorsal prostate epithelial cells exhibited diffuse cytoplasmic prolactin binding often confined to large apical blebs (Fig. 2). Luminal material of the lateral prostate showed intense prolactin-dependent immunostaining which was reduced in dorsal prostate and nonexistent in ventral prostate or any of the other male reproductive structures examined (Figs. 1,2). We found that lateral lobe had the most prolactin binding activity of the prostatic lobes examined which is consistent with several reports that this is the most responsive of prostatic zones to the hormone [23–25]. It is of interest that the pattern of prolactin binding which we observed in lateral lobe is similar to the distribution of zinc in this region [26] and that the uptake of zinc by the dorsolateral prostate is apparently stimulated by prolactin both in the presence and absence of androgen [27,28]. Intraluminal prolactin binding activity in dorsolateral prostate may have relevance in the observations from other laboratories of immunoreactive prolactin accumulation in seminal fluid which is apparently derived from sex accessory structures rather than spermatozoa or testicular fluid [29,30]. Our observations by immunohistochemistry of significant prolactin binding activity in dorsolateral prostate, which as cited above are consistent with physiological observations, do not agree with a report that the binding of ^{125}I-labelled-ovine prolactin to crude membrane-rich pellets of rat dorsolateral prostate is negligible compared to ventral prostate [31]. The reason for this discrepancy is not known but may be related to the fact that in our immunohistochemical studies uniodinated rat hormone was used in contrast to

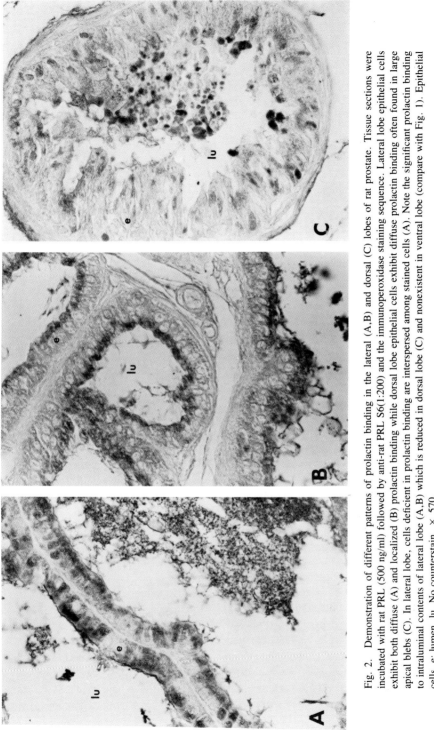

Fig. 2. Demonstration of different patterns of prolactin binding in the lateral (A,B) and dorsal (C) lobes of rat prostate. Tissue sections were incubated with rat PRL (500 ng/ml) followed by anti-rat PRL S6(1:200) and the immunoperoxidase staining sequence. Lateral lobe epithelial cells exhibit both diffuse (A) and localized (B) prolactin binding while dorsal lobe epithelial cells exhibit diffuse prolactin binding often found in large apical blebs (C). In lateral lobe, cells deficient in prolactin binding are interspersed among stained cells (A). Note the significant prolactin binding to intraluminal contents of lateral lobe (A,B) which is reduced in dorsal lobe (C) and nonexistent in ventral lobe (compare with Fig. 1). Epithelial cells, e; lumen, lu. No counterstain. × 570.

the radiolabelled heterologous hormone of radioreceptor studies. In addition to the striking differences in the distribution of prolactin binding sites among the ventral, lateral, and dorsal lobes of the prostate we also observed significant tinctorial differences among these regions using hematoxylin-Gomori's trichrome stain [32]. The functional significance of differences in prolactin binding patterns and histology among the three zones of rat prostate are as yet unexplained but of continuing interest.

We recently observed regional differences in the testicular dependence of prostatic prolactin binding. A marked diminution in prolactin binding of ventral prostate epithelial cells was observed within 4 days postcastration which continued to diminish with time. This agreed with the time course of changes in prostatic prolactin binding activity reported by others using radioreceptor methods [6–8]. In dorsolateral prostate, on the other hand, prolactin binding was undiminished 8 days postcastration and still evident after 3–4 weeks [15]. Similarly, we observed that the cytologic regression of ventral prostate occurred more rapidly than dorsolateral prostate. The data from this castration study as well as from androgen replacement experiments currently in progress suggest that prolactin binding activity is intimately associated with the functional status of the prostate epithelial cell. It is also of interest and of possible importance to note that while the rat ventral lobe is the model of choice for most studies on the prostate, the rat dorsal and lateral lobes which may be governed by different endocrine control mechanisms are homologous to their counterparts in man and the ventral lobe apparently is not [33].

As a logical extension of our work on normal rat prostate we attempted to test for and to localize prolactin binding activity in the Dunning R3327 transplantable cancer line which is derived from the dorsolateral prostate of an aged Copenhagen rat [13,34]. Diffuse intracytoplasmic prolactin binding activity was observed in cells of both differentiated and undifferentiated regions of the tumors we examined (Fig. 3). In contrast to normal dorsolateral prostate tissue, which exhibited significant intraluminal prolactin binding activity, we saw little evidence of prolactin binding to luminal contents of R3327 prostatic cancers (Fig. 3). However, extracellular prolactin binding was observed in less well-differentiated regions of the tumor. A significant degree of variation in the proportion of cells with prolactin binding activity was observed within and between tumor specimens and the degree of prolactin binding activity in this initial study involving only 16 individual tumor specimens did not appear to be associated with tumor size [13]. There have been relatively few attempts at associating prolactin with prostatic cancer and these have been reviewed in a previous publication from our laboratory [13]. Recently, Rosoff et al reported that perphenazine administration which produces hyperprolactinemia retarded the growth of R3327 tumors suggesting an inhibitory effect of prolactin on the proliferation of this tumor line [35]. More extensive studies are currently in progress in our laboratory

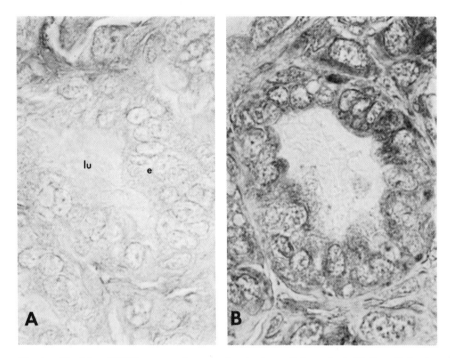

Fig. 3. Gland from R3327 rat prostatic cancer showing intracellular prolactin binding. A) Section exposed to PBS-BSA, followed by anti-rat PRL S3(1:200) and the immunoperoxidase staining sequence. Section is unstained although diffraction patterns reveal cellular features and intraluminal material. B) Same gland from another section exposed to rat PRL (5 μg/ml) followed by anti-rat PRL S3(1:200) and the immunoperoxidase staining sequence. Prolactin-dependent staining is distributed throughout the cytoplasm of cells within the alveolus and also in cells outside of the alveolus (upper right). Note that intraluminal contents do not exhibit prolactin binding activity. Epithelial cells, e; lumen, lu. × 1430.

to determine whether the degree of prolactin binding activity in this tumor line is associated (in a negative or positive sense) with the rate tumor growth.

Prolactin Binding in Normal and Diseased Human Prostate Tissue

Patterns of hormone binding. We have examined a limited number of human prostate specimens (3 normal, 5 benign prostatic hypertrophy, and 2 carcinoma) and have observed a variety PRL binding of patterns [14]. For the localization of prolactin binding sites in human tissue specimens we have used rat prolactin, human prolactin, and human placental lactogen (HPL) and their respective antisera. The rat hormone-antiserum combination was used because

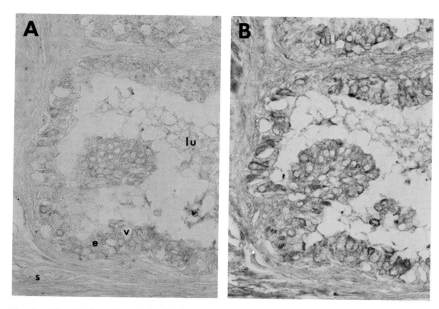

Fig. 4.   Visualization of prolactin binding in normal human prostate. Specimen was obtained at autopsy and stored in nutrient medium for 48 hours prior to fixation and embedding. A) Section was exposed to PBS-BSA then to anti-human PRL (1:2400) prior to the immunoperoxidase staining sequence. Section is unstained but diffraction patterns reveal epithelial cells (e), stroma (s), and intraluminal contents (lu). B) Adjacent section showing same field exposed to human PRL (250 ng/ml) then to anti-human PRL (1:2400) and the immunoperoxidase staining sequence. Diffuse intra-epithelial cell prolactin binding is observed. Prolactin-dependent staining is also found in stroma and to luminal contents. Large vacuoles (v) are also in the epithelial cell layer of this specimen, presumably associated with the storage of the specimen in nutrient medium prior to tissue processing. × 416.

it is well characterized immunohistochemically and appears to work on human tissue. Human hormones were used because they seem more appropriate for studies involving human specimens. Human placental lactogen (also called human chorionic somatomammotropin, HCS), which is secreted during pregnancy, is chemically very similar to human growth hormone and exhibits significant lactogen-like biological activity including prostatotrophic effects [36,37]. Diffuse intracytoplasmic epithelial cell prolactin binding predominated in normal and diseased human prostate specimens (Figs. 4,5,8), although discrete binding in the cytoplasm was occasionally seen in benign prostatic hypertrophy [14]. Intraluminal prolactin binding was seen in specimens of normal prostate (Fig. 4) and benign prostatic hypertrophy [14]. Binding of hormone to the nucleus was also observed in several specimens and predominated in a specimen of multifocal

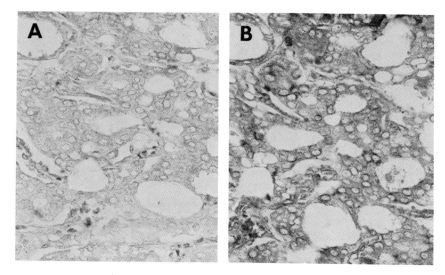

Fig. 5.   Specimen of prostatic carcinoma which had metastasized to the vertebral column (obtained at autopsy). A) Section was exposed to PBS-BSA followed by anti-human PRL (1:2400) and the immunoperoxidase staining sequence. Section is lightly stained and reveals nuclei and back to back glandular arrangement of tissue. B) Adjacent section exposed to human PRL (250 ng/ml) followed by anti-human PRL (1:2400) prior to the immunoperoxidase staining sequence. Diffuse intracytoplasmic prolactin binding is demonstrated. × 416.

prostatic carcinoma (Fig. 6). In normal and hypertrophied specimens, hormone-dependent cytoplasmic staining of myoepithelial cells was also observed (Fig. 7).

A considerable degree of heterogeneity with respect to prolactin-dependent immunostaining was observed in human prostate specimens. Cells that were intensely stained were often found interspersed among less stained or unstained cells or vice versa. This heterogeneity was very evident in a specimen of benign prostatic hypertrophy in a region where squamous metaplasia had occurred (Fig. 8). In the specimens of normal and hypertrophied prostate examined we observed

Fig. 7.   Normal human prostate (obtained at autopsy and shipped in nutrient medium) showing prolactin binding in myoepithelial cells, as well as secretory epithelial cells. A) Section exposed to PBS-BSA then to anti-human PRL (1:2400) and the immunoperoxidase staining sequence. Section is unstained although diffraction patterns reveal epithelial cells (e) as well as large vacuoles (v) between cells. B) Another section showing same field of cells exposed to human PRL (250 ng/ml) then to anti-human PRL (1:2400) and the immunoperoxidase staining sequence. Diffuse prolactin-dependent staining is observed in epithelial cells. More intense prolactin-dependent staining of myoepithelial cells is observed subjacent to the epithelial cell layer. × 416.

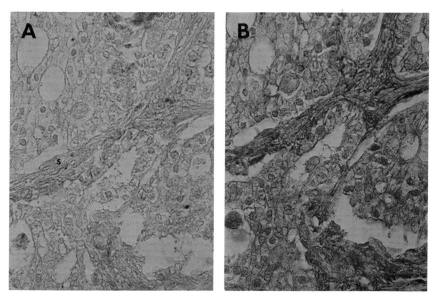

Fig. 6.   Specimen of multifocal prostatic carcinoma showing prolactin binding to nuclei. A) Section was exposed to PBS-BSA followed by anti-human PRL (1:2400) and the immunoperoxidase staining sequence. Section is unstained although diffraction patterns reveal neoplastic cells. B) Same field of cells from an adjacent section which was exposed to human PRL (250 ng/ml) followed by anti-human PRL (1:2400) and the immunoperoxidase staining sequence. In addition to nuclear staining, prolactin binding was also observed in stroma (s). × 416.

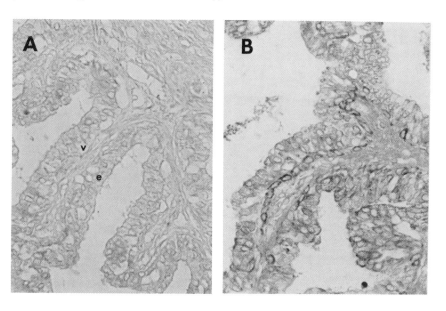

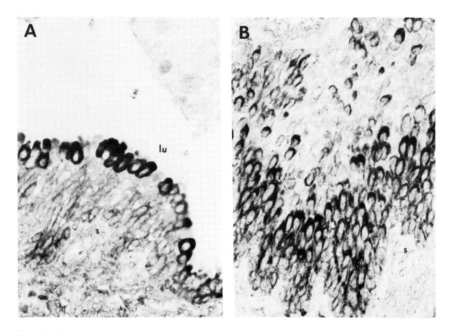

Fig. 8. Benign prostatic hypertrophy (obtained through biopsy) showing heterogeneity among individual cells in their ability to bind prolactin. In this region of the specimen, squamous metaplasia was observed. Tissue section was exposed to human PRL (2.5 μg/ml) followed by anti-human PRL (1:2400) and the immunoperoxidase staining sequence. A) Field shows individual cells which are intensely stained adjacent to the lumen (lu). B) Another field in which the more intensely stained cells were observed in the more basal layers of the squamous metaplasia adjacent to the stroma (s). No counterstain. × 570.

what appeared to be considerable interglandular heterogeneity where some alveoli seemed to bind prolactin more intensely than others (Fig. 9). Some of the specimens, particularly those received in nutrient medium, exhibited significant hormone binding to stromal elements (Fig. 4). It is not known whether this extraglandular prolactin binding activity is a product of connective tissue cells or alveolar contents which seeped to the stroma in the course of tissue handling (surgical extirpation and/or storage in nutrient media for extended periods). With the exception of myoepithelial cell prolactin dependent staining reported above, the hormone binding patterns seen in human prostate specimens were observed in normal and neoplastic rat prostate tissue. The existence of prolactin binding in human prostate has also been recently reported by Keenan et al using radio-receptor methods [38].

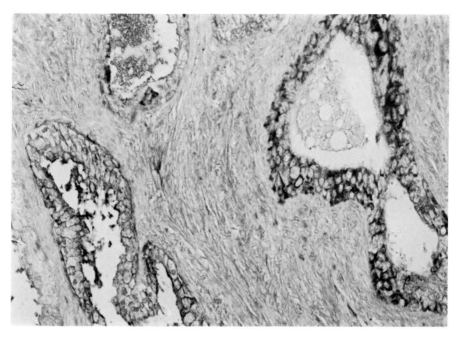

Fig. 9. Benign prostatic hypertrophy (obtained through biopsy) showing differences in the degree of prolactin binding activity between alveoli. The section was exposed to human PRL (250 ng/ml) followed by anti-human PRL (1:2400) and the immunoperoxidase staining sequence. Alveolus on the right exhibits more intense cell staining than the two alveoli on the left. No counterstain. × 285.

Characterization of lactogenic hormone binding in human prostate specimens. We are currently extending our studies on human prostate to optimize assay conditions and to determine whether these prolactin binding sites exhibit characteristics associated with a specific hormone receptor, namely high affinity for hormone, saturability, and biological specificity. These studies on human specimens are a continuation of similar experiments conducted on rat ventral prostate which will be reported elsewhere [16]. In order to enhance the sensitivity of the binding procedure for human tissues we have implemented modifications indicated in the Materials and Methods section (ie, small sections, osmication and the use of more recent lots of anti-rat PRL). When human hormones are involved we use anti-HPL and anti-human PRL at dilutions of 1:1600 and 1:2400, respectively.

In the past, suitable visualization of prolactin binding sites for most human

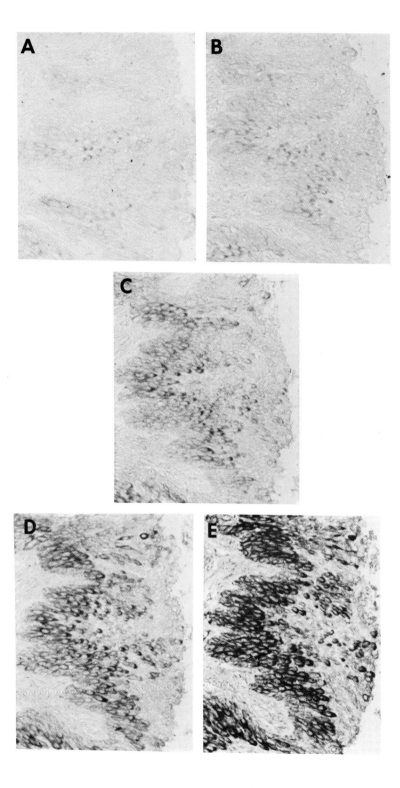

specimens required hormone incubation concentrations in the microgram per milliliter range. Currently we are able to consistently visualize hormone binding sites in human specimens at 100–250 ng/ml (Fig. 10). The fact that higher amounts of hormone are required for the visualization of prolactin binding in human prostate than in rat ventral prostate [16] may reflect species differences or the differing conditions under which the specimens were removed (ie, laboratory versus morgue and operating room). Prolactin binding in human prostate specimens is saturable since a hormone concentration is reached at which tissue staining no longer increases (Fig. 11).

The immunohistochemical localization of a binding site requires that a very strong association be established between ligand and tissue. This is because the hormone that binds to the tissue section must then be exposed for up to 24 hours to the primary antiserum solution which is virtually hormone free. Under these conditions, one would expect most of the hormone to leave the tissue and diffuse into the incubating solution and yet significant hormone-dependent immunostaining occurs. The affinity of the hormone for its binding site was further examined by incubating the section in PBS for 24 hours between hormone exposure and the application of primary antiserum. Under these conditions, we still observed significant hormone-dependent immunostaining (Fig. 12) indicating that the hormone-binding site interaction in human prostate is quite strong.

In radioreceptor experiments hormone binding to particulate fractions is considered specific only if excess unlabelled ligand displaces tracer amounts of its labelled counterpart. Since radiolabelled hormones are not used in immunohistochemical experiments this test for displacement was not possible. Alternatively, we tested for specificity of hormone binding in human prostate specimens by coincubating the hormone in question with excess amounts of different hormones which were lactogenic in biological action but unreactive with the primary antiserum. The hormone combinations we used were rat PRL (250 ng/ml) with 400-fold excess amounts (100 μg/ml) of porcine PRL (NIAMDD, SP 162C) or HPL, combinations which were studied initially in rat ventral prostate [16]. Neither HPL nor porcine PRL appeared to cross react with the primary antiserum, anti-rat PRL. If rat PRL were displaced from its binding site by excess competitor one would expect a diminution in hormone-dependent immunostaining since the displacing ligand now on the prolactin binding site would be undetected by the primary antiserum. Under these conditions, porcine PRL produced a marked

Fig. 10. Demonstration of dose-related prolactin binding in specimen of benign prostatic hypertrophy (obtained through biopsy). Prior to anti-human PRL (1:2400) and the immunoperoxidase staining sequence, serial tissue sections were exposed to one of the following treatments: A) PBS-BSA; B) human PRL, 25 ng/ml; C) human PRL, 100 ng/ml; D) human PRL, 250 ng/ml; E) human PRL, 2.5 μg/ml. The field in the photograph is squamous metaplasia. Prolactin binding of individual cells is demonstrable at 100 ng/ml and is dose-related up to 2.5 μg/ml. × 300.

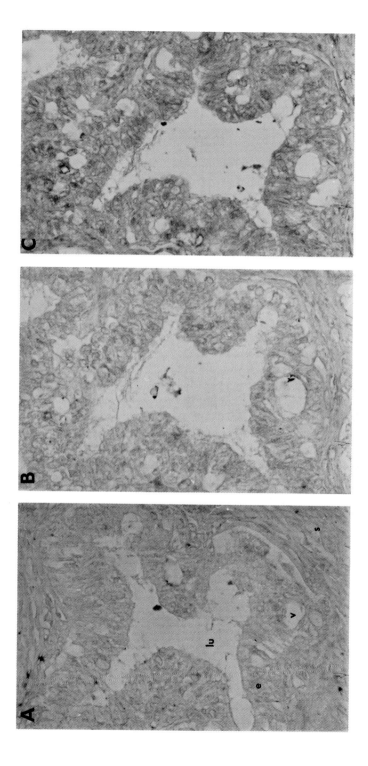

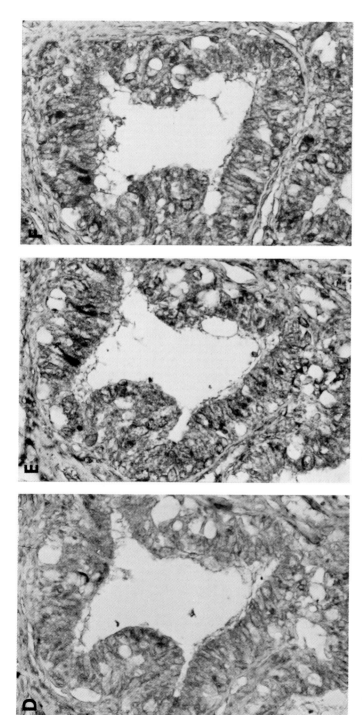

Fig. 11. Demonstration that prolactin binding sites in human prostate specimens are saturable. A single alveolus of normal prostate tissue is depicted (obtained through autopsy and stored in nutrient medium). Prior to exposure to anti-human PRL (1:2400) and the immunoperoxidase staining sequence, serial sections were exposed to one of the following treatments: A) PBS-BSA; B) human PRL, 100 ng/ml; C) human PRL, 250 ng/ml; D) human PRL, 500 ng/ml; E) human PRL, 2.5 μg/ml; F) human PRL, 10 μg/ml human PRL. Between human PRL doses of 2.5 μg/ml and 10 μg/ml binding sites appear saturated since staining no longer intensifies. Epithelial cells, e; lumen, lu; stroma, s; vacuoles, v. × 570.

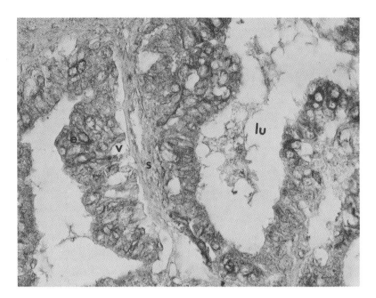

Fig. 12. Demonstration that prolactin binding sites in human prostate tissue have a strong affinity for the hormone. This specimen is normal human prostate obtained through autopsy and stored in nutrient medium. The tissue section was first exposed to human PRL (250 ng/ml) for 24 hours and then incubated in hormone-free medium (PBS) for another 24 hours prior to application of anti-human PRL (1:2400) and the immunoperoxidase staining sequence. Prolactin-dependent staining is still demonstrable in epithelial cells (e) after prolonged exposure to PBS. Lumen, lu; stroma, s; vacuoles, v. No counterstain. × 416.

diminution in rat PRL-dependent immunostaining while the effects of HPL were equivocal (Fig. 13). Similarly, porcine PRL was more effective than HPL in displacing rat PRL from its Golgi localized binding site in rat ventral prostate [16]. The porcine prolactin may be more effective than HPL in displacing rat PRL from its binding site because of its closer homology to the rat PRL molecule. In addition, porcine PRL may have a higher affinity for the prolactin binding site in human prostate tissue than HPL. Species differences in the affinities of hormones for a tissue receptor have been reported [39,40].

CONCLUSIONS

The characteristics of prolactin binding sites which we observe in human prostate (visualization after incubation of sections with small amounts of hormone, saturability, high affinity, and apparent specificity) confirm our findings in rat ventral prostate tissue and appear consistent with biochemical criteria for a specific hormone receptor. For the tissue to retain these characteristics after having undergone tissue processing seems remarkable. In addition, the conditions

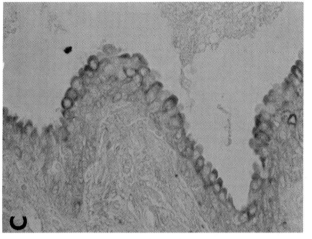

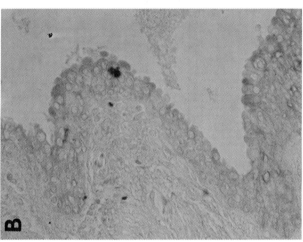

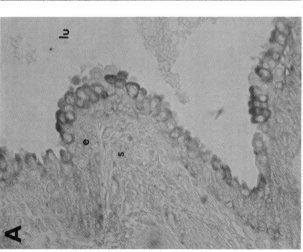

Fig. 13. Demonstration that rat PRL can be displaced from its binding site on human prostate tissue by another lactogenic hormone. The specimen is benign prostatic hypertrophy in a region of squamous metaplasia. Prior to exposure to anti-rat PRL S7 (1:200) and the immunoperoxidase staining sequence, tissue sections were exposed to one of the following treatments: A) rat PRL, 250 ng/ml; B) rat PRL (250 ng/ml) + porcine PRL (100 μg/ml); C) rat PRL (250 ng/ml) + human placental lactogen (HPL, 100 μg/ml). Porcine PRL coincubated with rat PRL markedly diminishes rat PRL-dependent staining of individual cells; HPL shows little or no effect. Squamous epithelial cells, e; stroma, s; lumen, lu. No counterstain. × 416.

of the immunohistochemical procedure where the binding site is immobilized in a tissue section while ligand is in the liquid phase are less than optimal for the demonstration of hormone-receptor site interactions. Nevertheless, the immunogenicity of many cell substances are preserved after tissue processing [11], and other laboratories have demonstrated that fixed tissue sections can bind exogenous hormone [41–43].

In our studies, intracellular prolactin binding was the prevalent feature and we saw little evidence of hormone binding on the cell surface. At the time of our initial report of intracellular prolactin binding sites in rat ventral prostate in 1977, it was generally believed that peptide hormones did not enter cells. Since that time, a growing body of evidence has accumulated that peptide hormones enter the cells of many target tissues [44]. However, it has not been resolved whether internalization of a peptide hormone is essential for an endocrine effect. In the case of prolactin, which has yet to be associated with a second messenger, hormone entry may be quite significant. Our immunohistochemical demonstration of intracellular prolactin binding sites in prostate cells, although consistent with the concept of peptide hormone internalization, does not prove that prolactin enters this cell. Under conditions of our procedure the internal components of the cell are exteriorized by tissue sectioning and therefore the cell membrane offers no barrier to the exogenously applied hormone. Binding of hormone to intracellular components as observed in our studies as well as in radioreceptor experiments might reflect in situ hormone receptors or the site where cell surface receptors are manufactured [45]. Experiments are currently underway in our laboratory in an attempt to determine whether immunoreactive prolactin is internalized in vivo by prostatic epithelial cells.

The immunohistochemical approach offers an alternative strategy for the study of hormone-receptor interactions. With the immunoperoxidase method, which has application at the ultrastructural level, it is possible to define the loci of hormone binding in relation to cell, tissue, and organ structure. This is rather important in heterogeneous tissues such as prostate which contain numerous elements in addition to secretory epithelial cells. Since the immunoperoxidase method capitalizes on the immunoactivity of a substance, radioiodinated hormones are not required and the problems inherent in their use, such as impaired or altered biological activity [46,47], can be avoided. It should be reiterated that the results obtained thus far with immunohistochemistry on prolactin binding in prostate tissue, for the most part, parallel data obtained by others using radio-receptor techniques, appear to satisfy biochemical criteria for hormone receptors, and are quite consistent with physiological information obtained from a variety of sources.

If prolactin plays a significant role in prostatic cancer, be it stimulatory or inhibitory, the advantages of a therapy for prostatic carcinoma based upon manipulation of this hormone seem obvious when one considers the current alternatives of castration or estrogen treatment. Therefore, an immunohistochemical assay for prolactin binding activity in prostate tissues may be of value in the diagnosis and treatment planning of prostatic disease as well as for restrospective studies. At present we have examined too few human prostate specimens to indicate the clinical value of the immunohistochemical approach to prolactin binding, although several provocative staining patterns were observed. Similar patterns of prolactin-dependent immunostaining have been seen by El Etreby et al in normal and experimentally induced abnormal canine prostate [48,49]. Immunohistochemical studies on large numbers of human specimens may reveal an association between hormone binding patterns, the degree of hormone binding, and prostatic disease. In addition, with the implementation of microdensitometry, the immunoperoxidase approach to hormone binding could evolve into a quantitative procedure.

ACKNOWLEDGMENTS

The author wishes to thank the NIAMDD Pituitary Hormone Distribution Program and Dr. A.F. Parlow for the gifts of hormones and primary antisera. The gifts of tumor-bearing rats from Dr. Norman Altman in association with the National Prostatic Cancer Project is also appreciated.

The author is grateful to Dr. Myron Tannenbaum, Department of Pathology, College of Physicians and Surgeons of Columbia University, for providing preembedded biopsy specimens of human prostate and to Dr. Theodore I. Malinin and Ms Nancy Castigleone, Department of Surgery, University of Miami in association with the National Prostatic Cancer Project for providing unembedded prostate tissue. The author also thanks Dr. Charles W. Moncure, Department of Pathology, Medical College of Virginia for providing preembedded autopsy specimens of human prostate and for providing assistance in the histological examination of abnormal prostate tissue.

Special thanks are also due to Ms Leanne Haskin for her outstanding technical work and to Ms Pat Holland for her excellent secretarial assistance.

This investigation was supported by grant 1R26 CA 23653 awarded by the National Cancer Institute, Department of Health and Human Services.

REFERENCES

1. Grayhack JT, Bunce PL, Kearns JW, Scott WW: Influence of the pituitary on prostate response to androgen in the rat. Johns Hopk Hosp Bull 96:154–163, 1955.
2. Huggins C, Russell PS: Quantitative effects of hypophysectomy on testis and prostate of dogs. Endocrinology 39:1–7, 1946.
3. Vanderlaan WP: Observations on the hormonal control of the prostate gland. Lab Invest 9:185–190, 1960.
4. Yamanaka H, Kirdani RY, Saroff J, Murphy GP, Sandberg AA: Effects of testosterone and prolactin on rat prostatic weight, 5α-reductase and arginase. Am J Physiol 229:1102–1109, 1975.

5. Sonenberg M, Money W: The fate and metabolism of anterior pituitary hormones. Rec Prog Horm Res, 11:43–82, 1955.
6. Aragona C, Friesen HG: Specific prolactin binding sites in the prostate and testis of rats. Endocrinology 97:677–684, 1975.
7. Hanlin NL, Yount AP: Prolactin binding in the rat ventral prostate. Endocrinol Res Commun 2:489–502, 1975.
8. Kledzik GS, Marshall S, Campbell GA, Gelati M, Meites J: Effects of castration, testosterone, estradiol and prolactin on specific prolactin-binding in ventral prostate of male rats. Endocrinology 98:373–379, 1976.
9. Nolin JM, Witorsch RJ: Detection of endogenous immunoreactive prolactin in rat mammary epithelial cells during lactation. Endocrinology 99:949–958, 1976.
10. Witorsch RJ, Smith JP: Evidence for androgen-dependent intracellular binding of prolactin in rat ventral prostate gland. Endocrinology 101:929–938, 1977.
11. Sternberger LA: Immunocytochemistry, 2nd Ed, New York: John Wiley and Sons, 1979.
12. Witorsch RJ: Immunohistochemical studies of prolactin-binding in sex accessory organs of the male rat. J Histochem Cytochem 26:565–580, 1978.
13. Witorsch RJ: Immunohistochemical localization of prolactin-binding sites in R3327 rat prostatic cancer cells. Hormone Res 10:268–281, 1979.
14. Witorsch RJ: The application of immunoperoxidase methodology for the visualization of prolactin binding sites in human prostate tissue. Hum Path 10:521–532, 1979.
15. Witorsch RJ, Robertson AT, Lord AC: Regional variations in prolactin binding activity and its androgen dependence in rat prostate gland. Proc 62nd Annual Meet Endocrinol Soc p 252, 1980 (abstr).
16. Witorsch RJ: Immunohistochemical evidence that Golgi-localized prolactin binding sites in rat ventral prostate are specific hormone receptors. Proc 63nd Annual Meet Endocrinol Soc p 220, 1981 (abstr).
17. Witorsch RJ: Evidence for human placental lactogen immunoreactivity in rat pars distalis. J Histochem Cytochem 28:1–9, 1980.
18. Moore CR, Price D, Gallagher TF: Rat-prostate cytology as a testis-hormone indicator and the prevention of castration changes by testis-extract injections. Am J Anat 45:71–107, 1930.
19. Price D, Williams-Ashman HG: The accessory reproductive glands of mammals. In Young WC (ed): "Sex and Internal Secretions." Baltimore: Williams and Wilkins, 1961, pp 366–448.
20. Lasnitski I: The effect of prolactin on rat prostate glands in organ culture. In Boyns AF, Griffiths K, (eds): "Prolactin and Carcinogenesis, Fourth Tenovus Workshop." Cardiff; Alpha Omega Alpha, 1972, pp 200–206.
21. Brandes D: The fine structure and cytochemistry of male sex accessory organs, In D Brandes (ed): "Male Accessory Sex Organs." New York: Academic Press, 1974, pp 18–114.
22. Shain SA, Boesel RW: Aging-associated diminished rat prostate androgen receptor content concurrent with decreased androgen dependence. Mech Ageing Dev, 6:219–232, 1977.
23. Grayhack JT, Lebowitz A: The effect of prolactin on citric acid of lateral lobe of prostate of Sprague-Dawley rats. Invest Urol 5:87–94, 1967.
24. Holland JM, Lee C: Effects of pituitary grafts on testosterone stimulated growth of rat prostate. Biol Reprod 22:351–355, 1980.
25. Kolbusz WE, Lee C, Grayhack JT: Delay in castration induced regression in rat prostate: Effect of prolactin. Proc 61st Annual Meet Endocrinol Soc p 292, 1979 (abstr).
26. Rixon RH, Whitfield JF: The histochemical localization of zinc in the dorsolateral prostate of the rat. J Histochem Cytochem 7:262–266, 1959.
27. Gunn SA, Gould TC, Anderson WAD: The effect of growth hormone and prolactin preparations on the control of intestinal cell-stimulating hormone of uptake of ^{65}Zn by the rat dorsolateral prostate. J Endocrinol 32:205–214, 1965.

28. Moger WH, Geschwind II: The action of prolactin on the sex accessory glands of the male rat. Proc Soc Exp Biol Med 141:1017–1021, 1972.
29. Sheth AR, Mugatwala PP, Shah GV, Rao SS: Occurrence of prolactin in human semen. Fertil Steril 26:905–907, 1975.
30. Luqman W, Smith M, Plymate S: Inherent ranges of seminal prolactin in pre- and postvasectomy subjects. Int J Fertil 24:286–288, 1979.
31. Aragona C, Bohnet HG, Friesen HG: Localization of prolactin binding in prostate and testis: The role of serum prolactin concentration on the testicular LH receptor. Acta Endocrinol 84:402–409, 1977.
32. Witorsch RJ: Unpublished observations.
33. Price D: Comparative aspects of development and structure in the prostate. Natl Cancer Inst Monogr 12:1–27, 1963.
34. Dunning WF: Prostate cancer in the rat. Natl Cancer Inst Monogr 12:352–369, 1963.
35. Rosoff B, Gaspar J, Diamond EJ: Perphenazine increases prolactin secretion and inhibits growth of the Dunning prostatic adenocarcinoma in rats. Fed Proc 39:858, 1980 (abstr).
36. Handwerger S, Sherwood LM: Comparison of the structure and lactogenic activity of human placental lactogen and human growth hormone. In Josimovich JB, Reynolds M, Cobo E (eds): "Lactogenic Hormones, Fetal Nutrition and Lactation." New York: John Wiley and Sons, 1974, pp 33–47.
37. Neri P, Arezzini C, Fruschelli C, Muller EE, Fioretti P, Genazzani AR: Effects of human chorionic somatomamanotropin on the male reproductive apparatus of rodents and on placental steroids during pregnancy. In Pecile A, Muller EE (eds): "Growth Hormone and Related Peptides." New York: American Elsevier, 1976, pp 345–368.
38. Keenan EJ, Kemp ED, Ramsey EE, Garrison LB, Pearse HD, Hodges CV: Specific binding of prolactin by the prostate gland of the rat and man. J Urol 122:43–46, 1979.
39. Shiu RPC, Kelly PA, Friesen HG: Radioreceptor assay for prolactin and other lactogenic hormones. Science 180:968–971, 1973.
40. Lesniak MA, Gorden P, Roth J: Reactivity of non-primate growth hormones and prolactins with human growth hormone receptors on cultured human lymphocytes. J Clin Endocrinol Metab 44:838–849, 1977.
41. DalLago A, Bortolussi M, Galli S, Marini G: Effects of picric acid-formaldehyde fixation on the LH(HCG) receptors' binding activity in the rat testis. Histochemistry 52:129–143, 1977.
42. Petrusz P: Demonstration of gonadotropin binding sties in the rat ovary by an immunoglobulin-enzyme bridge method. Eur J Obstet Gynecol Reprod Biol 4:S3–S9, 1974.
43. Sternberger LA, Petrali JP: Quantitative immunocytochemistry of pituitary receptors for luteinizing hormone-releasing hormone. Cell Tiss Res 162:141, 1975.
44. Schlessinger J: The mechanism and role of hormone-induced clustering of membrane receptors. Trends Biochem Sci 5:210–214, 1980.
45. Bergeron JJM, Evans WH, Geschwind II: Insulin binding to rat liver Golgi fractions. J Cell Biol 59:771–776, 1973.
46. Frantz WL, Turkington RW: Formation of biologically active ^{125}I-prolactin by enzymatic radioiodination. Endocrinology 91:1545–1548, 1972.
47. Salih M, Murthy GS, Friesen HG: Stability of hormone receptors with fixation: Implications for immunocytochemical localization of receptors. Endocrinology 105:21–26, 1979.
48. El Etreby MF, Mahrous AT: Immunocytochemical technique for detection of prolactin (PRL) and growth hormone (GH) in hyperplastic and neoplastic lesions of dog prostate and mammary gland. Histochemistry 64:279–286, 1979.
49. El Etreby MF, Friedreich E, Hasan SH, Mahrous AT, Schwarz K, Senge Th, Tunn U, Neumann F: Role of the pituitary gland in experimental hormonal induction and prevention of benign prostatic hyperplasia in the dog. Cell Tiss Res 204:367–378, 1979.

The Prostatic Cell: Structure and Function
Part B, pages 115-128
© 1981 Alan R. Liss, Inc., 150 Fifth Avenue, New York, NY 10011

The Immunocytochemical Detection of Growth Hormone and Prolactin in Human Prostatic Tissues

M.E. Harper, P.E.C. Sibley, W.B. Peeling, and K. Griffiths

INTRODUCTION

Although the androgen dependency of prostatic tissue is well documented [1,2], the role that pituitary protein hormones play in the growth and functioning of the gland is uncertain. The possibility that abnormal levels of pituitary protein hormones might be involved in the aetiology of prostatic hyperplasia and neoplasia has also been intimated [3–7]. Concentrations of various hormones in plasma from tumour-bearing patients and from normal subjects were not shown to be significantly different.

Animal experimentation has indicated that prolactin has a direct, yet synergistic action with androgen on prostatic tissue, influencing both growth and biochemistry [8–10]. Prolactin binding to prostatic tissue has been demonstrated by several groups [11,12], consistent with the suggested direct action of the hormone, but little attention has been directed to the possible binding of other protein hormones such as growth hormone and follicle stimulating hormone (FSH). Growth hormone has to some extent been implicated in the pathogenesis of prostatic cancer [13], and there is a need to identify possible relationships that may exist between the localization of these hormones in prostatic tissue and any consequent biochemical effects. Such an objective may be facilitated using immunocytochemical techniques [14]. Identification and localization of the protein hormones in the pituitary gland has been well established by such procedures [15–17], although their application to the study of target tissues for hormones has met with greater problems, largely due to the lower hormonal concentrations in these tissues. There is good evidence to suggest that protein hormones elicit their effects by binding to membrane-bound receptors [18], and therefore it would be anticipated that the localization should be at these sites. Recent autoradiographic and biochemical studies have indicated, however, the presence of protein hormones within cells [19,20], which is in agreement with immunocytochemical data recently described [21,22].

Studies on the topographical distribution of protein hormones by immuno-cytochemical techniques are presently limited by the availability of specific antisera and highly purified antigens. The immunocytochemical specificity of the antisera was checked by localizing protein hormones in specific cells of the human pituitary gland. Possible changes in the antigenicity of the tissues during routine histological processing have been investigated by comparing results obtained in both frozen and wax-embedded tissue sections. A further indication of the specificity of protein hormone localization in prostate tissues has been gained from absorption control experiments by admixing the antisera with pure hormonal preparations.

MATERIALS AND METHODS

Tissues, Antisera, Antigens

Benign prostatic hyperplastic (BPH) tissue was obtained by open prostatectomy operations, and prostatic carcinoma specimens were acquired by means of cold punch or 'Trucut' needle biopsies. Confirmation of the histological diagnosis of BPH or prostatic carcinoma was obtained prior to inclusion in this study. Bouin's fixed, wax-embedded serial sections allowed direct comparison of all experimental and control immunocytochemical procedures. Some tissues were divided into portions and snap frozen in liquid nitrogen or processed routinely. Serial frozen sections were cut and fixed in Bouin's fluid prior to inclusion in the immunocytochemical procedures. Serial sections of formal-saline fixed human pituitaries were also used to test the specificity of the antisera. In each experiment, one of the serial sections was stained with haematoxylin and eosin for morphological comparison.

Antisera raised in rabbits against human growth hormone (M153) and FSH (M91/1), both gifts of Professor W. Butt, Birmingham and Midland Hospital for Women, U.K., were used in these studies. The cross reactivities of these antisera with other hormones were less than 1%, as assessed by radioimmunoassay. An antiserum (7110) raised in the Tenovus Institute to a pituitary extract and used to assay prolactin had less than 1% cross reactivity with LH and FSH [23]. This antiserum contained two separate populations of antibodies, one specific for prolactin and one specific for growth hormone. The dilutions of these antisera for immunodetection ranged from 1/100 to 1/500. Another prolactin antiserum (G/R/51-IIAB), provided by Professor V. Marks, University of Surrey, Guildford, U.K., which crossreacted less than 1% with LH, FSH, and growth hormone was utilized in later experiments. Additional methodological requirements included a wide spectrum second antibody, sheep anti-rabbit serum [24] and peroxidase antiperoxidase (PAP), which was prepared as outlined by Mason and Sammons [25].

Purified preparations of protein hormones extracted from human pituitary glands were used in absorption control experiments. Human prolactin (WHO hPRL 75/504) and human growth hormone (MRC 69/46) were obtained from the National Institute for Biological Standards and Control, and purified human FSH was the gift of Professor W. Butt, Birmingham and Midland Hospital for Women, U.K.

Immunocytochemical Staining Procedures

The unlabelled antibody enzyme method [14] was chosen for these studies; the methodological procedures are outlined in Table I. This involved the overnight incubation of tissue with either the antiserum under investigation or control preparations, followed by incubation with sheep anti-rabbit serum and PAP. Finally the substrate containing 3,3'-diaminobenzidine-tetrahydrochloride (DAB 4HCl; 0.05% w/v) and hydrogen peroxide (0.01%) in Tris-HCl buffer (0.05 M, pH 7.6) were added to complete the staining sequence, the former being converted to a dark brown reaction product. Prior incubation with nonimmune sheep serum was used to block nonspecific binding of the sheep anti-rabbit serum. Each addition was preceded by copious washing procedures.

Controls

Methodological controls involved replacement of the appropriate antiserum with phosphate-buffered saline or a nonimmune rabbit serum, and the endogenous peroxidase activity was monitored by incubating sections with enzyme substrate alone. Specificity or "absorption" controls were prepared by admixing the hormonal antiserum and a purified hormone preparation for 24 hours at 4°C, prior

TABLE I. Sequence of incubations for immunocytochemical localization: Unlabelled antibody enzyme method

1)	Preincubation with nonimmune sheep serum	30 min
2)	Incubation of protein hormone antiserum (or control serum preparations)	15 hr
3)	Three washes with fresh PBS	1 hr
4)	Incubation of sheep anti-rabbit serum	2 hr
5)	Three washes with fresh PBS	1 hr
6)	Incubation of PAP	30 min
7)	Three washes with fresh PBS	1 hr
8)	Incubation of substrate (DAB4HCl + H_2O_2)	6 min
9)	Final wash with PBS to terminate reaction	1 hr
10)	Counterstaining at this stage, if required, prior to mounting sections using UV inert aqueous mounting medium.	

to inclusion in the immunocytochemical procedure. A rat pituitary section with a rat prolactin antiserum [26] was included in each experiment as a reagent control.

An evaluation of the specificity of the hormonal antisera was also gained from a series of experiments using serial human pituitary sections. Due to the high concentration of hormones within this gland, very dilute antisera could be utilized to demonstrate staining which consequently required small amounts of purified protein hormones for the absorption controls. Specific cell populations were stained by the individual hormonal antisera, and those cells stained by the FSH antiserum could be absorbed by FSH but not by the growth hormone and prolactin preparations. Cells stained by the growth hormone antiserum could be absorbed with growth hormone but not with prolactin or FSH preparations. The prolactin antiserum (7110) stained two populations of cells in the pituitary, one of which was identical to growth hormone-containing cells and could be absorbed with growth hormone, but neither were absorbed with FSH.

RESULTS

BPH Tissues

Prostatic tissue sections from 13 patients with BPH were examined. Staining, attributable to the binding of the growth hormone antiserum was predominently confined to stromal areas, particular stromal regions showing more intense staining than others (Fig. 1c). The reaction product was located in capillaries, some blood cells, and in acellular elements of the stroma. Epithelial cells were rarely stained.

When the prolactin antiserum (7110) was included in the immunocytochemical procedure, apparent intracellular staining of prolactin was observed in the vast majority of epithelial cells (Fig. 1d). The epithelial localization was cytoplasmic and not confined to any particular region of the cytoplasm, with the nuclei noticeably unstained. Reaction product was also seen in the acini secretions. Intense stromal staining was noted in capillaries, blood cells, and fibromuscular elements, similar to the results obtained with the growth hormone antiserum.

Fig. 1. a–d) Consecutive sections of an acinus taken from a patient with BPH ($\times$ 405). a) Haematoxylin and eosin (H & E) showing a glandular acinus, surrounded by stroma. b) Human FSH antiserum (1/100): Strong intracellular cytoplasmic staining of particular epithelial cells. c) Human growth hormone antiserum (1/100): Reaction product is visible only in the stroma. d) Human prolactin antiserum (7110) (1/500): Reaction product is located intracellularly in the cytoplasm of epithelial cells—the nuclei are clearly unstained. Acellular elements and capillaries in the stroma are stained. e,f) Consecutive frozen sections taken from a patient with BPH, counterstained with haematoxylin to ascertain the tissue morphology ($\times$ 160). e) Human growth hormone antiserum (1/100): Reaction product (arrowed) observed solely in the stroma. f) Human prolactin antiserum (7110) (1/500): Staining is located intracellularly in the cytoplasm of epithelial cells and also in the stroma (arrowed).

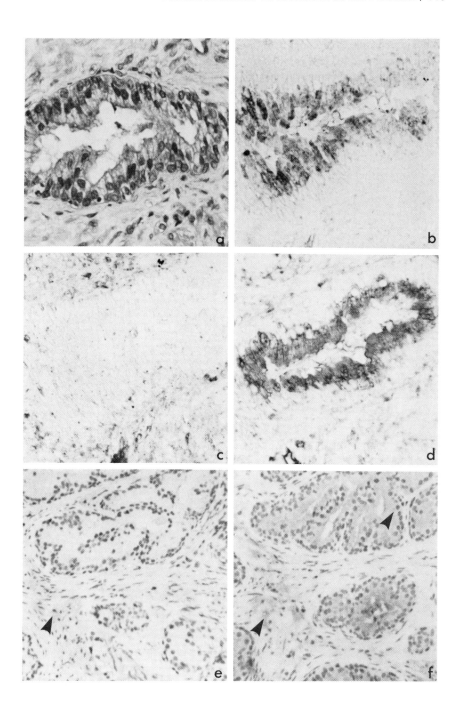

Recently, a second human prolactin antiserum (G/R/51-IIAB) was utilized which did not contain a separate population of growth hormone antibodies. When used in both wax-embedded and frozen sections of BPH tissue, albeit at a low dilution (1/10), the immunolocation of reaction product was seen in the epithelial cells and not in the stroma.

Staining, attributable to the FSH antiserum, was demonstrated in the cytoplasm of epithelial cells lining acini and also in their secretions (Fig. 1b). The majority of cystic acini were intensely stained, but only a proportion of the epithelium in glandular acini displayed immunoreactive FSH localization. The amount of staining observed in the cytoplasm varied, even between adjacent epithelial cells. Stromal areas, except for the occasional capillary, were blank. This pattern of cytoplasmic epithelial FSH localization was present in the tissue from all 13 patients. A small amount of stromal staining, mostly of capillary origin, was observed in tissue from four of the prostatic tumours.

Identical results were obtained in frozen sections of tissue from patients with BPH as had been observed with the various protein hormone antisera in the wax-embedded tissues. Staining was detected in stromal areas of the sections in the presence of both the growth hormone and prolactin antiserum (7110) (Fig. 1e, f), but was only seen in the epithelial cell cytoplasm with the prolactin antiserum (7110) (Fig. 1f). The nuclei of these frozen sections were counterstained with haematoxylin for ease of histological examination.

Only a limited number of absorption control experiments were undertaken on BPH sections due to the scarcity of purified protein hormone preparations. Prior absorption of the FSH antiserum with FSH (20 μg/ml) resulted in negative staining of epithelial cells in an acinus, which in a serial section exhibited positive staining with the same dilution of nonabsorbed FSH antiserum (Fig. 2a, b). Admixing the FSH antiserum with growth hormone (100 μg/ml) did not affect the result. The stromal staining observed with the growth hormone antiserum (Fig. 2c) could be eliminated by prior absorption of the antiserum with growth hormone (100 μg/ml) (Fig. 2d). Similarly this amount of growth hormone absorbed the stromal but not the epithelial cell staining obtained with the prolactin antiserum (7110) (Fig. 2e, f).

Fig. 2.   a–f) Absorption control experiments on sections taken from a patient with BPH (× 405): a) Human FSH antiserum (1/250): Intracellular, cytoplasmic staining of particular epithelial cells. b) Human FSH antiserum (1/250) absorbed with FSH (20 μg/ml): The specific immunolocalization has been completely absorbed. c) Human growth hormone antiserum (1/250): Reaction product is located in the stroma (arrowed). d) Elimination of staining by application of human growth hormone antiserum (1/250) absorbed with growth hormone (100 μg/ml). e) Human prolactin antiserum (7110) (1/500): Epithelial cytoplasm and stroma are stained. f) The stromal-staining component is absent when the human prolactin antiserum (7110) (1/500) is absorbed by growth hormone (100 μg/ml).

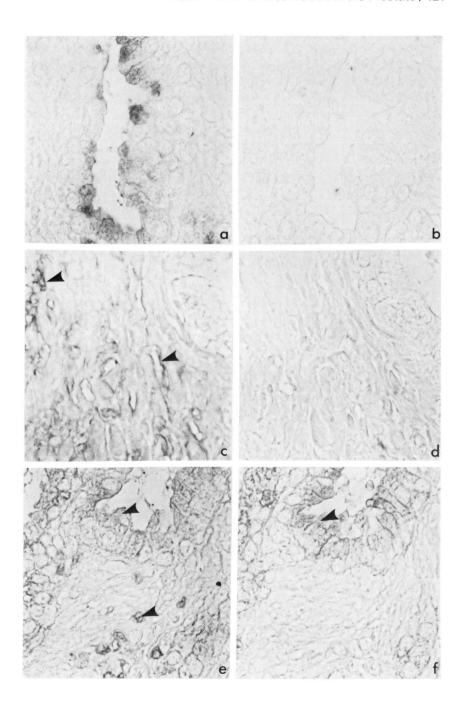

Prostatic Carcinoma Tissues

Cold punch or 'Trucut' needle biopsy prostatic tissue specimens from eight patients with histologically proven prostatic cancer were examined in this study. The majority of the tumours demonstrated marked variation in differentiation which necessitated evaluation of tissue sections from different regions of the specimen. Some characteristics of the protein hormone antiserum binding which had been observed in BPH specimens were present in the carcinomas, but additional morphological features were stained in several tumours.

Growth hormone antiserum gave positive stromal staining which was often more intense in areas adjacent to infiltrating carcinoma cells. Additional staining of epithelial cell nuclei and some epithelial cell cytoplasms was encountered in particular specimens (Fig. 3c). Even within a small area of tumour, marked variation in immunocytochemical staining was observed: Adjacent cells exhibited negative staining, cytoplasmic, nuclear, or cytoplasmic and nuclear staining (Fig. 4e). In another area of the same specimen only stromal staining was apparent (Fig. 4a).

Use of the prolactin antiserum (7110) in the prostatic carcinoma specimens resulted in intense staining of many areas. Positive staining was seen in the epithelial cytoplasm of all eight tumours (Fig. 3d, Fig. 4b, f). Nuclear staining of epithelial cells was noted in some regions particularly in the more anaplastic areas. Stromal staining of the tumours was extensive and often made the precise location of the reaction product difficult to ascertain (Fig. 4f).

Positive staining with the FSH antiserum was rarely encountered, but when present it was located in epithelial cell cytoplasm (not illustrated).

Occasional capillary staining was observed in the carcinoma tissues with nonimmune rabbit serum used at a similar dilution to the hormonal antisera in the immunocytochemical procedure (Figs. 3b, 3f, 4d).

DISCUSSION

Antisera to protein hormones were used in this study to locate the presence of the endogenous hormones in sections of prostatic tissue removed from patients with BPH or carcinoma of the prostate. The problems concerned with the interpretation of immunocytochemical data are mainly due to the relatively poor specificity of the available antisera, coupled with the lack of definitive controls

---

Fig. 3.   a–d) Consecutive sections taken from a prostatic cancer patient (H.H.) (× 260). Sections counterstained with haematoxylin for morphological comparison. a) H & E. b) Nonimmune rabbit serum (1/100) control section: No reaction product visible. c) Human growth hormone antiserum (1/100): Cytoplasm, nuclei, stroma stained (arrowed). d) Human prolactin antiserum (7110) (1/500): Cytoplasm, nuclei, stroma stained (arrowed). e,f) Prostatic cancer patient (A.R.) (× 350). e) H & E. f) Nonimmune rabbit serum (1/100) control counterstained with fast green (see also Fig. 4 a,b).

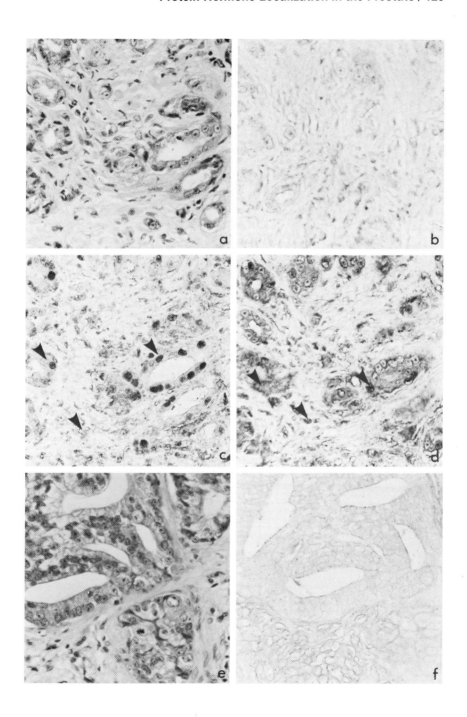

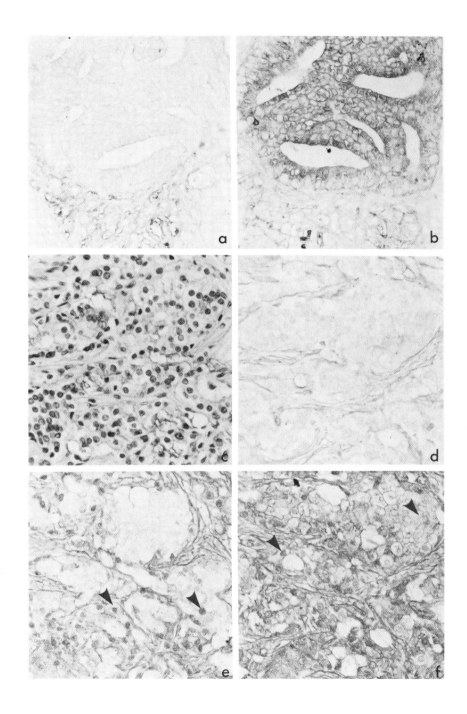

[27]. The preparation of antisera by monoclonal methods would probably ensure a greater specificity of the results. Using the antisera presently available, however, protein hormones appear to have been located in a variety of cellular components of prostatic tumours.

An evaluation of the immunocytochemical specificity of the antisera was obtained by the positive staining of specific cells of human pituitary glands, which could be absorbed only with their appropriate antigens. The results described in this communication include data obtained from both frozen and wax-embedded BPH tissues. In addition, the specificity of FSH and growth hormone staining in prostatic tissues was demonstrated by prior absorption of the antisera with purified protein hormones.

The immunocytochemical detection of prolactin in the cytoplasm of epithelial cells was interesting, as several reports have described the internalization of hormones or hormone receptor complexes in the cytoplasm of particular target tissues [28,29]. Prolactin has been shown to have direct effects on prostatic growth and metabolism, and the cellular localization is in agreement with these biochemical data. Although membrane localization of the protein hormones may have been anticipated, this was not apparent in the present study, probably due to the low concentration of endogenous hormone present on such structures. In the limited information previously available on the visualization of prolactin in human prostatic tissue [21], reaction product was only detected in epithelial cytoplasm after a prior incubation with prolactin.

Nuclear localization of staining product was rarely encountered and was not seen in the BPH specimens with any of the protein hormones antisera tested, ie, prolactin, growth hormone, FSH, LH, TSH, and βHCG. Particular areas of prostatic carcinoma tissues, however, exhibited positive nuclear staining with prolactin and growth hormone antisera. This intriguing observation obviously requires further investigation as there is little evidence for direct interaction of protein hormones on nuclear function. These data would agree with the nuclear immunocytochemical localization of growth hormone and prolactin described in canine prostate tissue [22].

Studies with growth hormone antiserum on tissue from the dog prostate have indicated membrane staining [22], but the method again included preincubation of the section with growth hormone and, in consequence, more than endogenous

Fig. 4. a,b) Prostatic cancer patient (A.R.). Sections counterstained with fast green ($\times$ 350). a) Human growth hormone antiserum (1/100): stromal staining. b) Human prolactin antiserum (7110) (1/500): Intracellular, cytoplasmic, and stromal staining (see also Fig. 3 e,f). c–f) Different area of same tumour ($\times$ 350). c) H & E. d) Nonimmune rabbit serum control (1/100). e) Human growth hormone antiserum (1/100): Stained nucleus and cytoplasm (arrowed). f) Human prolactin antiserum (7110) (1/500): Stained nucleus and cytoplasm (arrowed).

hormone has been detected. In contrast, the studies now reported have shown a complete lack of growth hormone staining in epithelial cells in BPH tissues, although the staining of many of the stromal components was a characteristic of all the BPH specimens examined. Although the stroma exhibited positive growth hormone localization in the carcinoma specimens, some tumour cells also displayed diffuse cytoplasmic staining. In a study using prolactin or human placental lactogen antisera in human and rat prostate, stromal localization of these hormones has not been reported [21,30].

Studies on the dog prostate have indicated prolactin in some fibromuscular elements but the presence of growth hormone in these areas was not observed. The results reported here indicate that although the prolactin antiserum (7110) produced staining in both epithelial cells and some stromal components, the latter was possibly due to growth hormone antibodies in the preparation, as these were absorbed with growth hormone. Also, immunolocalization with a second prolactin antiserum (G/R/51-IIAB) was observed only within epithelial cells of BPH tissues.

The presence of growth hormone in the stromal areas may be of importance when considering the interrelationships of the stroma and epithelium in the growth and dissemination of prostatic tumours. Of interest in this respect is the reported increased levels of growth hormone in prostatic cancer patients with metastases compared to those without metastatic spread [13].

The heterogeneity of prolactin and growth hormone antiserum staining in the prostatic carcinomas may be an expression of tumour cell clones having different abilities to bind and perhaps respond to these hormones.

Detection of immunoreactive FSH in prostatic epithelium was surprising, since neither receptors for FSH, nor autoradiographic localization of this hormone have previously been reported. Furthermore, direct effects of FSH on prostatic biochemistry have not been described and a possible role for FSH in the prostate might be worth further investigation, especially when considering the increasing concentration of this hormone in the elderly male.

Apart from the accompanying changes in protein hormone concentrations which occur in the aging male, many of the major therapies for prostatic cancer drastically alter plasma protein hormones [5]. It would therefore seem pertinent to investigate their binding and significance in prostatic tumours. Immunocytochemical procedures to localize more precisely both endogenous hormone and also hormone receptor distribution, offer advantages over most other methods involving cell-free systems, especially when dealing with the heterogeneous population of cells generally present in most tumours. It is hoped that such data may provide a valuable insight into the role of protein hormones in prostatic pathogenesis.

CONCLUSIONS

The immunocytochemical detection of prolactin, growth hormone, and FSH in both BPH and prostatic carcinoma tissues has been described. Limitations imposed on the interpretation of results due to the specificity of the antisera have been discussed. The distribution of staining in the BPH tissue was consistently found in particular cellular components. Growth hormone localized in stromal regions: FSH in the epithelial cell cytoplasm of approximately 30% of the acini and prolactin uniformily present in epithelial cell cytoplasm and in various stromal components. Prostatic carcinoma tissues displayed more diverse staining of cellular elements. Tumour cell nuclei and cytoplasm often showed reaction product deposition attributable to growth hormone and prolactin in addition to stromal staining. FSH was rarely found in the carcinomatous areas. The heterogeneity of the localization might be a consequence of the degree of tumour cell differentiation and this requires additional investigation. The immunocytochemical results are consistent with internalization of fragments of whole protein hormone molecules within prostatic cells and their significance needs further evaluation.

ACKNOWLEDGMENTS

The authors would like to acknowledge the generous financial support of the Tenovus Organization. We would also like to thank Mr. C. Smith for excellent photographic assistance.

REFERENCES

1. Dorfman R I, Shipley R A: Androgens. Biochemistry, Physiology and Clinical Significance. New York: John Wiley and Sons, 1956.
2. Griffiths K, Davies P, Harper M E, Peeling W B, Pierrepoint C G: The etiology and endocrinology of prostatic cancer. In Rose D P (ed): Endocrinology of Cancer. Florida: CRC Press, Vol 2, 1979, pp 1–55.
3. Geller J, Baron A, Kleinman S: Pituitary luteinizing hormone reserve in elderly men with prostatic disease. J Endocrinol 48: 289–290, 1970.
4. Asano M: Studies on urinary prolactin with special reference to carcinoma of the prostate. Jpn J Urol 53: 901–918, 1962.
5. Harper M E, Peeling W B, Cowley T, Brownsey B G, Phillips M E A, Groom G, Fahmy D R, Griffiths K: Plasma steroid and protein hormone concentrations in patients with prostatic carcinoma, before and during oestrogen therapy. Acta Endocrinol (Kbh) 81: 409–426, 1976.
6. Hammond G L, Kontturi M, Maattala P, Puukka M, Vihko R: Serum FSH, LH and prolactin in normal males and patients with prostatic disease. Clin Endocrinol 7: 129–135, 1977.
7. Bartsch W, Horst H J, Becker H, Nehse G: Sex hormone binding globulin capacity, testosterone, 5 alpha-dihydrotestosterone, oestradiol and prolactin in plasma of patients with prostatic carcinoma under various types of hormonal treatment. Acta Endocrinol (Kbh) 85: 650–664, 1977.

8. Gunn S A, Gould T C, Anderson W A: The effect of growth hormone and prolactin preparations on the control by interstitial cell-stimulating hormone of uptake of 65-Zn by the rat dorsolateral prostate. J Endocrinol 32: 205–214, 1965.

9. Grayhack J T, Lebowitz J M: Effect of prolactin on citric acid of lateral lobe of prostate of Sprague-Dawley rat. Invest Urol 5: 87–94, 1967.

10. Chase M D, Geschwind I I, Bern H A: Synergistic role of prolactin in response of male rat sex accessories to androgen. Proc Soc Exp Biol NY 94: 680–683, 1957.

11. Aragona C, Friesen H G: Specific prolactin binding sites in the prostate and testis of rats. Endocrinology 97: 677–684, 1975.

12. Kledzik G S, Marshall S, Campbell G A, Gelato M, Meites J: Effects of castration, testosterone, estradiol and prolactin on specific prolactin-binding activity in ventral prostate of male rats. Endocrinology 98: 373–379, 1976.

13. British Prostate Study Group: Evaluation of plasma hormone concentrations in relation to clinical staging in patients with prostate cancer. Br J Urol 51: 382, 1979.

14. Sternberger L A: The unlabeled antibody enzyme method. In: Osler A, Weiss L (eds): Foundations of Immunology Series. Englewood Cliffs, New Jersey: Prentice-Hall Inc.: 129–171, 1974, pp 129–171.

15. Nakane P K: Classifications of anterior pituitary cell types with immunoenzyme histochemistry. J Histochem Cytochem 18: 9–20, 1970.

16. Moriarty G C: Adenohypophysis: ultrastructural cytochemistry. A review. J Histochem Cytochem 21: 855–894, 1973.

17. el-Etreby M F, el-Bab M R: The utility of antisera to canine growth hormone and canine prolactin for immunocytochemical staining of the dog pituitary gland. Histochemistry 53: 1–15, 1977.

18. Catt K J, Dufau M L: Interactions of LH and hCG with testicular gonadotrophin receptors. Adv Exp Med Biol 36: 379–418, 1973.

19. Conn P M, Conti M, Harwood J P, Dufau M L, Catt K J: Internalization of gonadotrophin-receptor complex in ovarian luteal cells. Nature 274: 598–600, 1978.

20. Rajaniemi H J, Manninen M, Huhtaniemi I T: Catabolism of human [^{125}I]iodochorionic gonadotrophin in rat testis. Endocrinology 105: 1208–1214, 1979.

21. Witorsch R J: The application of immunoperoxidase methodology for the visualization of prolactin binding sites in human prostatic tissue. Hum Pathol 10: 521–532, 1979.

22. el Etreby M F, Mahrous A T: Immunocytochemical technique for detection of prolactin (PRL) and growth hormone (GH) in hyperplastic and neoplastic lesions of dog prostate and mammary gland. Histochemistry 64: 279–286, 1979.

23. Groom G V: The measurement of human gonadotrophins by radioimmunoassay. J Reprod Fertil 51: 273–286, 1977.

24. Joyce B G, Read G F, Fahmy D R: Enzymeimmunoassay for progesterone and oestradiol: a study of factors influencing sensitivity. International symposium on radioimmunoassay and related procedures in medicine: IAEA (Vienna) 1: 289–295, 1978.

25. Mason D Y, Sammons R: Rapid preparations of peroxidase: anti-peroxidase complexes for immunocytochemical use. J Immunol Meth 20: 317–324, 1978.

26. Sibley P E C, Harper M E, Joyce B G, Griffiths K G: Immunocytochemical staining obtained with a rat prolactin antiserum in various rat tissues. J Endocrinol 85: 58–59P, 1980.

27. Heyderman E: The immunoperoxidase technique in histopathology: application, methods and controls. J Clin Pathol 32: 971–978, 1979.

28. Nolin J M, Witorsch R J: Detection of endogenous immunoreactive prolactin in rat mammary epithelial cells during lactation. Endocrinology 99: 949–958, 1976.

29. Nolin J M: Intracellular prolactin in rat corpus luteum and adrenal cortex. Endocrinology 102: 402–406, 1978.

30. Witorsch R J, Smith J P: Evidence for androgen-dependent intracellular binding of prolactin in rat ventral prostate gland. Endocrinology 101: 929–938, 1977.

CARCINOGENS AND ENZYME INDUCTION

The Prostatic Cell: Structure and Function
Part B, pages 131–163
© 1981 Alan R. Liss, Inc., 150 Fifth Avenue, New York, NY 10011

Uptake and Secretion of Carcinogenic Chemicals by the Dog and Rat Prostate

Emil R. Smith and Miasnig Hagopian

INTRODUCTION

Information about the interactions of carcinogenic chemicals and the prostate of animals is important for at least two reasons. First, it might provide the basis for the experimental development of chemically induced prostatic tumors in animals, and an animal model of prostatic adenocarcinoma might, among other things, further our practical knowledge concerning the pathogenesis, diagnosis, and treatment of human prostatic cancer whatever its cause(s). In addition, such information would seem an important component of any attempt to evaluate the role of chemicals in the etiology of human prostatic adenocarcinoma.

Our present knowledge suggests that the prostate of both domestic and laboratory animals is relatively insensitive to the carcinogenic effects of chemicals. While spontaneous prostatic adenocarcinoma has been observed, albeit rarely, in rats, hamsters, dogs, and monkeys [1], the finding of such tumors at least makes it clear that the prostatic epithelium of these species is capable of malignant transformation, whatever the causes of such spontaneous tumors might be. Despite this, experimental attempts to produce such tumors using chemicals have not been generally successful [2]. Moreover, it is significant that among the published studies on chemical carcinogenesis involving hundreds of compounds being administered systemically to thousands of animals for prolonged periods of time, there do not appear to be any reports of chemically induced prostatic adenocarcinomas. While obviously the majority of such studies were not specific attempts to produce prostatic tumors, and in many the prostates were not examined or may have received only a cursory examination, the general conclusion to be reached is that while the prostatic epithelium might not be completely insensitive to carcinogens, it certainly would seem to be relatively insensitive; otherwise, one might expect that prostatic adenocarcinomas would have been found after treatment with some chemicals, even if their appearance were incidental to the major purpose of the experiment, or if they appeared in only a small proportion of animals being studied.

Two things suggest, however, that the insensitivity of the prostatic epithelium of animals is more relative than absolute. Prostatic adenocarcinomas have been produced by putting the polycyclic hydrocarbons benzypyrene, dimethylbenzanthracene and 3-methylcholanthrene directly into the prostate gland of mice, rats, and hamsters [2]. In addition, some carcinogenic chemicals are able to transform prostatic epithelium in vitro [5,6].

One reason for the insensitivity of the prostate to carcinogenic chemicals might be an inability of such chemicals to enter the prostate. In this regard, it has been widely held within the medical profession that drugs penetrate poorly into the prostate [7].

Contrary to this belief, in the past few years a variety of antibiotics have been found to rapidly enter both the prostate gland and prostatic fluid of the dog, although none has been found to be highly concentrated within the tissue or the fluid [8–11]. More recently, similar observations have been made on the penetration of antibiotics into the human prostate and prostatic fluid [11–13]. However, since the penetration of chemicals into the prostate and its secretion should be determined by the physical-chemical properties of the particular compound rather independently of its biological effects, and the antibiotics which have been found to penetrate into the prostate are all weak acids or bases, these observations do not preclude the possibility that carcinogens with other physical-chemical properties might not enter the prostate either more or less readily than antibiotics.

Accordingly, we decided to assess the ability of some carcinogenic chemicals to enter both the prostate and prostatic fluid of dogs and rats. Rather than conduct extensive studies on a few compounds we decided to make less extensive observation on a larger number of compounds and to select compounds with diverse physical-chemical properties. Because of the technical demands associated with the precise measurements of small amounts of chemicals in small biological samples, the choice of substances for study was based also upon the availability of relatively uncomplicated methods for their direct measurement or upon the availability of ^{14}C-labelled material. From the onset we were aware that while the use of ^{14}C-labelled chemicals was technically expedient, it complicated interpretation of results since ^{14}C-counting does not distinguish between ^{14}C-labelled unchanged chemical and its ^{14}C-labelled metabolites.

Bearing these considerations in mind, the following eight compounds were selected for study: 3-methylcholanthrene, 7,12-dimethylbenz[a]anthracene, N-hydroxyurethane, aflatoxin B_1, 3-amino-1,2,4-triazole, 2-acetylaminofluorene, N-methyl-N'-nitro-N-nitrosoguanidine, and cadmium.

MATERIALS AND METHODS
Chemicals

Experiments were performed using 3-methylcholanthrene-6-^{14}C, 3-amino-1,2,4-triazole-5-^{14}C, N-acetyl-2-aminofluorene-9-^{14}C, and N-methyl-N'-nitro-N-nitrosoguanidine (methyl-^{14}C) obtained from New England Nuclear Corp.;

7,12-dimethylbenz[a]-anthracene-12-^{14}C obtained from Amersham/Searle Corp.; N-hydroxyurethane and aflatoxin B_1 obtained from Aldrich Chemical Co.; and $CdCl_2 \cdot 2.5H_2O$ obtained from Fisher Scientific Company. The radiochemical purity of all ^{14}C-material was determined by thin layer chromatography to be greater than 96%. All animals were treated with formulations prepared on the day of the experiment; all intravenous injection were given over periods of five minutes. In experiments with labelled material all groups of animals were treated with commerically obtained, unlabelled chemicals given in doses dependent on body weight but containing a total amount of ^{14}C-material of about 5–50 μCi and 50–200 μCi for dogs and rats, respectively.

Experiments in Dogs

Tissue distribution. Male mongrel dogs were fasted overnight, were treated with the chemical and were then returned to their cages. Before and at selected intervals after treatment blood samples were taken for analysis, and at some time after treatment the animals were sacrificed using intravenous doses of pentobarbital sodium, and samples of the prostate and selected organs and tissues were taken for analysis.

Prostatic secretion. The secretion of chemicals by the prostate of the dog was studied in unanesthetized animals with prostatic fistulas which allowed the collection of uncontaminated prostatic fluid. The fistulas were prepared surgically as described by Mason et al [14] and experimentation was begun only after the animals had fully recovered from the surgery. In some cases the dogs were castrated and given daily subcutaneous doses of 5 mg of testosterone, while some dogs remained intact and were not treated with testosterone. In most experiments samples of the resting or basal secretion, which is produced at about 0.5 ml/hr, were collected as well as samples of fluid secreted in response to the rapid administration of 0.7 mg/kg of pilocarpine hydrochloride. In all experiments samples of blood and prostatic fluid were taken both before and at intervals after treatment; in some experiments the animals were then sacrificed and samples of the prostate and selected organs and tissues were taken for analysis.

Experiments in Rats

Tissue distribution. The plasma and tissue levels of chemicals were determined in male Sprague Dawley rats (Charles River Breeding Laboratories). Groups of animals were treated and returned to their cages where food and water were continuously available. At intervals after treatment rats were anesthetized with ether, a blood sample was taken by direct cardiac puncture and then selected organs and tissues, including the prostate, were taken for analysis. For purposes of these experiments separate analyses were conducted upon the paired, discrete ventral lobes of the prostate (the ventral prostate) and upon the remainder of the gland (the dorsolateral prostate).

Prostatic secretion. The secretion of chemicals in the prostatic fluid of the rat was studied in acute experiments conducted on male Sprague Dawley rats (retired breeding stock, Charles River Breeding Laboratories). The rats were anesthetized by the intraperitoneal (IP) administration of 60 mg/kg of pentobarbital sodium, an endotracheal tube was put in place and the pelvic organs exposed via a laparotomy. The penis and the vas deferens were ligated and the seminal vesicles and the coagulating glands were ligated and removed. The ureters were cut to prevent urine from reaching the bladder and then one end of an 18-cm length of polyethylene tubing (PE-240) was passed through a stab wound in the bladder and fixed in place in the neck of the bladder with its opening at the level of the prostatic urethra. Finally, a saline-filled catheter was tied into the jugular vein to allow the intravenous (IV) administration of chemicals and/or supplemental doses of pentobarbital sodium, if needed.

In each experiment the secretion of prostatic fluid was monitored by recording the distance traveled by the meniscus of the fluid in the polyethylene tube draining the prostatic urethra, the volume of a unit length of tubing having previously been determined. At the termination of all experiments, the prostatic fluid was weighed, a sample of heparinized blood was taken by cardiac puncture, and selected tissues, including the prostate, were taken for analysis.

In some experiments the effects of chemicals on the rate of secretion was assessed by comparing the rate of secretion of prostatic fluid in saline-treated rats with that of the animals treated with the chemical.

Analytical Methods

Determination of radioactivity in tissues and fluids. For measuring their ^{14}C content, tissues were homogenized in four volumes of distilled water and the radioactivity of aliquots of each homogenate was measured in a liquid scintillation counter after preparation of the samples in Bio-Solv BBS-3 (Beckman Instruments) as described in Beckman Technical Report 551. Plasma and prostatic fluid samples were counted directly in the above cocktail. Fully realizing that some of the radioactivity recovered after treatment probably represented metabolites of the ^{14}C-labelled chemicals, the results of these analyses were nevertheless expressed as the amount of administered material equivalent to the radioactivity recovered.

Determination of N-hydroxyurethane. The concentration of N-hydroxyurethane in tissues and fluids was determined by thin-layer chromatography as previously described [15].

Determination of aflatoxin B_1. For the determination of aflatoxin B_1 the individual fresh or frozen organs or samples of plasma or prostatic fluid were homogenized in, or mixed with, 10–30 ml of an azeotropic mixture of acetone, chloroform, and water (58:38:4). The samples were filtered through a plug of glass wool and the filtrates were concentrated to near dryness in a rotary evaporator in vacuo at 40°C. The residues were recovered in 10 ml of methanol–water (80:20) and washed two times with 10 ml of normal hexane to remove the lipids. The aqueous methanol phase was again concentrated in vacuo, the residues were quantitatively transferred to graduated centrifuge tubes with chloroform, and the volume of each extract was adjusted to 4 ml.

The concentration of aflatoxin B_1 was estimated by thin-layer chromatography on silica gel plates. Adsorbasil-5 20 $\times$ 20 cm plates (Applied Science Laboratories) were activated for 30 minutes at 110°C before use. The chromatograms were developed in a solvent system of chloroform-acetate-methanol (80:20:3). The aflatoxin B_1 zones in the developed chromatograms were readily detected because of their intense fluorescence under ultraviolet irradiation at approximately 360 nm.

A series of aliquots from each sample were spotted along with known amounts of aflatoxin B_1 standards. It was determined in preliminary experiments that the best estimation of aflatoxin B_1 levels could be made by visual comparison with standards applied in amounts near the threshold of visibility (0.5–2.5 ng). Accordingly, appropriate dilutions of the samples were made, when necessary, in order to determine this extinction level.

Determination of cadmium. The levels of cadmium in plasma, prostatic fluid, and tissues were determined by atomic absorption spectroscopy (Model 303 spectrophotometer, Perkin-Elmer Corporation) using the general analytical procedures recommended by the manufacturer. Samples of tissues were prepared for analysis by digesting them overnight at room temperature in a mixture of 20:1 (v/v) concentrated nitric acid and 70% perchloric acid. The resultant digest was then gently heated until clear and adjusted to a predetermined known volume. Plasma and prostatic fluid samples were prepared by mixing them with equal volumes of 10% trichloroacetic acid and removing the resultant protein precipitates.

Statistical Analysis

In all cases the calculated group means are presented with the estimated standard error. Group means were compared using unpaired t tests.

RESULTS

3-Methylcholanthrene (3-MCA)

The results of our experiments with 3-MCA have already been published [16].

Dogs. In three fistula-dogs given intraperitoneal doses of 0.5 mg/kg of [^{14}C]-3-MCA, the levels of radioactivity in the plasma rose slowly, peaked at about 48 hours, and then declined very slowly. During the first few hours after treatment the ^{14}C-levels in the resting prostatic secretion were about 2–20 times higher than in plasma, but with time they fell to values below that in plasma.

These initial high levels might have reflected the ability of unchanged 3-MCA not only to enter but actually to concentrate to some extent in prostatic fluid, while the falling levels could have reflected the ongoing metabolism of 3-MCA, either within the gland or elsewhere, with the metabolites not partitioning to the same extent into prostatic fluid. In keeping with these possibilities, the metabolites of 3-MCA are more polar than the parent compound [17], and it is generally observed that polar compounds penetrate biological membranes less readily than their less polar counterparts.

In the same experiments the levels of radioactivity in prostatic fluid fell precipitously, but briefly, when the rate of prostatic secretion was transiently increased by intravenous pilocarpine. Presumably the rate of penetration of ^{14}C-labelled material was sufficiently fast that at low rates of prostatic secretion its partitioning into the fluid was at or near a steady state, but at higher rates of secretion the rate of penetration of the ^{14}C-labelled material from plasma to prostatic fluid was not fast enough to maintain these levels and they fell.

The levels of radioactivity were also measured in the plasma, prostate gland, and other tissues of four dogs at 50 hours after single IP doses of 0.5 mg/kg of [^{14}C]-3-MCA. At that time the levels in the prostate were about one fourth that of plasma.

Rats. In four rats in which prostatic fluid was collected during the 2-hour interval between 24 and 26 hours after the IP administration of 5 mg/kg of [^{14}C]3-MCA, the levels of radioactivity in the prostatic fluid was only slightly less than that in plasma. At 26 hours after treatment, levels within the prostate itself were 3–5 times higher than in plasma.

7,12-Dimethylbenz[a]anthracene (DMBA)

Dogs. In two fistula-dogs the IP administration of 2.5 mg/kg of [^{14}C]-DMBA was followed by the appearance of radioactivity in both plasma and the resting prostatic secretion (Figs. 1, 2), and while the levels in prostatic fluid varied somewhat they were about equal to the plasma levels. As with 3-MCA, and presumably for the same reasons, when one dog was given an IV dose of pilocarpine, the levels of radioactivity fell in the prostatic fluid samples collected at high rates of secretion (Fig. 2).

The levels of radioactivity in the prostate and other tissues of these two fistula-dogs and the two similarly treated nonfistula dogs were determined at 50 hours after treatment (Table I). The highest levels were found in the pancreas and liver, with lower levels in fat and kidney, and even lower levels in the prostate and testis; the levels in the prostate averaged 0.44 times that in plasma.

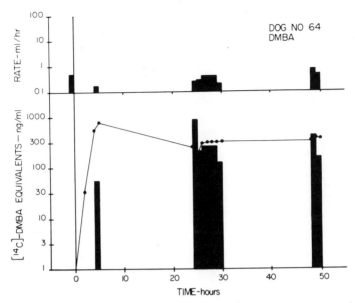

Fig. 1. Secretion of [^{14}C]-DMBA in canine prostatic fluid. Results of an experiment on one dog. The abscissa represents the time after an intraperitoneal injection of 2.5 mg/kg of [^{14}C]-DMBA. Upper portion: The height of each column represents the mean rate of secretion of prostatic fluid over the period of time indicated by the width of the column. Lower portion: Each point represents the level of radioactivity in a plasma sample taken at the indicated time after treatment while the height of each column represents the level of activity in the sample of prostatic fluid collected over the period of time indicated by the width of the column.

The chemical nature of the radioactivity found in the prostates of the two fistula-dogs was examined and it was found that 7% and 25% of this radioactivity could be extracted from alkaline alcoholic suspensions by hexane using the method described by Levine [18] and, hence, probably represented unchanged [^{14}C]-DMBA.

Rats. Prostatic fluid was collected from rats between 24 and 26 hours after treatment with single IP doses of 5 mg/kg of [^{14}C]-DMBA (Table II). During this 120-minute interval the rate of secretion of fluid was comparable in three [^{14}C]-DMBA-treated rats and six rats treated with the vehicle. The mean weights of the fluid samples collected were 0.078 ± 0.033 and 0.146 ± 0.050 gm for the two groups, respectively; these means are not statistically different (P >0.05).

Radioactivity was present in the prostatic fluid samples from all three [^{14}C]-DMBA-treated rats. The levels found were similar to, or higher than, the levels in plasma samples taken at the end of the collection period, the individual prostatic fluid to plasma ratios being 0.53, 1.91, and 3.64 (mean ± SE = 2.03 ± 0.90).

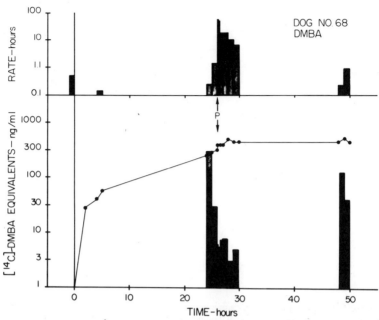

Fig. 2. Secretion of [^{14}C]-DMBA in canine prostatic fluid before and after administration of pilocarpine. Results of an experiment in one dog. The abscissa and ordinates are the same as for Figure 1. P represents the time of intravenous administration of 0.7 mg/kg of pilocarpine hydrochloride.

TABLE I. Levels of radioactivity in the plasma and selected tissues of dogs after the intraperitoneal administration of 2.5 mg/kg of [^{14}C]-DMBA

Fluid or tissue	[^{14}C]-DMBA-equivalents (ng/gm or ml)
Plasma	
2 hr[a]	32 ± 3
4 hr	55 ± 6
24 hr	247 ± 12
26 hr	283 ± 20
48 hr	352 ± 36
50 hr	365 ± 43
Tissues: 50 hr	
prostate	164 ± 25
liver	1507 ± 234
kidney	658 ± 100
testis	87 ± 20
pancreas	1614 ± 390
fat	842 ± 166

[a]Time after administration of [^{14}C]-DMBA.

TABLE II. Levels of radioactivity in the plasma, prostatic fluid, and selected tissues from anesthetized rats 24 and 26 hours after the intraperitoneal administration of 5 mg/kg of [^{14}C]-DMBA

Fluid or tissue	[^{14}C]-DMBA-equivalents (μg/gm)	
	Three animals sacrificed 24 hr after treatment	Three animals sacrificed 26 hr after treatment
Plasma	0.43 ± 0.09	0.33 ± 0.12
Prostatic fluid[a]	—	0.60 ± 0.36
Ventral prostate	0.85 ± 0.14	0.42 ± 0.21
Dorsolateral prostate	0.66 ± 0.30	0.32 ± 0.14
Liver	2.89 ± 0.38	2.44 ± 1.16
Kidney	1.01 ± 0.26	1.11 ± 0.36
Pancreas	52.68 ± 9.53	41.90 ± 21.88
Abdominal fat	6.48 ± 1.65	3.02 ± 1.59

[a]Samples collected over the 2 hours prior to sacrifice.

Among the tissues, the highest levels of radioactivity were found in the pancreas, with lower levels in fat, liver, kidney, and the prostate (Table II). The relative contribution of unchanged [^{14}C]-DMBA and of metabolites to the radioactivity in the prostates of these six rats were examined by partition characteristics [18]. An average of 74 ± 6% of the radioactivity of the ventral prostates and 30 ± 7% of the radioactivity in the dorsolateral prostates was extracted from alkaline alcoholic suspensions of tissue homogenates by hexane and probably represented unchanged [^{14}C]-DMBA.

N-Hydroxyurethane

A full report of our experiments on N-hydroxyurethane has already been published [15].

Dogs. Four fistula-dogs were given IV doses of 100 mg/kg of N-hydroxyurethane and as expected following intravenous administration the plasma concentrations were highest immediately after treatment and then fell rapidly; the plasma half-life was about 40 minutes. N-hydroxyurethane was found in prostatic fluid of all four dogs where its level was generally proportional to the plasma level. In one animal given IV pilocarpine the level of N-hydroxyurethane in prostatic fluid did not change when the rate of secretion markedly increased.

When the relationship between the concentration of N-hydroxyurethane in plasma and in prostatic fluid was examined in more detail, the concentration of the chemical in prostatic fluid was found to be directly proportional to the mean plasma concentration. The correlation between these parameters (excluding one aberrant value) was highly significant (n = 9, r = 0.95, P < 0.01); the mean prostatic fluid-to-plasma ratio was 0.95 ± 0.10.

Rats. The concentration of N-hydroxyurethane was followed in the plasma, prostatic fluid, and tissues of rats for up to 6 hours after the IV administration of 100 mg/kg of N-hydroxyurethane. This dose of N-hydroxyurethane did not modify the rate of secretion of prostatic fluid.

Treatment led to readily detectable but rapidly declining concentrations of N-hydroxyurethane in plasma; the plasma half-life was 22 minutes. Furthermore, N-hydroxyurethane was found in all samples of prostatic fluid which were analyzed and these concentrations slowly fell during the six hours. The calculated prostatic fluid-to-plasma ratio was 0.97 ± 0.10. In animals sacrificed 2, 60, and 120 minutes after treatment, N-hydroxyurethane was detected in the prostates and the mean prostate-to-plasma levels were about 0.5, 0.8 and 2.4, respectively.

N-Hydroxyurethane was detected in some of the tissues from these animals. As soon as two minutes after treatment detectible quantities were found in the ventral and dorsolateral prostates, and over the period of the first 2 hours after treatment the mean gland-to-plasma ratios were 1.33 and 0.91, respectively. N-Hydroxyurethane was also found in the kidneys of these animals but it was not detected in the liver or fat of any of the animals at any time.

Aflatoxin B₁

Dogs. In plasma samples collected both before and for up to 5 hours after two dogs with fistulas were each given IV doses of 0.1 mg/kg of aflatoxin B₁, the levels of aflatoxin B₁ peaked immediately after injection and declined rather rapidly, with half-lives of 23 and 88 minutes. At the same time, aflatoxin B₁ was present in samples of prostatic fluid collected from both dogs over the first and second hours after treatment but not in samples collected thereafter.

Figure 3A summarizes the results of one of these experiments and Figure 3B summarizes the results of a third experiment in which the same animal was given an intravenous dose of pilocarpine 1 hour after similar treatment with aflatoxin B₁ in order to stimulate the secretion of larger quantities of fluid for analysis. In both cases the peak plasma levels of aflatoxin B₁ were similar, as were rates of decline of these levels. Also, in both experiments the levels in prostatic fluid were similar, being about one tenth of the plasma levels. Of particular interest, it was found that the prostatic fluid levels were not altered when the rate of secretion of prostate was very markedly increased.

In four final experiments two dogs with fistulas and two dogs without fistulas were given intravenous doses of 0.1 mg/kg of aflatoxin B₁, and after following plasma and prostatic fluid levels for 120 minutes the animals were sacrificed for tissue level determinations. The plasma levels were of similar magnitude and

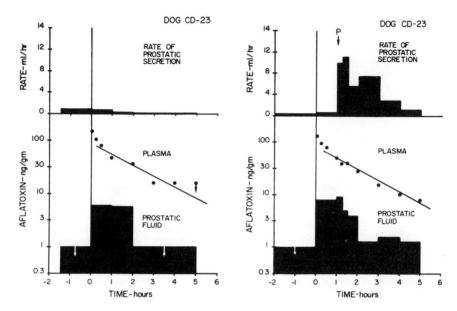

Fig. 3. Secretion of aflatoxin B_1 in canine prostatic fluid. Results of two experiments on one dog. In each case the abscissa represents time after termination of an intravenous injection of 0.1 mg/kg of aflatoxin B_1 given over five minutes. Upper portion: The height of each column represents the mean rate of secretion of prostatic fluid over the period of time indicated by the width of the column. Lower portion: The points represent the concentration of aflatoxin B_1 in plasma samples taken at various times after treatment, while the height of each column represents the concentration of aflatoxin B_1 in the sample of prostatic fluid collected over the period of time indicated by the width of the columns. Circles or columns with downward directed arrows indicate plasma and prostatic fluid samples in which the concentration of aflatoxin B_1 was below the indicated level. P represents the intravenous administration of 0.7 mg/kg of pilocarpine hydrochloride.

declined at about the same rates as in the first three experiments. Aflatoxin B_1 was found in only the first sample of prostatic fluid collected after treatment, and again the levels were about one tenth that of plasma. In the tissues, low levels of aflatoxin B_1 were found in the prostate, liver, kidney, and testis of one of the dogs but was not detected in any of these same tissues from the other three dogs. In addition, aflatoxin B_1 was not detected in fat samples from the four dogs.

In the seven experiments, measurable levels of aflatoxin B_1 were found in 13 prostatic fluid samples and these levels were correlated with the mean plasma levels for the same periods of time ($r = 0.567$; $P < 0.05$). Figure 4 is a plot of these data, and the line in the figure is drawn with a slope equivalent to the calculated mean fluid-to-plasma ratio of 0.10 (SE $= 0.01$).

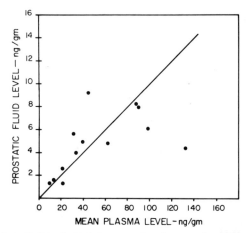

Fig. 4. The partitioning of aflatoxin B_1 between canine plasma and prostatic fluid. The ordinate represents the concentration of aflatoxin B_1 in prostatic fluid, while the abscissa represents the mean plasma concentration over the period of collection of the prostatic fluid sample. Each point represents the results of a single prostatic fluid analysis. The line is drawn with a slope equivalent to the calculated mean fluid-to-plasma ratio of 0.10.

For the six dogs the mean plasma half-life of aflatoxin B_1 was 44 ± 12 minutes, and the mean apparent volume of distribution was 1.00 ± 0.13 l/kg.

Also of particular interest, during the thin-layer chromatographic determination of the aflatoxin B_1 content of the plasma and prostatic fluid samples, a second spot, presumably a metabolite of aflatoxin B_1, was sometimes present and, although it was not positively identified, it had a mobility similar to that described for aflatoxin M_1 [19].

Rats. Because aflatoxin B_1 could not be detected in either the plasma or prostatic fluid of rats given IV doses of 0.1 mg/kg of aflatoxin, experiments were conducted in which rats were given IV doses of 1 mg/kg. In these experiments the mean rate of secretion in six rats after aflatoxin B_1 was 0.137 ± 0.040 gm/hr and in nine rats after IV saline was 0.039 ± 0.012 gm/hr; the difference between these means was statistically significant (P < 0.05).

Aflatoxin B_1 was present in plasma and prostatic fluid from these animals (Fig. 5). As expected, the levels in plasma were highest immediately after treatment and declined thereafter. The decline appeared to follow first-order kinetics with a half-life of 20 minutes; the apparent volume of distribution was 1.43 l/kg. As in the dog, the level of aflatoxin B_1 in prostatic fluid was proportional to the level in plasma (Fig. 6); again the correlation was highly significant (n = 6; r = 0.98; P < 0.01).

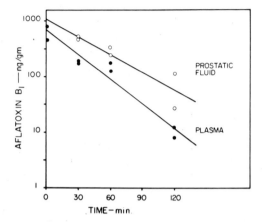

Fig. 5. Secretion of aflatoxin B_1 in rat prostatic fluid. The abscissa represents time after the intravenous injection of 1 mg/kg of aflatoxin B_1 and the ordinate represents the concentration of aflatoxin in either plasma or prostatic fluid. The values for plasma are plotted at the time the samples were taken, while the values for prostatic fluid are plotted at the times the collections of fluid were terminated. The straight lines were fit by the method of least squares.

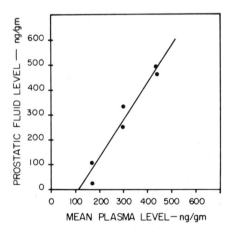

Fig. 6. The partitioning of aflatoxin B_1 between rat plasma and prostatic fluid. The ordinate represents the concentration of aflatoxin B_1 in prostatic fluid, while the abscissa represents the mean plasma concentration over the period of collection of the prostatic fluid sample. Each point represents the results of a single prostatic fluid analysis. The line was fit by the method of least squares.

When the animals were sacrificed at 2, 30, 60, and 120 minutes after treatment, aflatoxin B_1 was found in all organs examined, including the prostate (Table III). The mean gland-to-plasma ratios for the ventral and dorsolateral prostates were 1.84 ± 0.50 and 3.34 ± 1.08, respectively, while for the liver and fat, the ratios were 5.27 ± 1.08 and 1.24 ± 0.39, respectively.

The thin-layer chromatograms revealed the presence of a second spot, perhaps aflatoxin M_1, in all of the samples of rat plasma, prostatic fluid and tissue.

3-Amino-1,2,4-trizaole (ATA)

Dogs. The levels of radioactivity in both plasma and resting prostatic fluid was followed for 240 minutes after the IV treatment of one fistula-dog with 1.25 mg/kg of $[^{14}C]$-ATA (Fig. 7), and it was found that after a brief initial drop in plasma radioactivity, the levels of radioactivity declined according to first-order kinetics with a half-life of 118 minutes. The levels of radioactivity in the prostatic fluid samples was much lower than, but generally parallel to, that of plasma, with the ratios for levels in prostatic fluid to mean levels in plasma over the period of collection of the same sample varying from 0.020–0.032, with a mean value of 0.024.

In a similar experiment on a second fistula-dog given the same treatment with $[^{14}C]$-ATA, but followed 60 minutes later by IV pilocarpine to increase the rate of secretion, the plasma levels of radioactivity declined in a manner similar to those in the first dog (Fig. 8). Similarly, the level of radioactivity in a sample of prostatic fluid collected after treatment with $[^{14}C]$-ATA but before pilocarpine treatment was much lower than that mean plasma level over the same time period, the prostatic fluid-to-plasma ratio being 0.097. However, following pilocarpine administration, when prostatic fluid was being secreted at an accelerated rate, the levels of radioactivity in the prostatic fluid samples rose sharply to levels near those in plasma, the prostatic fluid-to-plasma ratios for six such samples ranging from 0.890–0.995, with a mean value of 0.926.

The experiments on four other dogs, one of which was a fistula-dog, are summarized in Table IV. For 120 minutes after treatment with IV doses of 1.25 mg/kg of $[^{14}C]$-ATA, the plasma and prostatic fluid levels were similar to those obtained in the first pair of experiments. Examination of selected tissues of radioactivity at 120 minutes after treatment revealed relatively high levels in the liver, with lower levels in the prostate, kidneys, and testis, and even lower levels in fat. For these tissues, the mean tissue-to-plasma levels in order of descending ratios were as follows: liver, 5.24 ± 0.80; kidneys, 1.74 ± 0.19; testis, 0.05 ± 0.15; prostate, 0.95 ± 0.03; fat, 0.25 ± 0.06.

Because the levels of radioactivity in the prostatic fluid samples from the experiment shown in Figure 8 rose with the rate of secretion, the exact relationship between secretory rate and the level of radioactivity in fluid was ex-

TABLE III. Levels of aflatoxin B₁ in the plasma and tissues of rats after the intravenous administration of 1 mg/kg of aflatoxin B₁

	Aflatoxin B₁ (ng/gm wet weight)[a]								
Fluid or tissue	2 min		30 min		60 min		120 min		
Plasma	450	790	182	181	120	176	8	9	15
Ventral prostate	380	715	270	231	73	230	11	46	55
Dorsolateral	430	422	310	258	280	236	77	67	71
Liver	1540	2614	1040	760	500	400	46	120	79
Kidney	160	1600	660	400	270	240	190	820	400
Fat	160	300	121	175	67	233	6	36	33

[a]Each value represents the results of the determination of aflatoxin B₁ in fluids or tissues from a single animal.

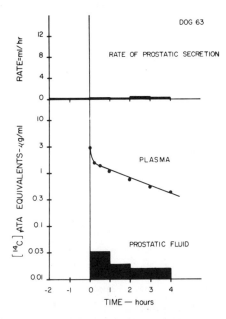

Fig. 7. Secretion of [^{14}C]-aminotriazole (ATA) in resting canine prostatic fluid. Results of an experiment in one dog. The abscissa represents time after termination of an intravenous injection of 1.25 mg/kg of [^{14}C]-aminotriazole over five minutes. Upper portion: The height of each column represents the mean rate of secretion of prostatic fluid over the period of time indicated by the width of the column. Lower portion: Each point represents the level of radioactivity in plasma samples taken at the indicated time after treatment while the height of each column represents the level of radioactivity in the sample of prostatic fluid collected over the period of time indicated by the width of the column. The linear portion of the plasma curve was fit by the method of least squares.

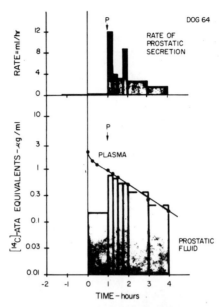

Fig. 8.   Secretion of [¹⁴C]-aminotriazole (ATA) in resting and pilocarpine-induced canine prostatic fluid. Results of an experiment in one dog. The abscissa and ordinates are the same as for Figure 8. P represents the time of intravenous administrations of 0.7 mg/kg of pilocarpine hydrochloride.

amined further by plotting the prostatic fluid-to-plasma ratio of each prostatic fluid sample from each dog against the mean rate at which the sample was secreted. This plot, seen in Figure 9, shows a distinctive relationship between these variables. Interestingly, this flow-dependence is remarkably similar to the flow-dependence of the sodium and chloride concentration of canine prostatic fluid itself [20,21].

Finally, the kinetics of the plasma decline in radioactivity in all six dogs were analyzed; the mean plasma half-life was 158 ± 28 minutes, and the apparent volume of distribution was 0.66 ± 0.67 l/kg.

Rats.   Prostatic fluid was collected from four rats over the first 120 minutes after IV treatment with 1.25 mg/kg of [¹⁴C]-ATA (Table V). The mean weight of fluid secreted was 0.097 ± 0.039 gm and was not different from that of a comparable group of six saline-treated control animals which secreted 0.096 ± 0.021 gm over the same period of time.

Radioactivity was recovered from the prostatic fluid samples of all four of these rats, although the levels were lower than the levels in plasma samples collected over the same time period. The levels of radioactivity in the tissues of these rats were generally similar to the plasma level at the time of sacrifice.

TABLE IV. Levels of radioactivity in the plasma, prostatic fluid, and tissues of dogs after the intravenous administration of 1.25 mg/kg of [^{14}C]-aminotriazole

Fluid or tissue	[^{14}C]-Aminotriazole-equivalent (μg/ml or μg/gm)
Plasma	
2 min[a]	2.75 ± 0.42
15 min	2.16 ± 0.34
30 min	1.94 ± 0.32
60 min	1.74 ± 0.31
120 min	1.46 ± 0.30
Prostatic fluid	
0–60 min	1.01[b]
60–120 min	1.32[b]
Tissues: 120 min	
prostate	1.37 ± 0.27
liver	6.95 ± 0.57
kidney	2.40 ± 0.32
testes	1.69 ± 0.48
fat	0.33 ± 0.07

[a]End of the injection of [^{14}C]-aminotriazole = 0 minutes.
[b]n = 1.

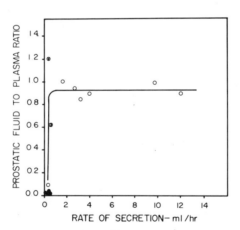

Fig. 9   Relationship between the level of [^{14}C]-aminotriazole in prostatic fluid and the rate of prostatic secretion. The prostatic fluid to plasma ratio associated with 13 prostatic fluid samples from three dogs is plotted (ordinate) against the rate of secretion of the particular sample (abscissa). Each dog is represented by a different symbol. The line was drawn by eye with the horizontal component corresponding to 0.92, the mean ratio for the six nearest open circles.

TABLE V. Levels of radioactivity in the plasma, prostatic fluid, and tissues of rats after the intravenous administration of 1.25 mg/kg of [^{14}C]-aminotriazole

Samples and times after treatment	[^{14}C]-Aminotriazole-equivalent (μg/gm or μg/ml)
Plasma	
15 min	1.35 ± 0.33[a]
60 min	1.44 ± 0.06[a]
120 min	1.65 ± 0.26
Prostatic fluid: 0–120 min	0.61 ± 0.10
Tissues: 120 min	
ventral prostate	1.02 ± 0.10
dorsolateral prostate	1.40 ± 0.20
liver	1.61 ± 0.15
kidney	2.14 ± 0.62
abdominal fat	0.23 ± 0.10

[a]n = 3.

The mean tissue-to-plasma ratio for those tissues examined were as follows: kidney, 1.34 ± 0.44; liver, 1.01 ± 0.09; dorsolateral prostate, 0.92 ± 0.20; ventral prostate, −0.66 ± 0.12; abdominal fat, 0.15 ± 0.07.

2-Acetylaminofluorene (2-AAF)

A full report of our experiments on 2-AAF has already been published [22].

Dogs. Three fistula-dogs were given single IP doses of 0.16–0.26 mg/kg of [^{14}C]-2-AAF, and the levels of radioactivity in plasma and samples of resting prostatic fluid was followed in one dog for 166 hours and in the remaining two dogs for six hours. Following treatment the levels of radioactivity in plasma rose rapidly, peaked at about 1 hour, and then fell slowly, following first-order kinetics. In all three dogs the levels of radioactivity in resting prostatic fluid was quite variable, with fluid-to-plasma ratios ranging from 0.14–2.54.

Radioactivity was found in the prostate glands of two of these dogs at 6 hours after treatment. The tissue-to-plasma ratios for the prostate gland were 0.22 and 0.26; lower levels were found in fat and pancreas and higher levels in kidney and liver.

Rats. Prostatic fluid was collected from four rats over the interval between 25 and 29 hours after single IP doses of 2 mg/kg of [^{14}C]-2-AAF. Radioactivity was found in secretion of all four rats and the concentrations were much lower than those in plasma at the end of each experiment. The prostatic fluid-to-plasma ratios for these four animals varied from 0.09–0.13 with a mean of 0.12 ± 0.01.

In a separate series of experiments the levels of radioactivity were measured in unanesthetized rats sacrificed 4–140 hours after single IP doses of 1.8 mg/kg of [^{14}C]-2-AAF. Plasma radioactivity was maximal at 4 hours after treatment, the earliest time examined, and fell steadily thereafter. At the same time, radioactivity was readily detected in the ventral and dorsolateral lobes of the prostate and in the liver, kidney, testis, and pancreas.

N-Methyl-N'-nitro-N-nitrosoguanidine (MNNG)

Dogs. Four dogs with prostatic fistulas were given IV doses of 0.3 mg/kg of [^{14}C]-MNNG and plasma and prostatic fluid levels of radioactivity were followed for 120 minutes, and then levels in selected organs were determined (Table VI). The mean resting rate of secretion of prostatic fluid by these animals prior to treatment was 0.22 ± 0.075 gm/hr; over the first 60 minutes after treatment it was 0.206 ± 0.078 gm/hr, and over the last 60 minutes it was 0.092 ± 0.033 gm/hr. Since there was a statistically significant difference between the pretreatment rate of secretion and the rate over the last collection period (P < 0.05), the treatment may have partially inhibited secretion.

As expected following IV treatment, the plasma levels of radioactivity were maximal in the first sample taken, at 2 minutes after treatment, and then fell steadily; the decline appeared to follow first-order kinetics with a mean half-life of about 290 minutes. Radioactivity was detected in all eight of the prostatic

TABLE VI. Levels of radioactivity in the plasma, prostatic fluid, and selected tissues of dogs after the intravenous administration of 0.3 mg/kg of [^{14}C]-MNNG

Fluid or tissue	[^{14}C]-MNNG-equivalent (ng/ml or ng/gm)
Plasma	
2 min	512 ± 20
15 min	435 ± 23
30 min	411 ± 23
60 min	372 ± 25
120 min	333 ± 21
Prostatic fluid	
0–60 min	192 ± 53
60–120 min	1493 ± 771
Tissues: 120 min	
prostate	326 ± 19
liver	449 ± 18
kidney	620 ± 42
testis	312 ± 23
fat	50 ± 12

fluid samples collected from these dogs. However, contrary to the consistency of the plasma levels from these dogs, two of the prostatic fluid samples contained inordinately and inexplicably high levels of radioactivity when compared to the other six samples of fluid. When the partition of radioactivity between prostatic fluid and plasma was calculated after estimating the mean plasma levels over the period of collection of each sample, six of the prostatic fluid-to-plasma ratios were between 0.14 and 0.68, with a mean of 0.48, while the other two ratios were 7.66 and 9.63.

Upon analysis of the tissues from these animals, intermediate levels of radioactivity were found in the prostate glands. Higher levels were found in the liver and kidneys, while more comparable levels were seen in the testis, and much lower levels were present in fat.

Rats. In experiments on three anesthetized rats in which prostatic fluid was collected for 120 minutes after treatment with IV doses of 0.3 mg/kg of [^{14}C]-MNNG, the rate of secretion was not altered; the weights of the fluid samples secreted by the three treated animals were 0.072, 0.105, and 0.108 gm while those secreted by three saline-treated animals were 0.042, 0.090, and 0.180 gm. The mean levels of radioactivity in the plasma at 15 and 120 minutes after treatment were 310 ± 25 and 278 ± 28 ng/gm [^{14}C]-MNNG-equivalent, and in the prostatic fluid samples collected over this time interval the mean level was 136 ± 19 ng/gm; the mean fluid-to-plasma ratios, estimated from the levels in each prostatic fluid sample and the mean plasma level over the period of 15–120 minutes, were 0.31, 0.60, and 0.49, respectively; the mean ratio was 0.47.

At 120 minutes after treatment the mean level of radioactivity in the ventral and dorsolateral prostate was 39 ± 4 and 153 ± 9 ng/gm. Levels were higher in abdominal fat (203 ± 20 ng/gm), liver (315 ± 27 ng/gm, and kidney (509 ± 47 ng/mg).

Cadmium

Dogs. In experiments on nonfistula dogs, four animals were each treated with a single subcutaneous (SC) dose of 10 mg/kg of $CdCl_2 \cdot 2.5\ H_2O$ and two went untreated. Blood samples were taken periodically from all animals for determination of cadmium levels and at either 2 or 24 hours after the start of the experiment, the dogs were sacrificed and selected tissues taken for analysis. The results of these analysis are shown in Table VII. Cadmium was found in the renal cortex of one of the untreated dogs and in several tissues of the other untreated dog, the highest level being in the renal cortex. After treatment with cadmium both blood and plasma levels of cadmium were detectable within 10 minutes and the peak levels occurred between 10 and 45 minutes after treatment.

TABLE VII. Cadmium content of plasma and selected tissues of dogs treated with single subcutaneous doses of 10 mg/kg of $CdCl_2 \cdot 2.5$ H_2O

	Level of cadmium (μg/ml or μg/gm wet weight)					
	Untreated		2 Hours		24 Hours	
Fluid or tissue	dog 24	dog 35	dog 19	dog 25	dog 21	dog 36
Plasma						
0 min	NDa	ND	ND	ND	ND	ND
10 min	ND	ND	0.1	0.5	0.3	1.5
20 min	ND	ND	0.4	0.4	0.8	2.2
30 min	ND	ND	0.5	0.4	0.7	1.7
60 min	ND	ND	0.8	0.2	0.6	1.0
120 min	ND	ND	0.4	ND	0.2	0.4
240 min	—	—	—	—	0.1	0.2
24 hours	—	—	—	—	ND	0.4
Tissues						
prostate gland	ND	0.2	1.1	ND	1.4	1.6
liver	ND	0.5	24.7	6.7	35.1	38.6
renal cortex	0.4	1.4	6.3	2.5	18.1	12.4
renal medulla	ND	1.2	2.4	ND	3.0	3.7
testis	ND	0.2	1.5	ND	1.5	0.5
heart (ventricle)	ND	0.2	2.2	0.1	3.6	2.6
lung	ND	0.1	4.3	ND	1.4	1.2
diaphragm	ND	0.3	2.9	ND	0.6	0.2
pancreas	ND	0.2	10.0	2.1	11.7	9.9

aND, not detected: < 0.1 μg/ml or μg/gm wet weight.

Cadmium appeared to localize in the liver to a greater extent than any of the other tissues. Among the tissues examined, the prostate gland, possessed the lowest, or nearly the lowest, concentration of cadmium.

Studies were also conducted in three dogs with fistulas (Table VIII). All three dogs were given a single SC dose of 30 mg/kg of $CdCl_2 \cdot 2.5$ H_2O and samples of plasma and both basal and pilocarpine-induced prostatic fluid were collected over the ensuing 120–150 minutes and analyzed for cadmium. One of these three dogs was sacrificed 120 minutes after treatment for analysis of the cadmium levels in the prostate gland and other tissues. The remaining two dogs died approximately 24 and 120 hours after treatment, and tissues from these animals were also analyzed.

The plasma levels of cadmium in these three dogs during the first 120–150 minutes after treatment were higher than those seen after doses of 10 mg/kg. Nevertheless, cadmium was not found in either basal or pilocarpine-induced prostatic fluid; that is, the levels were less than 0.1 μg/ml. In the dog sacrificed

TABLE VIII. Cadmium content of plasma and selected tissues of dogs treated with single subcutaneous doses of 30 mg/kg of $CdCl_2 \cdot 2.5 \ H_2O$

	Level of cadmium (μg/ml or μg/gm wet weight)		
Fluid or tissue	Dog 8 (sacrificed at 2 hr)	Dog 15 (died at 24 hr)	Dog 32 (died at 120 hr)
Plasma			
0 min	ND[a]	ND	ND
15 min	0.9	3.2	2.3
30 min	1.9	3.2	1.8
60–75 min	1.5	8.1	2.0
120–150 min	1.7	1.1	—
48 hr	—	—	0.4
Tissues			
prostate gland	0.5	4.5	4.3
liver	42.8	32.0	32.6
renal cortex	6.4	15.6	30.3
testis	—[b]	—[b]	1.2
heart (ventricle)	2.2	6.3	5.6
lung	4.6	4.9	3.9
diaphragm	0.8	1.4	5.0
pancreas	7.3	8.9	8.7[c]

[a]ND, not detected: $< 0.1 \ \mu$g/ml or μg/gm wet weight.
[b]Had been castrated and treated daily with single subcutaneous doses of 5 mg of testosterone.
[c]Severely hemorrhagic.

120 minutes after treatment, cadmium was not found in either of the two serial 1-hour samples of the basal secretion collected between treatment and sacrifice. In the second dog, which died approximately 24 hours after treatment, cadmium was not found in basal fluid collected over the first 150 minutes after treatment. The third dog was given an IV dose of 0.7 mg/kg of pilocarpine hydrochloride immediately after treatment with cadmium and the more copious prostatic secretion which resulted was collected over the ensuing 75 minutes as three serial 5-minute samples followed by four serial 15-minute samples; cadmium could not be detected in any of these seven samples of fluid.

Although cadmium could not be detected in the prostatic fluid of these dogs, it was found in the prostate glands of all three dogs (Table VIII). As seen in the experiments on nonfistula dogs, levels of cadmium were highest in the liver and renal cortex, with lower levels being found in other tissues.

Rats. Levels of cadmium were determined in plasma and tissues of unanesthetized rats before and at intervals for up to 24 hours after treatment with single subcutaneous doses of 30 mg/kg of $CdCl_2 \cdot 2.5 \ H_2O$ (Table IX). Of

TABLE IX. Levels of cadmium in the plasma, prostate, and selected tissues of unanesthetized rats after single subcutaneous doses of 30 mg/kg of $CdCl_2 \cdot 2.5\ H_2O$

| After treatment | Rat number | Cadmium (μg/ml or μg/gm wet weight) | | | | | | |
		Plasma	Ventral prostate	Dorsolateral prostate	Testis	Liver	Kidney	Pancreas
0	1	ND[a]	ND	0.2	0.3	ND	ND	ND
	2	0.3	0.9	1.0	0.3	ND	0.1	ND
15 min	3	1.8	0.7	0.9	0.3	2.2	0.6	—
	4	3.3	1.4	2.6	0.4	6.1	1.5	1.5
30 min	5	2.2	1.4	2.1	0.5	8.6	2.1	2.7
	6	2.0	0.9	1.4	0.4	12.1	2.2	2.4
1 hr	7	1.4	1.6	2.1	0.5	13.7	3.0	2.7
	8	1.2	1.2	1.6	0.6	17.0	4.7	4.9
2 hr	9	1.2	1.0	1.4	0.5	12.5	3.0	4.4
	10	2.0	1.6	2.8	0.6	14.0	4.8	30.0
4 hr	11	0.5	1.1	1.3	0.6	18.1	3.2	7.2
	12	0.8	0.8	1.7	0.5	19.4	5.7	6.6
24 hr	13	0.8	1.6	2.1	0.6[b]	25.7	14.6	9.7
	14	0.3	1.2	2.3	0.6[b]	27.7	9.4	11.3

[a]ND, not detectable: $< 0.1\ \mu$g/ml or μg/gm.
[b]Grossly hemorrhagic.

particular interest, low levels of cadmium were found in the plasma, prostate, testes, and kidney in one or both of the untreated, control animals. With respect to treatment, the plasma levels were highest immediately after treatment and then declined slowly, while the levels of cadmium in both the ventral and dorsolateral lobes of the prostate rose rapidly after treatment and were sustained. At the same time, levels of cadmium in the liver, kidney, and pancreas rose slowly and steadily over the 24 hours after treatment. The levels of cadmium could not be followed for longer intervals after treatment because animals began to die at about 24 hours after treatment with this dose of cadmium.

Levels of cadmium also were measured in the plasma, prostatic fluid, prostate gland, and other tissues of four anesthetized rats at 24–26 hours after single SC doses of 3 mg/kg of $CdCl_2 \cdot 2.5\ H_2O$. In these experiments, cadmium was consistently present in the liver and kidneys, but it was detectable in the dorsolateral prostate of only two of the four rats, and it was not found in measurable amounts in the plasma, ventral prostate, or abdominal fat of any of the animals. With respect to prostatic fluid, it was not found in the prostatic fluid secreted by the first rat studied, nor was it found in a sample of fluid formed by pooling the prostatic secretions of the remaining three rats. Attempts to perform additional, similar experiments using higher doses of cadmium were unsuccessful as rats treated with 10 mg/kg of $CdCl_2 \cdot 2.5\ H_2O$ died soon after being given anesthesia-producing doses of pentobarbital sodium.

DISCUSSION

Theoretical Considerations

Before discussing the results of these experiments, there are some theoretical considerations about the penetration of chemicals into the prostate and its secretion which should be emphasized. Smith [8] has already discussed some aspects of those factors which control the passive diffusion of substances into prostatic fluid but did not consider penetration into the gland per se.

For substances which passively enter the gland and its secretion from the circulation, as after systemic administration, two important determinants of penetration are the plasma level of the chemical and its lipid solubility. The plasma level is important because it provides the driving force for the diffusion from plasma into the tissue and fluid. Since under experimental conditions the plasma level of any substance can be expected to vary widely depending upon dose of chemical administered, nature of the adminstered material, route of administration, time after treatment, etc, when studying the penetration of substances from plasma into the gland and/or the fluid it is necessary to determine the levels of the substances in plasma and to relate tissue and fluid levels to these plasma levels. In practice, this is conventionally done by calculating the ratio of the concentration in tissues to the concentration in plasma or the ratio of the concentration in fluid to the concentration in plasma; ie, the tissue-to-plasma and/or fluid-to-plasma ratios.

The lipid solubility of the chemical is important because the passage from plasma into cells and hence into prostatic fluid necessitates traversing several cell walls or membrane barriers which are lipid in nature and, hence, would be penetrated more readily by lipid soluble substances. In this regard, nondissociable, nonpolar molecules should penetrate more readily than charged or highly polar molecules.

Partitioning of nondissociating substances. With these two considerations in mind, it is possible to prepare schematics for the penetration of nondissociable and dissociable molecules into the prostate and prostatic fluid. Figure 10 is such a schematic for nondissociating substances of sufficiently high lipid solubility. As can be seen in this figure, at equilibrium the penetrating substance would be found in all three compartments and probably in two states in each compartment. Some material in each compartment might be bound to protein or other constituents while some would probably be unbound or "free." Notice that at steady state the concentration of unbound chemical in all three

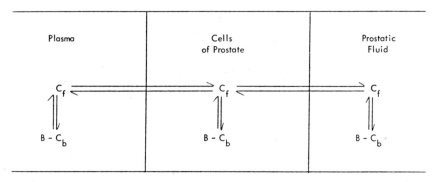

Fig. 10. The partitioning of nondissociable chemicals between plasma, the prostate gland, and prostatic fluid. C_f, free or unbound chemical; C_b, bound chemical; B, binding sites on proteins or other constituents.

compartments would be equal, and the tissue-to-plasma and prostatic fluid-to-plasma ratios for unbound material would be *one*. However, in terms of the overall distribution of such chemicals, the possible binding to protein and/or other constituents of plasma, cells and prostatic fluid cannot be ignored and while the binding of foreign chemicals to proteins or other substances in prostatic fluid has not been studied, binding to cellular constitutents undoubtedly occurs. The nature and extent of this binding probably varies widely among substances. Notice, however, that measurements of the concentration of the chemical in any of these three compartments usually involves the determination of both unbound and bound substances indiscriminately. It might be anticipated, therefore, that at steady state the tissue-to-plasma ratio or the prostatic fluid-to-plasma ratio might vary from unity; the variation would reflect in part the difference in binding. For example, because tissues might afford a greater potential for binding than plasma, the tissue-to-plasma ratios among a variety of substances might be expected to commonly exceed one, while on the other hand prostatic fluid contains smaller amounts of many constituents than does plasma, it might be expected that the prostatic fluid-to-plasma ratios might commonly be less than one.

It is obvious on the basis of these considerations that it would be desirable to determine the levels of the unbound and bound material separately, rather than measuring them together. While this would certainly simplify the interpretation of studies on partitioning, it presents technical difficulties. Using dialysis techniques it is possible to study binding to plasma components and these same techniques could be applied to prostatic fluid samples, although this would be made much more difficult by the very small volumes of fluid available. On the other hand, there are no techniques for differentiating between unbound and bound chemicals in tissues. In view of the lack of methods suitable for tissues and the technical difficulties imposed by the small volumes of prostatic fluid available, studies of this kind cannot be pursued at this time. Nevertheless, binding cannot be overlooked as an important factor determining the partitioning of chemicals between plasma, the prostate and prostatic fluid.

Partitioning of dissociating substances. The theoretical considerations governing the penetration of substances which are either weakly acidic or basic are somewhat more complicated than for nondissociable molecules, because if they dissociate at the physiological pH range, then one must be concerned with the partitioning of both the uncharged and charged forms of the chemical. The behavior of these two forms can be quite different because the charged form may not pass cell membranes and barriers as readily; also it may be more or less susceptible to binding at various sites.

Figure 11 is a schematic showing some aspects of the partitioning of a weak acid and base between plasma, the prostate, and prostatic fluid. This schematic is based upon the general observations that biological membranes are generally much more permeable to the uncharged form of a molecule than to its charged counterpart [8]. Thus, the figure shows that the uncharged acid, HA, and base, B, penetrate into both the gland and the fluid while the charged moieties, A$^-$ and BH$^+$, do not.

In systems such as these, when either weak acids or bases are allowed to equilibrate between compartments of differing pH, the acidic substances tend to accumulate in the more alkaline compartments while the basic substances tend to accumulate in the more acid compartment [23]. Since we have no knowledge about the internal pH of the cells of the prostate, no conclusion can be drawn about the role of dissociation in the tendency of substances to accumulate in the prostate and hence to determine tissue-to-plasma ratios. On the other hand, since prostatic fluid of the dog normally is slightly acidic [8], it can be predicted that basic chemicals, but not acidic substances, would concentrate more readily in prostatic fluid.

Stamey et al [24] have described the concepts underlying this phenomenon and its potential application to studies on the prostate. Assuming a plasma pH of 7.4 and a prostatic fluid pH of 6.6, they calculated the theoretical ratios of prostatic fluid-to-plasma which should be attained at steady state following administration of both acids and bases of varying pK$_a$s. For relatively strong acids (pK$_a$ ≤ 6), the theoretical ratios were very low, on the order of 0.2; for the weaker acids (pK$_a$ ≥ 9) and the weaker bases (pK$_a$ ≤ 6), the calculated ratios were 1; for the stronger bases (pK$_a$ ≥ 9) the ratios were about 6. Thus, the concentration of strong acids in prostatic fluid would be very low in comparison with the levels in plasma, while the concentrations of weak acids and bases would approximate those of plasma and the strong bases would accumulate in the fluid.

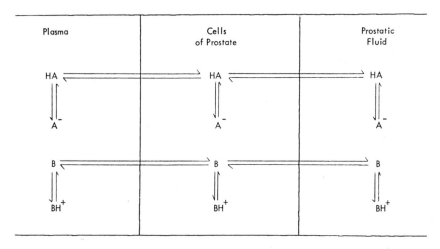

Fig. 11.   The partitioning of weak acids and bases between plasma, the prostate gland, and prostatic fluid. HA, acid; B, base.

In experiments on dogs there is excellent agreement between the expected and observed partitioning of antibiotics between plasma and prostatic fluid [9,24], thus confirming the assumption that it is the uncharged and not the charged forms of acids and bases that penetrate the cellular barriers and enter prostatic fluid.

It will be quickly recognized that the scheme shown in Figure 11 is incomplete in that provisions are not given for the possible binding of either the undissociated or dissociated forms of either the acid or base to the constituents of each compartment. The figure could have shown two theoretical binding sites in each compartment, one for each molecule species. However, it is not difficult after examining Figure 10 to appreciate the role of such binding sites to the distribution of acids and bases as shown in Figure 11.

It should also be recognized that the above discussions have not considered the presence of bulk lipid stores, such as in fat cells, for although this would play an important role in the tissue accumulation of many chemicals, such stores do not occur in the prostate.

Role of metabolism.   Figures 10 and 11 could also have been expanded to show the possible outcomes of metabolic alteration of the chemicals under consideration. Following systemic administration many substances are metabolized in the liver or other tissues and the metabolites circulate in plasma. Thus, one or more metabolites might penetrate from plasma into the prostate and prostatic fluid. Alternatively, it is possible that the prostate itself might metabolize some chemicals. In this case the metabolites might diffuse from the prostatic cells into plasma or into prostatic fluid. Moreover, there are a variety of enzymes in prostatic fluid, and it is possible that a substance might penetrate from plasma into the gland and then into the secretion where it is metabolized, and the metabolite might then pass back into the cells of the gland and back into plasma.

While metabolism will not contribute at all to the partitioning behavior depicted in Figures 10 and 11, it is important for two other reasons. First, in studying the distribution of radiolabelled material it must be fully appreciated that the radioactivity being measured may represent an admixture of unchanged chemical and metabolites or that it may represent only unchanged chemical or only metabolites.

The metabolic modifiction of chemicals is especially important in the area of chemical carcinogenesis for it is now clear that many substances are not carcinogenic themselves but rather because they are metabolized to active metabolites which interact with cells in some manner as to provoke tumor development. In this regard, it is extremely important to point out that many, if not all, such ultimate carcinogens are highly reactive, positively charged, electrophilic molecules [25]. As such these substances would probably act at or near their sites of generation. In the first place, their charged nature probably limits their ability to penetrate cell membranes. Moreover, they are so reactive that unless generated near their site of action they may be consumed in noncarcinogenic reactions.

Uptake by Prostate Gland

All eight of the substances which were studied were taken up by the prostate gland of both the rat and dog. For most substances the tissue-to-plasma ratios were about 0.2–1.0 in both species. There were a few notable exceptions, however. In the rat, the tissue-to-plasma ratios after 3-MCA, DMBA, and aflatoxin B_1 were higher, about 1–5. These substances may concentrate by binding to cellular constituents.

Cadmium represented an interesting case, for soon after treatment the levels in the rat prostate rose and remained high even when the plasma levels fell; thus, the tissue-to-plasma ratio increased with time from values of less than one to values greater than two. Possibly this reflects the penetration of cadmium at high plasma levels, followed by relatively irreversible binding to cellular constituents and a resultant failure to reenter plasma as the plasma levels declined. The strong binding of cadmium to the prostate might also explain its failure to appear in prostatic fluid.

Secretion in Prostatic Fluid

Basal secretion. In our experiments the penetration of chemicals and/or their metabolites into prostatic fluid was studied in two different conditions. The penetration into the basal or resting secretion of both dogs and rats was studied, as well as the penetration into the more copious pilocarpine-induced secretion of the dog. With the exception of cadmium, all of the substances and/or their metabolites penetrated from plasma into the basal secretion. Moreover, in both species the levels of most substances in prostatic fluid rose very rapidly as the plasma levels rose after treatment, suggesting that there was no overwhelming barrier to the diffusion of substances from plasma to prostatic fluid.

Of the substances studied, 3-MCA appeared to concentrate to a greater extent in the resting prostatic secretion of the dog than the other compounds. The prostatic fluid-to-plasma ratios for radioactivity after treatment with [^{14}C]3-MCA were highest immediately after treatment, the ratios being about 2-20, and they subsequently declined, perhaps as the 3-MCA was metabolized. If the declining ratios with time reflect changes due to the metabolism of 3-MCA then the initial prostatic fluid-to-plasma ratios, at 2–20, may in fact represent the partitioning of 3-MCA itself between these fluid compartments.

In rats, the highest prostatic fluid-to-plasma ratio observed was in the radioactivity levels after treatment with [^{14}C]-DMBA. In this case the ratio was about 2.0.

Cadmium represented the opposite end of the spectrum. It could not be detected in resting prostatic secretion of either dogs or rats even after lethal doses of cadmium were administered. Finally, all of the other substances studied represented intermediate cases, with prostatic fluid-to-plasma ratios in both dogs and rats being in the range of 0.1–1.0.

Pilocarpine-induced secretion. The effects of pilocarpine-induced stimulation of prostatic secretion on the levels of some chemicals and/or metabolites in prostatic fluid were striking. The stimulation of secretion produced marked decreases in the prostatic fluid-to-plasma ratios of radioactivity after [^{14}C]-3-MCA and [^{14}C]-DMBA, did not appreciably alter the ratios for N-hydroxyurethane or aflatoxin B_1, and markedly increased the ratio of radioactivity after [^{14}C]-ATA.

The reason why the partitioning of some of these substances is flow dependent is not known although some explanations can be offered. First, with respect to an increasing ratio for ATA after pilocarpine, it can be pointed out that the secretion of both sodium and chloride follow a similar pattern [21,22], and a similar explanation can be offered for both—that the primary secretion of the acinar epithelium is modified as the fluid passes through the ductile portions of the gland. In the case of sodium and chloride, the modification might represent reabsorption of both substances. At low rates of secretion, this reabsorption would significantly reduce the concentration of sodium and potassium in the secretion, while at high rates of secretion the reabsorptive capacity would be overwhelmed and the concentration of sodium and chloride in the secretion would rise and become equal to that of the primary acinar secretion. If this explanation also pertains to the secretion of radioactivity in [^{14}C]-ATA-treated animals, then the ductile portion of the gland must reabsorb or bind ATA and/ or its metabolites, at least to some limited degree. Obviously, this is only one possibility. Further study will be needed in order to more fully understand those factors controlling the appearance of ATA and/or its metabolites in prostatic fluid and why the fluid-to-plasma ratio rises with an increase in secretory activity.

The pilocarpine-induced decreases in the prostatic fluid-to-plasma ratios of radioactivity after $[^{14}C]$-3-MCA and $[^{14}C]$-DMBA could indicate that the secretion of prostatic fluid and penetration of radioactivity into prostatic fluid are relatively independent events, and that the partitioning of these substances between plasma and prostatic fluid only slowly approaches a steady-state. Accordingly, at low rates of secretion the partitioning of ^{14}C-labelled material between plasma and prostatic fluid would approach steady state, and relatively high levels would be found in samples of such fluid. At high rates of secretion, however, the fluid might be secreted so rapidly that the time available for diffusion of these chemicals into the fluid might be impinged upon, and lower concentrations are found in the secretion.

Relationship Between Uptake and Secretion

The present experiments have demonstrated that there is no simple or consistent relationship between the uptake and the secretion of foreign chemicals by the prostate. This is an important conclusion because one might speculate that analysis of human prostatic fluid samples could be used to estimate the exposure of the prostate to such chemicals. While this may be true for some compounds, it obviously is not true for all chemicals. The most striking example of this is cadmium which enters the prostate but not prostatic fluid. On the other hand, those compounds which displayed relatively constant tissue-to-plasma ratios (most readily seen in rat experiments) and relatively constant prostatic fluid-to-plasma ratios (most readily seen in dog experiments), one might expect that the levels in resting prostatic fluid would closely mirror the levels in the gland itself.

Uptake and Carcinogenic Effects

While there do not appear to be any published reports of the induction of prostatic tumors following systemic administration of carcinogenic chemicals, the present experiments make it clear that there is no absolute barrier to the penetration of carcinogenic substances into the prostate. Not only have we observed that all eight of the substances tested entered the glands of both species, but we also have found direct or indirect evidence of metabolites of some of these substances in these glands. The apparent relative refractoriness of the prostate to carcinogenic chemicals must be explained in terms other than the failure of substances to enter the gland.

One obvious explanation is that although these substances penetrate into the gland, the concentrations in the gland are insufficient to produce tumors. This has experimental support. In experiments where 3-MCA and DMBA have been placed directly into the prostate gland, some tumors did develop after treatment [26–30]. Even so, the doses of chemicals used were very high and the local concentration within the gland must have been extremely high. For example, doses of 3–5 mg of 3-MCA per gland have been employed in some rat studies [26–28], while in one mouse study the prostate was removed, wrapped around crystals of pure 3-MCA, and then transplanted under the skin of a host animals [29]. Doses of 0.05 mg of DMBA have also been injected into the prostate gland of the hamster [30]. While these procedures produced tumors although usually few if any adenocarcinomas, because of the massive amounts of chemicals involved one must still conclude that the prostate is relatively insensitive to carcinogenic chemicals.

A possible explanation for this relative insensitivity, and one which can be approached experimentally, can be based upon the observation that many or most carcinogens act after metabolic conversions to metabolites which in turn provoke the carcinogenic response by actions near their site of production. Accordingly, the prostate may be refractory to the carcinogenic effects of chemicals because it has a limited capacity to metabolize chemicals and hence generate carcinogenic metabolites near the target cells. In this regard, it is noteworthy that both the rat and mouse prostates have at least some capacity to metabolize 3-MCA in vitro [31]. However, more information is needed before any reasonable attempt can be made at evaluating the role of prostatic metabolism of foreign chemicals in prostatic carcinogenesis.

Secretion and Carcinogenic Effects

Lastly, the possibility should not be overlooked that the prostatic secretion could play a role in prostatic carcinogenesis. Studies on chemical carcinogens have often shown that tumors of the epithelial linings of hollow structures often develop from chemicals which enter from the luminal surface rather than from the circulation. An example are tumors of the upper gastrointestinal tract produced by the drinking or eating of carcinogenic substances. Further examples would be tumors of the lower gastrointestinal tract related to chemicals excreted in bile and tumors of the bladder resulting from substances excreted in urine. It is very possible that prostatic tumors could result from chemicals reaching prostatic fluid and the prostate by a retrograde penetration up the glandulars duct from the urethra. This approach to the prostate is of further interest because it is well known that microorganisms commonly ascend the prostatic ducts and subsequently produce prostatitis. It is conceivable that these microorganisms might produce carcinogenic substances which could enter the gland or they might convert chemicals from other sources into carcinogenic metabolites.

SUMMARY

Because the prostate of laboratory animals seems relatively resistant to the carcinogenic effects of systematically administered chemicals—an observation of some significance in attempts to establish the etiology of human prostatic adenocarcinoma and to produce animal models of prostatic cancer—we studied the penetration of eight carcinogenic chemicals into both the prostate gland and the prostatic secretion of the dog and the rat. The eight chemicals were 3-methylcholanthrene, 7,12-dimethylbenz[a]anthracene, N-hydroxyurethane, aflatoxin B_1, 3-amino-1,2,4-triazole, 2-acetylaminofluorene, N-Methyl-N'-nitro-N-nitrosoguanidine, and cadmium. In both species all eight substances and/or their metabolites were found to rapidly enter the prostate, and all except cadmium were recovered from prostatic fluid. Thus, although the levels in prostatic fluid did not always reflect levels in the gland, there was little if any barrier to the penetration of these chemicals into the gland. The apparent relative refractoriness of the prostate to systematically administered carcinogenic chemicals cannot be due to failure of such substances to enter the gland.

ACKNOWLEDGMENTS

The authors would like to acknowledge the expert technical assistance of Linda Marshall, David McCracken, Richard Norlin, Howard Reister, and Bernard Schmall in the conduct of these experiments.

These studies were supported by National Cancer Institute Contract NO1-CP-23238 and grant 1 RO1 CA-21607.

REFERENCES

1. Rivenson A, Silverman J: The prostatic carcinoma in laboratory animals. A bibliographic survey from 1900 to 1977. Invest Urol 16:468–472, 1979.
2. Sandberg AA, Gaunt R: Model systems for studies of prostatic cancer. Semin Oncol 3:177–187, 1976.
3. Price D, Williams-Ashman HG: The accessary reproductive glands of mammals. In Young WC (ed): "Sex and Internal Secretions." Baltimore: Williams and Wilkins, Baltimore, 1961, pp 366–448.
4. Fingerhut B, Veenema RJ: An animal model for the study of prostatic adenocarcinoma. Invest Urol 15:42–48, 1977.
5. Marquardt H, Kuroki T, Huberman E, Selkirk JK, Heidelberger C, Grover PL, Sims P: Malignant transformation of cells derived from mouse prostate by epoxides and other derivatives of polycyclic hydrocarbons. Cancer Res 32:716–720, 1972.
6. Chopra DP, Wilkoff LJ: Inhibition and reversal by β-retinoic acid of hyperplasia induced in cultured mouse prostate tissue by 3-methylcholanthrene or N-methyl-N'-nitro-N-nitrosoguanidine. J Natl Cancer Inst 56:583–587, 1976.
7. Freedman LR, Epstein FH: Urinary tract infection, pyelonephritis, and related conditions. In Thorn GW, et al (eds): "Harrison's Principles of Internal Medicine." New York: McGraw-Hill, 8th Ed, 1977, pp 1460–1467.
8. Smith ER: The canine prostate and its secretion. In Thomas JA, Singhal RL (eds): "Molecular Mechanisms of Gonodal Hormone Action." Vol. 1: Advances in Sex Hormone Research." Baltimore: University Park Press, 1975, pp 167–204.

9. Kjaer TB, Madsen PO: Prostatic fluid and tissue concentrations of ampicillin after administration of ketacillin ester (BL-P1761). Invest Urol 14:57–59, 1976.

10. Baumueller A, Kjaer TB, Madsen PO: Prostatic tissue and secretion concentrations of rosamicin and erythromycin. Experimental studies in the dog. Invest Urol 15:158–160, 1977.

11. Madsen PO, Kjaer TB, Baumueller A: Prostatic tissue and fluid concentrations of trimethoprim and sulfamethoxazole. Experimental and clinical studies. Urology 8:129–132, 1976.

12. Litvak AS, Franks CD, Vaught SK, McRoberts JW: Cifazolin and cephalexin levels in prostatic tissue and sera. Urology 7:497–498, 1976.

13. Williams CB, Litvak AS, McRoberts JW: Comparison of serum and prostatic levels of tobramycin. Urology 8:598–591, 1979.

14. Mason MM, Keefe F, Boria T: Specialized surgery of the bladder and prostate. J Am Vet Med Ass 139:1007–1014, 1961.

15. Smith ER, Hagopian M, Norlin RD: The penetration of N-hydroxyurethane into the prostate and prostatic secretion of the rat and dog. Toxicol Appl Pharmacol 40:335–345, 1977.

16. Smith ER, Hagopian M: The uptake and secretion of 3-methylcholanthrene by the prostate glands of the rat and dog. J Natl Cancer Inst 59:119–122, 1977.

17. Sims P: The metabolism of 3-methylcholanthrene and some related compounds by rat liver homogenates. Biochem J 98:215–228, 1966.

18. Levine WG: Hepatic uptake, metabolism and biliary excretion of 7,12-dimethyl-benzanthracene in the rat. Drug Metab Dispos 2:169–177, 1974.

19. Steyn M, Pitant MJ, Purchase IFH: A comparative study on aflatoxin B_1 metabolism in mice and rats. Br J Cancer 25:291–297, 1971.

20. Smith ER: The secretion of electrolytes by the pilocarpine-stimulated canine prostate gland. Proc Exp Biol Med 132:223–226, 1969.

21. Smith ER, Lebeaux M: The composition of nerve induced canine prostatic secretion. Invest Urol 9:100–103, 1971.

22. Smith ER, Hagopian M, Reister HC: The uptake and secretion of 2-acetylaminofluorene by the rat and dog prostate. Toxicol Appl Pharmacol 40:185–191, 1977.

23. Shanker LS: Passage of drugs across body membranes. Pharm Rev 14:501–530, 1962.

24. Stamey TA, Meares EM Jr, Winningham DS: Chronic bacterial prostatitis and the diffusion of drugs into prostatic fluid. Trans Am Assoc Genito-Urinary Surgeons 61:27–34, 1969.

25. Miller JA: Carcinogenesis by chemicals: an overview—G.H.A. Clowes Memorial Lecture. Cancer Res 30:559–576, 1970.

26. Dunning WF, Curtis MR, Segaloff A: Methylcholanthrene squamous cell carcinoma of the rat prostate with skeletal metastases, and failure of the rat liver to respond to the same carcinogen. Cancer Res 6:256–262, 1946.

27. Wojewski A, Laska A: Experimental cancer in the rat. Urol Int 17:223–229, 1964.

28. Ishibe T, Fukushige M, Takenaka I, Mizaguchi M, Kazuta M: Hormonal effects on the enzyme activities of the prostate of the rat during 20-methylcholanthrene carcinogenesis. Endocrinol Jpn 15:181–187, 1968.

29. Horning ES, Melbourne MA: Induction of glandular carcinomas of the prostate in the mouse. Lancet 251:829–830, 1946.

30. Varkarakis MJ, Sampson D, Schoones R, Gaeta SF, Reynoso G, Mirand EA, Murphy GP: The effects of androgens and estrogens on induced prostatic tumor in the hamster. J Surg Oncol 1:48–59, 1972.

31. Lasnitski I, Bard DR, Franklin HR: 3-Methylcholanthrene uptake and metabolism in organ culture, Br J Cancer 32:219–229, 1975.

The Prostatic Cell: Structure and Function
Part B, pages 165–182
© 1981 Alan R. Liss, Inc., 150 Fifth Avenue, New York, NY 10011

Chlorinated Insecticides and Hormone Receptors of the Prostate

Willard J. Visek

The organochlorine insecticides include the chlorinated ethane derivatives, of which DDT is the best known example, the cyclodienes, which include chlordane, aldrin, dieldrin[1], hepatachlor, endrin, and toxaphene, and the hexachlorocyclohexanes, such as lindane. From the mid 1940s to the mid 1960s these insecticides were widely used for controlling agricultural insects and malaria. With continued use they fell into disfavor because their persistence caused them to accumulate in the environment and to affect target and nontarget species. As use of the chlorinated insecticides extended into the late 1960s, their biological accumulation, particularly of DDT, in natural food chains became a major concern. Such accumulation was found to cause reproductive failure in certain predatory species and much was written about its influence on vertebrate reproduction [1,2]. Subsequently, evidence also showed that mice fed dieldrin developed liver tumors in long-term studies [3,4]. However, its ability to cause cancer in other species remains controversial. The evidence that chlorinated hydrocarbon insecticides cause reproductive failure, particularly in predatory birds, led to our studies concerning the influence of dieldrin on the prostate. It is well known that the external secretion of the canine prostate is highly hormone-dependent [5], and it has been used as a means for evaluating the biological potency of hormonal-like compounds [6]. We therefore undertook investigations of possible hormone dieldrin[1] interactions in dogs fed concentrations of the insecticide found in human foods [7,8]. The mammalian toxicity of aldrin and its epoxide, dieldrin, have been reviewed by Hodge and associates [9].

---

[1]Dieldrin is the coined name for the product 1,2,3,4,10,10a-hexachlora-6,7,epoxy-1,4,4a,5,6,7,8,8a-octahydro-1,4,endoexo-5,8-dimethanapthalene. It has been known by other names and a common designation has been HEOD. A pure, odorless white crystalline material, it is stable to the action of alkali and has a melting point of 175–176°C. An oxidation product of aldrin, it is also a metabolite formed by microsomal enzymes from aldrin. It has been described as the most persistent toxic member of the cyclodiene insecticides. Characteristic of chlorinated hydrocarbon insecticides, dieldrin has a very high partition coefficient being over 5000 times more soluble in benzene than in water. It can enter the animal body via the skin, inhalation, or ingestion.

PHARMACOLOGICAL EFFECTS OF DIELDRIN

The organochlorines are less acutely toxic neurotoxins than the organophosphate or carbamate insecticides. Not much is known about dieldrin except that cyclodienes in general are not antienzymes but form complexes in neuromembranes to modify neurological activity. Although there is evidence that cyclodiene toxicity arises from actions on the autonomic nervous system, the consensus is that these agents affect both the central and peripheral nervous systems [1,10]. Studies with labeled dieldrin in blood show that it is found mainly in the plasma and erythrocytes and not in leukocytes, platelets, or stroma. It is bound to plasma albumen and some associates with α-globulins and another protein in blood [11].

METABOLISM OF DIELDRIN

Dieldrin is not readily metabolized and accumulates in body fat [10]. Food chains appear to be the most probable source of exposure but its accumulation in animals can arise via other routes. Much evidence shows that treatment of animals with foreign chemicals including halogenated hydrocarbon insecticides elicits several biochemical responses which include increased drug and steroid hydroxylating enzyme activity in liver microsomes, enhanced liver growth and synthesis of liver microsomal protein, proliferation of hepatic smooth endoplasmic reticulum, and enhanced metabolism of glucose via the glucuronide pathway [12,13]. Peakall and others have observed that injections of 10 ppm of DDT or 2 ppm of dieldrin induce increased rates of steroid metabolism and decreased fertility in birds [14]. Although dieldrin is stored mainly in adipose tissue, epoxides may be metabolized to more hydrophyllic substances such as the dihydrodiols which are conjugated and excreted in the urine. Biliary and fecal excretion of the cyclodienes also occurs [15].

INTERACTIONS OF PESTICIDES AND STEROIDS

According to Kupfer [16], interest in the possible effects of insecticides on steroid metabolism in mammals arose from the finding that the administration of technical grade DDD to dogs produced gross atrophy of the adrenals accompanied by decreased excretion of urinary 17-hydroxycorticoids and the observation that there is a striking similarity between the mixed function oxidase metabolizing enzymes and the steroid hydroxylases. Since most steroid hormones exert their effect in target tissue without prior chemical alteration, it was logical to postulate that the stimulation of microsomal enzyme activity reduced the available concentration of specific steroids for interaction with target tissue. It is not surprising that the evidence led to the hypothesis that the organochlorine insecticides were exerting their effects on reproduction through pathways of drug metabolism. However, our investigations into the possibility that dieldrin may act directly on hormonally dependent tissues came from evidence suggesting that dieldrin was influencing prostatic secretion in dogs at concentrations approximating those found in the human food chain and believed insufficient to stimulate drug-metabolizing activity.

Since the demonstration by Huggins [5] that the secretory rate of the prostate in the dog is highly correlated with androgen levels in the blood, many surgical procedures have been developed in order to test the hormonal properties of drugs in dogs. Our investigations employed this approach in an effort to characterize the effects on the canine prostate caused by steroid compounds and dieldrin when fed simultaneously.

EXPERIMENTS IN DOGS WITH CYSTOPREPUTIOSTOMIES

Adult mongrel dogs weighing 7–16 kg and ranging in age from 16–30 months were surgically modified according to the procedure of Mason et al [17], whereby the bladder neck and the prostatic urether were transected and closed and the inner sheath of the prepuce was sutured to an opening in the fundus of the urinary bladder to serve as an urinary conduit (Fig. 1). After a convalescence of about 2–3 weeks the animals were assigned to dry meal basal diet. The control animals were kept on the basal diet whereas experimental animals were fed the basal diet with 50 μg/kg body weight per day of chlormadinone acetate[2] (CAP) or 15 μg/kg body weight per day of recrystallized dieldrin singly or in combination [18]. CAP has potent anti-androgenic activity. Two separate experiments were

[2]6-chloro-17-acetoxypregna-4,6-diene-3,20-dione.

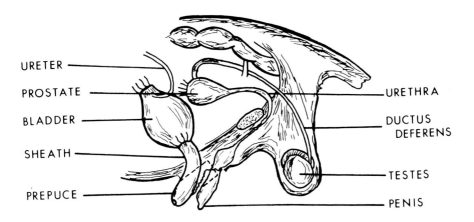

Fig. 1.   Diagram of cystopreputiostomy in dogs.

conducted. Experiment 1 employing 8 dogs began on September 1, 1968, and ended June 1, 1969, while Experiment 2, employing 16 dogs, started September 1, 1969, and lasted through March 21, 1970. Prostatic fluid was collected with the dogs in a standing position during 1-hour periods after 0.7 mg/kg of pilocarpine hydrochloride solution was administered intraveneously. Collections were made twice weekly for the first 3 weeks of each month in both experiments [19,20].

The body weight, food consumption, and general well being of animals exposed to these treatments were not observably changed by dieldrin and/or CAP feeding. Average prostatic fluid volume declined to about 1% of pretreatment volume during the fourth month of CAP feeding and remained so until the end of Experiment 1 (Table I). One animal fed CAP died after the fourth month so that subsequent data for this treatment came from only one animal. However, with CAP and dieldrin combined the decrease in prostatic fluid volume at 4 months was much smaller, being 59% of pretreatment volumes with only a 13% decline thereafter. When these treatments were applied again in Experiment 2, the prostatic fluid volume of CAP-fed dogs declined to 24% of their pretreatment volume during the fourth month of feeding. These reductions were found to be

TABLE I. Prostatic fluid volume as a percent of pretreatment volume in dogs fed 50 μg/kg body weight/day of chlormadinone acetate (CAP) and/or 15 μg/kg body weight/day of dieldrin

Treatment	Pretreatment period	Month number		
		2	3	4
		Experiment 1		
Control (2)[a]	—	100.0 ± 11.8^b	112.0 ± 2.0	124.0 ± 5.0
Dieldrin (2)	100.0 ± 6.0	121.6 ± 7.0	103.7 ± 4.0	114.8 ± 2.0
CAP (2)	100.0 ± 5.0	39.7 ± 4.0^d	$1.0 \pm 0.0^{c,e}$	0.7 ± 0.0^e
CAP + dieldrin (2)	100.0 ± 7.5	76.7 ± 7.0	58.7 ± 8.0	46.0 ± 3.0^d
		Experiment 2		
Control (4)	100.0 ± 15.0	94.0 ± 7.1	96.0 ± 12.0	100.0 ± 8.0
Dieldrin (3)	100.0 ± 20.0	90.0 ± 15.0	112.0 ± 7.0	118.0 ± 6.0
CAP (3)	100.0 ± 12.0	33.0 ± 15.0^d	24.0 ± 11.0^d	27.0 ± 3.0^d
CAP + dieldrin (4)	100.0 ± 16.0	50.0 ± 18.0^d	37.0 ± 15.0^d	41.0 ± 12.5^d

Pretreatment period = 6 weeks.
[a]Number of dogs per treatment group in parentheses.
[b]Each value is the percent of pretreatment volume for six collections ± SE.
[c]Data obtained for only one animal after the fourth month.
[d]$P < 0.05$, significantly different from pretreatment value for the group.
[e]$P < 0.01$.

statistically significant. Dogs fed CAP with dieldrin yielded volumes of prostatic fluid which were 37% of pretreatment volumes and statistical analysis of the 4-month data suggested an interaction between CAP and dieldrin. The acid phosphatase activity of prostatic fluid for control dogs and those fed CAP with dieldrin showed a statistically significant reduction also (Table II). However, in both experiments, total solids, pH, specific gravity, zinc concentrations, and osmolarity of the prostatic fluid showed no significant differences. The interesting finding in both experiments was that the CAP effect on the prostatic fluid volume was lessened when 0.5 ppm of dieldrin were fed simultaneously [19,20].

Animals of Experiment 2 were necropsied. No histological changes attributable to experimental treatment were observed in the liver, adrenal, or pituitary sections. Dieldrin alone at 0.5 ppm did not affect liver size, weight, or histological appearance. The alveolar structure of the prostatic parenchyma was dramatically changed in the medial sections of the central and dorsal lobes of the prostate from animals fed CAP or CAP plus dieldrin. Peripheral areas of these lobes seemed to be unresponsive to the treatment but the acini were slightly to moderately dilated. Prostates from dogs receiving dieldrin alone appeared nor-

TABLE II. Units of acid phosphatase activity/ml in prostatic fluid from dogs fed chlormadinone acetate (CAP) (50 μg/kg body weight) and/or dieldrin (15 μg/kg body weight)

Treatment	Pretreatment period	Month number		
		2	4	6
		Experiment 1		
Control (2)[a]	—	46.6 ± 5.0[b]	45.7 ± 10.0	61.0 ± 10.0
Dieldrin (2)	—	58.8 ± 5.0	77.4 ± 4.0	50.9 ± 10.0
CAP (2)	35.6 ± 5.0	19.0 ± 7.0	—	—
CAP + dieldrin	37.5 ± 5.0	42.8 ± 10.0	13.0 ± 4.0	18.9 ± 5.0
		Experiment 2		
Control (4)	134.6 ± 4.4	152.2 ± 4.7	138.4 ± 4.7	138.4 ± 4.7
Dieldrin (3)	92.5 ± 4.0	52.5 ± 4.7	91.5 ± 6.4	111.7 ± 7.1
CAP (3)	136.0 ± 4.7	65.4 ± 4.4	41.8 ± 4.0	37.5 ± 4.4
CAP + dieldrin (4)	61.2 ± 4.7	27.7 ± 4.2	29.7 ± 4.7	35.8 ± 5.1

Unit = the amount of phosphatase that will liberate 1 mmole of p-nitrophenol per hour under the specified conditions described in Sigma Technical Bulletin No. 104, Sigma Chemical Company, St. Louis, MO.
Pretreatment period = 6 weeks.
[a]Number of dogs per treatment in parentheses.
[b]Each value represents the mean of six determinations ± SE.

mal. In general, control and dieldrin-fed dogs showed normal spermatogenesis and typical testicular histology, whereas dogs receiving CAP and CAP plus dieldrin showed extreme degeneration of the germinal epithelium with complete destruction of spermatogenesis and no spermatozoa in the semiferous tubules or the epididymis (Figs. 2,3). As expected, concentrations of dieldrin were highest in the fat of males on treatment for 6 months and these were directly related to dieldrin intake. In general, the animals fed CAP with dieldrin had slightly higher concentrations of the insecticide than animals on other treatments, but the number of observations was insufficient for a definitive statement [19].

ORGAN CULTURE STUDIES OF PROSTATIC EXPLANTS

Since the concentrations of dieldrin in the feeding experiments were insufficient to cause significant changes in drug metabolizing enzyme activity we undertook organ culture studies to determine direct affects of dieldrin on prostate tissue. For these, V-shaped sections were taken from the right dorsal prostatic lobe of untreated mongrel dogs ranging in age from 9 months to 5 years, and about 1 mg explants of the gland trimmed free of connective tissue were transferred to Petri dishes where they were placed upon the surface of tea-bag paper lying over stainless steel grids and moistened by culturing medium. These were maintained in a humidified atmosphere of 95% air and 5% CO_2 for as long as 6 days. Dieldrin, at a concentration of 1 ppm, did not change the incorporation of progesterone, whereas dieldrin at concentrations of 10 ppm showed significantly decreased progesterone uptake. Dieldrin also inhibited the uptake of testosterone at 10 ppm but not at 1 ppm. The inhibition of testosterone uptake by dieldrin at 10 ppm was not as great as with progesterone at the same concentration. Dieldrin decreased the amount of cellular hypertrophy in explants exposed to progesterone [19].

DIELDRIN AND 5α-DIHYDROTESTOSTERONE[3] BINDING IN THE CYTOSOL AND NUCLEUS OF THE RAT VENTRAL PROSTATE

The androgen which preferentially binds to receptors in the prostate is 5α-dihydrotestosterone (5α-DHT) [21,22]. Fang and Liao [23] showed that the cyproterone acetate[4] is anti-androgenic and antagonizes the effects of 5α-DHT on the prostate in vivo and in vitro. This suggested that various combinations of cyproterone acetate with dieldrin might be useful in studying the binding of dieldrin and 5α-DHT by the rat ventral prostate.

Minced prostate tissues from adult Sprague-Dawley rats (240–350 gm) castrated 24 hours earlier were incubated at 37° for 30 minutes in 5 ml of medium containing tritiated 5α-DHT. Dieldrin (50 μg; 10 ppm) and cyproterone acetate (5 μM) were added to the medium of various treatments in a small volume of

[3]5α-androstan-17β-ol-3-one (5α-DHT).
[4]1,2α-Methylene-6-chloro-$\Delta^{4,6}$-pregnadien-17α-ol-3,20-dion-17α-acetate.

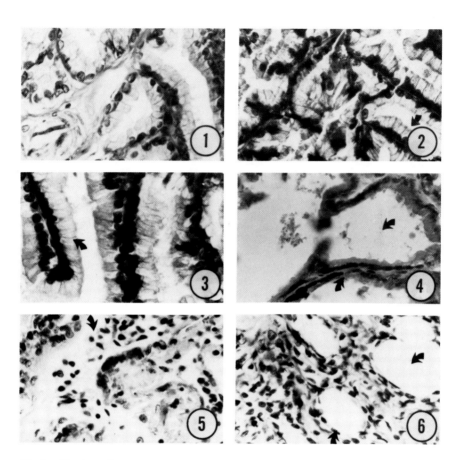

Fig. 2.   Histology of prostate and testes from dogs fed 50 μg/kg body weight/day of chlormadinone acetate and/or 15 μg/kg body weight/day of dieldrin [19]. 1) Prostate tissue from control dog #253 at surgery; 2) Prostate tissue from control dog #253 at necropsy; 3) prostate tissue from dog #257 at surgery prior to treatment; 4) prostate tissue from dog #257 after feeding of CAP for 6 months (Experiment 2) showing low cuboidal to squamous type of secretory epithelial cells and distended lumina; 5) prostate tissue from dog #260 at surgery; 6) prostate tissue from dog #260 after CAP + dieldrin feeding for 6 months. The secretory epithelial cells are reduced in size and the luminae are distended.

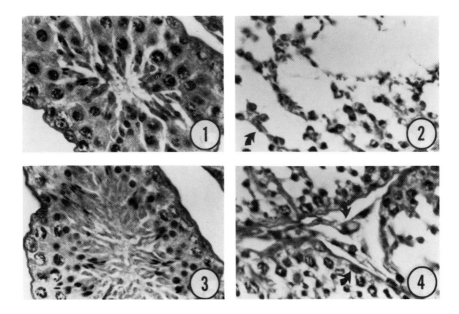

Fig. 3. Histology of prostate and testes from dogs fed 50 µg/kg body weight/day of chlormadinone acetate and/or 15 µg/kg body weight/day of dieldrin [19]. 1) Testicular tissue from dog #A-6 at surgery before treatment; 2) testicular tissue from dog #A-6 after feeding of CAP for 6 months; cellular degeneration is evident and no sperm cells are visible. 3) testicular tissue from dog #A-9 after dieldrin feeding for 6 months. Appearance is normal and sperm cells are visible; 4) testicular tissue from dog #A-6 after CAP feeding for 6 months (Experiment 2). Sperm cells are reduced in number. CAP fed dogs also showed fewer Leidig cells than the control animals.

acetone. After incubation the tissue was washed and homogenized. Purified nuclei were prepared. Samples of cytosol and nuclear extract were passed through Sephadex G-25 gel columns. Bound labelled 5α-DHT was collected in the void volume and free steroid was retained on the column. Cytosol and nuclear binding were assessed and specific activity expressed as DPM per mg protein of the eluted fraction. The cytosol and nuclear extracts were also subjected to enzymatic treatment to determine whether the binding was to protein or some other component. The nuclear membrane was removed with Triton X-100 or mixed detergents as described by Anderson et al [24]. Identical experiments were also conducted with nuclei exposed to a solution of two parts of 10% Tween 80 and one part of 10% deoxycholate [25].

The specific activity of the binding fraction eluted at the void volume of the Sephadex G-25 column showed that dieldrin significantly inhibited binding in both cytosol and nuclear fractions (Table III). Table IV shows the results of a similar series of studies with 4 μM cyproterone acetate in the medium and the percentage inhibition was in agreement with other published data. When cytosol and the nuclear fraction were incubated with Pronase there was a reduction in protein and activity of the binding fractions expressed as a percent of the corresponding control incubated under identical conditions without Pronase (Table V). The reduction in protein and radioactivity was highly significant and there were no significant differences in the effects of Pronase on the cytosol and nuclei. When the cytosol and nuclear fractions were incubated at 20°C for 90 minutes in the absence of enzymes, bound activity dropped as compared to the unheated control (Fig. 4). Both Pronase and lipase caused a large reduction in binding in

TABLE III. Inhibition of [³H]5α-dihydrotestosterone binding in rat ventral prostate by 10 ppm dieldrin

Component	dpm × 10⁻³ᵃ		% Inhibition
	Control	10 ppm Dieldrin	
Cytosol (6)ᵇ	48.2 ± 4.7	30.7 ± 3.3ᶜ	36.6 ± 1.8
Nucleus (7)	41.9 ± 3.5	27.8 ± 3.0ᵈ	33.6 ± 4.0

ᵃSpecific activity, dpm/mg protein of binding fraction eluted at the void volume of Sephadex column. Mean ± SE.
ᵇNumber of experiments in parentheses.
ᶜP < 0.05.
ᵈP < 0.001.

TABLE IV. Inhibition of binding of [³H]5α-dihydrotestosterone in rat ventral prostate by 4 μM cyproterone acetate

Component	dpm × 10⁻³ᵃ		% Inhibition
	Control	Cyproterone acetate	
Cytosol (5)ᵇ	42.6 ± 3.1	18.1 ± 2.7ᶜ	57.4 ± 6.2
Nucleus (4)	37.4 ± 3.9	12.4 ± 2.0ᶜ	67.2 ± 3.8

ᵃSpecific activity, dpm/mg protein of binding fraction eluted at the void volume of Sephadex column. Mean ± SE.
ᵇNumber of experiments in parentheses.
ᶜP < 0.01.

TABLE V. Effect of Pronase incubation on the binding of [³H]5α-DHT in the rat ventral prostate

	Percent of control ± SE[a]	
	Protein[b]	Radioactivity[b]
Cytosol (7)[c]	23.5 ± 3.8	9.1 ± 1.6
Nucleus (4)	29.3 ± 5.1	12.8 ± 3.6

[a]Control samples incubated for 90 minutes at 26°C.
[b]Percent of control after incubation for 90 minutes at 26°C with 100 μg/ml Pronase. Mean ± SE.
[c]Number of experiments in parentheses.

the cytosol fraction while DNase and RNase did not reduce binding significantly. The effects for nuclear fractions were qualitatively similar. Nuclei showed larger loss of bound radioactivity than the cytosol and DNase and RNase tended to further reduce binding with incubation at 26°C for 90 minutes. However, the reductions in bound radioactivity with Pronase and lipase were still greater. When the nuclear membrane was removed by detergent washing after incubation with dieldrin or 5α-DHT, the radioactivity associated with the nuclear fraction showed a larger percentage reduction. This was interpreted as evidence that dieldrin was preferentially associated with the nuclear membrane (Fig. 5).

Since the degree of binding inhibition was the same in both cytosol and nuclear fractions the evidence suggested that the effects were on the first stage of steroid binding believed to be temperature independent in cytosol and followed subsequently by a temperature-dependent transfer of the hormone protein complex into the nucleus [26]. An effect upon the plasma or nuclear membrane was not excluded, however. Although the separation of free and bound activity by gel filtration had been established as a method of choice for measurement of sex steroid binding protein interaction [22,27–29], the inhibition of cytosol and nuclear binding of 5α-DHT by cyproterone as measured in these studies agreed closely with the previous reports on the effect of this anti-androgen on the formation of 5α-DHT protein complexes in cytosol [20] and nuclei [23,31] of the rat prostate. Susceptibility of the binding fraction to Pronase and its resistance to hydrolysis by DNase and RNase supported the assumption that the binding was due predominantly to an interaction with cellular protein in agreement with Bruchovsky and Wilson [22] and Mainwaring [27,28]. The results of the detergent washing of nuclei labeled with C¹⁴-dieldrin and tritated 5α-DHT gave support to the hypothesis that the binding fraction may be associated with the nuclear membrane. The reduction of 5α-DHT associated with nuclei after the removal of the nuclear membrane by detergent washing suggested that the pro-

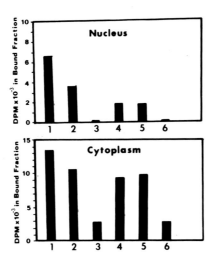

Fig. 4. Effect of incubation with hydrolytic enzymes on the cytoplasmic and nuclear binding of [1,2-³H]5α-dihydrostosterone. Treatments: 1) Nonincubated control; 2) incubated control, 26°C, 90 minutes; 3) 26°C, 90 minutes, 100 μg/ml Pronase; 4) 26°C, 90 minutes, 100 μg/ml RNase; 5) 26°C, 90 minutes, 100 μg/ml DNase; 6) 26°C, 90 minutes, 100 μg/ml lipase [25].

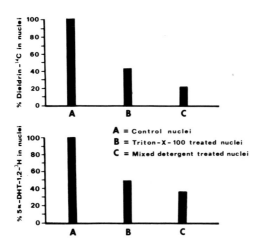

Fig. 5. Effects of Triton X-100 and mixed detergents on the binding of [1,2-³H]5α-dihydrotestosterone and [¹⁴C]dieldrin by prostate nuclei. The mixed detergent contained 2 parts of 10% Tween 80 and 1 part of 10% sodium deoxycholate [25].

cedure may have ruptured a significant portion of the nuclei releasing bound 5α-DHT into the soluble fraction. The possibility that a significant portion of the bound 5α-DHT was associated with nuclear membrane, however, was not excluded by our results and involvement of lipid in the binding was strongly indicated by the decrease in binding with detergent washing and lipase. Special precautions had been taken to assure that the lipase used in these studies was not contaminated by proteolytic enzymes [25].

INHIBITION OF 5α-DIHYDROTESTOSTERONE BINDING IN THE RAT VENTRAL PROSTATE BY DIELDRIN AND o,p'-DDT [32]

When cytosol fractions from the prostate of rats were incubated in the presence of 0.4 M KCl with C^{14}-dieldrin or o,p' C^{14} DDT and subjected to sucrose density gradient analyses, a binding peak sedimenting at the same distance from the origin as 5α-(^{3}H)-DHT was demonstrated (Fig. 6A) [32]. Polyacrylamide gel electrophoresis of similarly labeled cytosol showed that radioactivity of 5α(^{3}H)-DHT, (^{14}C) dieldrin, or o,p' (^{14}C) DDT migrated an identical distance in the gel. Sucrose density gradient analyses of cytosols showed that dieldrin and o,p'-DDT strongly inhibited binding of 5α-DHT by the 3.5S region. o,p'-DDT reduced binding by 80% at a concentration of 1.4×10^{-5} M (5 ppm), whereas the same percentage reduction in binding with dieldrin required a concentration of $2.6–3.9 \times 10^{-5}$ M (10–15 ppm) (Fig. 6B). Cyproterone acetate had no effect on the 3.5S binding which could be saturated by concentrations of 5α-DHT to 10^{-7} M. Similar 3.5S binding fractions for 5α-DHT were also present in serum and in liver and kidney cytosol. Thus the 3.5S binding peak was nonspecific and not characteristic of the high affinity specific hormone receptor in the prostate. Prior to our work, Mainwaring [27,28] reported a region of nonspecific binding at 3.5S and a region of specific binding at 8S in sucrose density gradient analysis of prostate cytosol incubated with 5α-DHT without 0.4 M KCl. Our evidence also showed these two binding regions in the rat prostate cytosol (Fig. 6B). Binding in the 8S region was abolished by parahydroxy-mercuribenzoate and was greatly reduced by cyproterone acetate. These two agents had little effect on slower 3.5S peak. We confirmed that the 3.5S peak was nonspecific and that the 8S peak represented specific binding. Increasing concentrations of 5α-DHT showed increased binding in the 3.5S region linearly with steroid concentrations up to 4.3×10^{-8} M, whereas binding in the 8S region was saturated at 2.4×10^{-8} (Fig. 7A).

At a concentration of 2.8×10^{-5} M (10 ppm) o,p'-DDT inhibited binding by 60% in the presence of a saturating concentration of 5α-DHT. The available concentration of 8S receptor was 2.4 and 2.9×10^{-10} mole/gm of cytosol protein in two control experiments and was reduced to 1.5×10^{-11} mole/gm in the presence of 2.8×10^{-5} or 10 ppm o,p'-DDT. When labeled o,p'-DDT

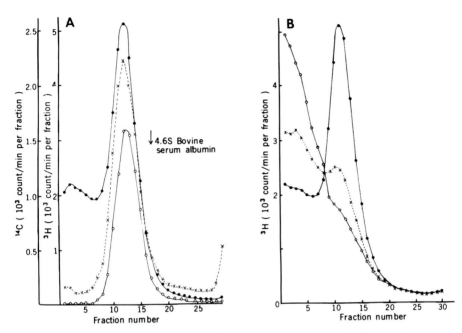

Fig. 6. A) The 3.5S binding protein for 5α-[³H]DHT in rat prostate cytosol. Prostates from rats castrated 24 hours previously were homogenized in three volumes of ice-cold HEPES (N–2–hydroxyethylpiperazine-N′–2–ethanesulfonic acid) buffer, pH 7.4, containing 1.5 mM EDTA and 2.0 mM mercaptoethanol (HEM). The cytosol fraction, prepared by centrifugation of the homogenate at 105,000g for 1 hour at 0°C, was mixed with an equal volume of HEM containing 0.8 M KCl and either 5α-[³H]DHT (●), or o,p′-[¹⁴C]DDT (X), or [¹⁴C]dieldrin (○), and held overnight at –20°C. After the mixture was thawed, 0.2 ml of each cytosol was analyzed by centrifugation on a linear sucrose gradient (5–15%), made up in HEM and containing 0.4 M KCl. Gradients were centrifuged at 45,000 rpm for 19 hours at 0°C (SW-50.1 rotor; Beckman L2-65B centrifuge). Sedimentation is from left to right in all cases. The position of bovine serum albumin is included as a marker. B) The effect of dieldrin and o,p′-DDT on the binding of 5α-[³H]DHT by the 3.5S fraction of rat prostate cytosol. The procedure was that described above except that all samples contained 5α-[³H]DHT and either 5 μl of ethanol (●), 5 μl of ethanol containing 2.6×10^{-5} M dieldrin (X), or 5 μl of ethanol containing 2.8×10^{-5} M o,p′-DDT (○). These molar concentrations correspond to 10 ppm for the insecticides.

replaced tritiated 5α-DHT in the incubation medium a peak of radioactivity was found in the 8S region.

Dieldrin in concentrations as high as 2.6×10^{-5} M (10 ppm) produced no significant inhibition of 5α-DHT binding in the 8S region in the presence of saturating concentrations of 5α-DHT. The binding of labeled dieldrin in the 8S

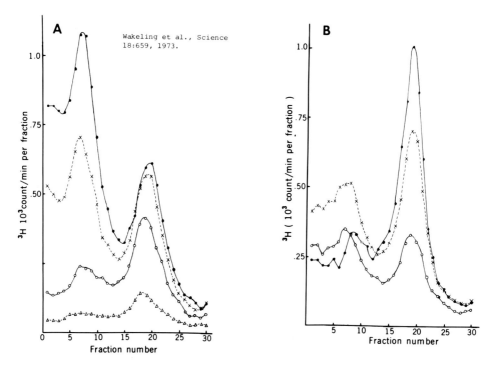

Fig. 7. A) The effect of increasing concentration of 5α-[³H]DHT on binding to rat prostate cytosol. Prostates were homogenized manually in an all-glass apparatus at 4°C in the cold room, in three volumes of 0.02 M phosphate buffer, pH 7.4, containing 1.5 mM EDTA and 2.0 mM mercaptoethanol (PEM). Cytosol was prepared as described (Fig. 6A). Portions of the cytosol were incubated with increasing concentrations of 5α-[³H]DHT added in 5 μl of ethanol. After incubation for 2 hours at 0°C, 0.2-ml portions were mixed with an equal volume of dextran-charcoal solution (0.25% dextran and 2.5% charcoal in PEM buffer) to remove unbound steroid. The charcoal was removed by centrifugation, and 0.2-ml portions of the supernatant were placed on linear sucrose gradients (5–20%) prepared in PEM buffer. The gradients were centrifuged at 30,000 rpm (SW-50.1 rotor) for 20 hours at 0°C, to give a sedimentation approximately one half that described in Fig. 6A and B. The total steroid concentrations were 4.3×10^{-8} M (●), 2.4×10^{-8} M (X), 5.9×10^{-9} M (○), and 1.4×10^{-9} M (△). B) The effect of o,p′-DDT upon binding of 5α-[³H]DHT by rat prostate cytosol. The procedure was that described above for samples containing 5α-[³H]DHT and 5 μl of ethanol, control (●), or 5 μl of ethanol containing o,p′-DDT to give a final concentration of 5.6×10^{-6} M (X) or 2.8×10^{-5} M (○).

region was detected after incubation of prostatic cytosol. However, in studies with a constant concentration (2.6×10^{-5} M, 10 ppm) of dieldrin and increasing concentrations of 5α-DHT, the available receptor concentration was reduced to 3.1×10^{-11} mole/gm cytosol protein compared to control.

The sucrose density gradient measurements of 5α-DHT binding to the specific receptor agreed with Agarose gel chromatography published by Notides et al [33]. The available receptor concentration of rat prostate cytosol measured by this technique was 1.2×10^{-10} mole/gm cytosol protein. This was significantly depressed by both dieldrin and o,p'-DDT, the inhibition being greater for o,p'-DDT. The association constant for prostate 8S 5α-DHT receptor was 2.0 and 1.9×10^{-9} M^{-1} as measured by sucrose density gradient and Agarose gel chromatography, respectively. These values were comparable to the various estimates for binding of 5α-DHT in rat epidydimis and for estradiol-17β in the uterus [34].

Thus our studies gave further evidence that chlorinated hydrocarbon insecticides inhibit binding of 5α-DHT to its specific receptor in the rat prostate cytosol. The results were characteristic of noncompetitive inhibition and probably resulted from a conformational change of the receptor protein induced by the insecticides. Direct competition of o,p'-DDT and dieldrin for hormone binding sites could not be excluded because of the concentrations of insecticides used relative to 5α-DHT.

The combination of studies that we carried out with dieldrin feeding and in vitro gave evidence that stimulation of liver microsomal steroid hydroxylase enzyme was not the complete explanation for the effects on reproduction seen when chlorinated insecticide are administered.

Chlorinated hydrocarbon insecticides have been shown to have both hormonal and antihormonal activity [1]. o,p'-DDT shows estrogenic activity in rats [35] and chickens [36], while evidence of interrupted estrous in rats has been obtained with aldrin [37]. o,p'-DDD, a metabolite of o,p'-DDT, produces atrophy of the zona fasciculata and zona reticularis of the adrenal cortex [38] and suppression of 17-hydroxycorticoid secretion [39]. It has been used in the treatment of adrenal corticoid carcinoma [40], Cushing syndrome [41], and cancer of the breast and prostate [42]. Administration of DDT has caused suppressed reproductive activity in male dogs [43] and retarded testicular growth and development of secondary facial characteristics in young cockerels [44,45]. Men exposed to organochlorine insecticides showed depression in sexual functions with return to normal after treatment with testosterone [46]. The influence of dieldrin and DDT on accumulation and biotransformation of testosterone by liver and sexual accessory glands of rodents have been studied extensively [47–50].

Our investigations were conducted in the early 1970s and little work appears to have been done to extend these observations. Part of the lack of interest in these particular agents probably stems from banning of their general use by regulatory agencies. More precise knowledge of their mechanisms of interaction remains for future investigations. Details of our experiments are given in other published reports [19,20,25,32].

ACKNOWLEDGMENTS

This research was partially supported by Grant ES 00094 of the Division of Environmental Health Sciences, U.S. Public Health Service and Toxicology Training Grant ES 00098 of the U.S. Public Health Service.

REFERENCES

1. Ecobichon D J: Clorinated hydrocarbon insecticides: Recent animal data of potential significance for man. Can Med Assoc J 103:711–716, 1970.
2. Dustman E H, Stickel L F: The occurrence and significance of pesticide residues in wild animals. Ann NY Acad Sci 160:162–172, 1969.
3. National Cancer Institute: Bioassays of aldrin and dieldrin for possible carcinogenicity. Tech Rep Ser No. 21, Washington, DC: DHEW Publication No. (NIH) 78-821, 1978.
4. National Cancer Institute: Bioassay of dieldrin for possible carcinogenicity. Tech Rep Ser No. 22, Washington, DC: DHEW Publication No. (NIH) 78-822, 1978.
5. Huggins C, Clark P J: Quantitative studies of prostatic secretion. II. The effect of castration and of estrogen injections on the normal and on the hyperplastic prostate glands of dogs. J Exp Med 72:747–762, 1940.
6. Rosenkrantz H, Mason M M: Bioevaluation of estrogenic compounds by the canine prostatic secretion method. Cancer Chemother Rep 20:33–39, 1962.
7. Robinson J, McGill A E J: Organochlorine insecticide residues in complete prepared meals in Great Britain during 1965. Nature 212:1037–1038, 1966.
8. Martinez-Manautou J, Maqueo-Topette M: Progestational and endometrial activity of 6 halo and 6 methyl derivatives of 17α-acetoxy progesterone. First Annual Meeting of the Mexican Society of Nutrition and Endocrinology, SanMiguel de Allende, Mexico, 1960.
9. Hodge H C, Boyce A M, Deichmann W B, Kraybill H F: Toxicology and no-effect levels of aldrin and dieldrin. Toxicol Appl Pharmacol 10:613–675, 1967.
10. O'Brien R D: Insecticides: Action and Metabolism. New York: Academic Press, 1967.
11. Hathway D E: The biochemistry of dieldrin and telodrin. A review of recent investigations related to the toxicity of these compounds in mammals. Arch Environ Health 11:380–383, 1965.
12. Gillette J R, Conney A H, Cosmides G F, Estabrooks R W, Fonts J R, Mannering G J (eds): Microsomes and Drug Oxidations. London: Academic Press, 1969.
13. LaDu B N, Mandel H G, Way E L: Fundamentals of Drug Metabolism and Drug Disposition. Baltimore: Williams and Wilkins Co., 1971.
14. Peakall D B: Pesticide-induced enzyme breakdown of steroids in birds. Nature 216:505–506, 1967.
15. Cole J F, Klevay L M, Zavon M R: Endrin and dieldrin: A comparison of hepatic excretion in the rat. Toxicol Appl Pharmacol 16:547–555, 1970.
16. Kupfer D: Influence of chlorinated hydrocarbons and organophosphate insecticides on metabolism of steroids. Ann NY Acad Sci 160:244–253, 1969.
17. Mason M M, Keefe F, Boria T: Specialized surgery of the canine bladder and prostate gland. J Am Vet Med Assoc 139:1007–1015, 1961.
18. Shane B S, Dunn H O, Kenney R M, Hansel W, Visek W J: Methyl testosterone-induced female pseudohermaphroditism in dogs. Biol Reprod 1:41–48, 1969.
19. Blend M J: In vivo and in vitro effect of low concentrations of dieldrin and steroid hormones on the dog prostate. Ph.D. Thesis, Cornell University, Ithaca, New York, 1970.
20. Blend M J, Visek W. J: Effects of low concentrations of dieldrin and chlormadinone acetate on canine prostatic fluid. Toxicol Appl Pharmacol 23:344–348, 1972.
21. Anderson K M, Liao S: Selective retention of dihydrotestosterone by prostatic nuclei. Nature 219:277–279, 1968.

22. Bruchovsky N, Wilson J D: The intranuclear binding of testosterone and 5α-androstan-17β-ol-3–one by rat prostate. J Biol Chem 243:5953–5960, 1968.

23. Fang S, Liao S: Antagonistic action of anti-androgens on the formation of a specific dihydro-testosterone-receptor protein complex in rat ventral prostate. Mol Pharmacol 5:428–431, 1969.

24. Anderson K M, Lee R M, Miyai K: Effects of androgen in vivo on some properties of isolated rat ventral prostate nuclei. Exp Cell Res 61:371–378, 1970.

25. Wakeling A E, Schmidt T J, Visek W J: Effects of dieldrin on 5α-dihydrotestosterone binding in the cytosol and nucleus of the rat ventral prostate. Toxicol Appl Pharmacol 25:267–275, 1973.

26. Jensen E V, Suzuki T, Kawashima T, Stumpf W E, Jungblut P W, Desombre E R: A two-step mechanism for the interaction of estradiol with rat uterus. Proc Natl Acad Sci USA 59:632–638, 1968.

27. Mainwaring W I P: The binding of [1,2-³H]-testosterone with nuclei of the rat prostate. J Endocrinol 44:323–333, 1969.

28. Mainwaring W I P: A soluble androgen receptor in the cytoplasm of rat prostate. J Endocrinol 45:531–541, 1969.

29. Puca G A, Nola E, Sica V, Bresciani F: Estrogen-binding proteins of calf uterus. Partial purification and preliminary characterization of two cytoplasmic proteins. Biochemistry 10:3769–3779, 1971.

30. Baulieu E E, Jung I: A prostatic cytosol receptor. Biochem Biophys Res Commun 38:599–606, 1970.

31. Fang S, Anderson K M, Liao L: Receptor proteins for androgens: on the role of specific proteins in selective retention of 17β-hydroxy-5α-androstan-3–one by rat ventral prostate in vivo and in vitro. J Biol Chem 244:6584–6595, 1969.

32. Wakeling A E, Visek W J: Insecticide inhibition of 5α-dihydrotestosterone binding in the rat ventral prostate. Science 181:659–661, 1973.

33. Notides A C, Hamilton D E, Rudolf J H: Estrogen-binding proteins of the human uterus. Biochem Biophys Acta 271:214–224, 1972.

34. Sanborn B M, Rao B R, Korenman S G: Interaction of 17-estradiol and its specific uterine receptor. Evidence for complex kinetic and equilibrium behavior. Biochemistry 10:4955–4962, 1971.

35. Welch R M, Levin W, Conney A H: Estrogenic action of DDT and its analogues. Toxicol Appl Pharmacol 14:358–367, 1969.

36. Bitman J, Cecil H C, Harris S J, Fries G F: Estrogenic activity of o,p′-DDT in the mammalian uterus and avian oviduct. Science 162:371–374, 1968.

37. Ball W L, Kay K, Sinclair J W: Observations on toxicity of aldrich. I. Growth and estrus in rat. Arch Ind Hyg 7:292–300, 1953.

38. Cazorla A, Moncloa F: Action of 1,1 dichloro–2–p–chlorophenyl–2–o–chlororphenylethane on dog adrenal cortex. Science 136:47, 1962.

39. Cueto C, Brown J H U: The chemical fractionation of an adrenocorticolytic drug. Endocrinology 62:326–333, 1958.

40. Bergenstal D M, Hertz R, Lipsett M B, Moy R H: Chemotherapy of adrenocortical cancer with o,p′-DDD. Ann Intern Med 53:672–682, 1960.

41. Southren A L, Tochimoto S, Strom L, Ratuschni A, Ross H, Gordon G: Remission in Cushing's syndrome with o,p′-DDD. J Clin Endocrinol 26:268–278, 1966.

42. Zimmermann B, Bloch H S, Williams W L, Hitchcock C R, Hoelscher B: Effect of DDD on the human adrenal. Cancer 9:940–948, 1956.

43. Deichmann W B, MacDonald W E, Beasley A G, Cubit D: Subnormal reproduction in beagle dogs induced by DDT and aldrin. Ind Med Surg 40:10–20, 1971.

44. Burlington H, Lindeman V F: Effect of DDT on testes and secondary sex characteristics of white leghorn cockerels. Proc Soc Exp Biol Med 74:48–51, 1950.

45. Ecobichon D J, Saschenbrecker P W: Pharmacodynamic study of DDT in cockerels. Can J Physiol Pharmacol 46:785–794, 1968.

46. Espir M L E, Hall J W, Shirreffs J G, Stevens D L: Impotence in farm workers using toxic chemicals. Br Med J 1:423–425, 1970.

47. Thomas J A, Lloyd J W, Smith M T, Mawhinney M G, Smith C G: Effect of dieldrin on the accumulation and biotransformation of radioactive testosterone by the mouse prostate gland. Toxicol Appl Pharmacol 26:523–531, 1973.

48. Schein L G, Thomas J A: Effects of dieldrin on the uptake and metabolism of testosterone-1,2-^{3}H by rodent sex accessory organs. Environ Res 9:26–31, 1975.

49. Schein L G, Thomas J A: Dieldrin and parathion interaction in the prostate and liver of the mouse. J Toxicol Environ Health 1:829–838, 1976.

50. Smith M T, Thomas J A, Smith C G, Mawhinney M G, Lloyd J W: Effects of DDT on radioactive uptake from testosterone-1,2-^{3}H by mouse prostate glands. Toxicol Appl Pharmacol 23:159–161, 1972.

The Prostatic Cell: Structure and Function
Part B, pages 183–190
© 1981 Alan R. Liss, Inc., 150 Fifth Avenue, New York, NY 10011

Aryl Hydrocarbon Hydroxylase Induction and Binding of Dimethylbenz(a)anthracene in Human Prostate

Myong Won Kahng, Mary W. Smith, and Benjamin F. Trump

INTRODUCTION

Spontaneous adenocarcinoma of the prostate is the most common malignant neoplasm in the adult male. Despite the importance of this disease there are no entirely satisfactory animal models at present time. In our laboratory, we reported details of a technique for maintenance of human prostate tissue in explant culture [1] and in vitro responses of normal human prostate to MNNG [2]. Explant and monolayer epithelial cell cultures of human prostate contained constitutive levels of AHH which was inducible by pre-exposure to PAH [3].

AHH converts procarcinogenic PAH to electrophiles that eventually bind to cellular informational molecules, DNA, RNA, and/or proteins during carcinogenesis [4]. Response of AHH to preexposure to BA, DMBA, and MNNG in human prostate in culture and the binding of DMBA to DNA were studied. The binding of DMBA to the target tissue was correlated to the binding of BP to DNA of monocytes, readily accessible cells, isolated from the blood of the same patient. The correlation, it is hoped, may prove useful in determining the host-risk factor for susceptibility to prostatic cancer in humans.

The role of environmental PAH in the etiology of prostatic cancer is not known. If it can be shown that human prostatic tissues are capable of metabolizing carcinogenic PAH and that the electrophilic metabolites of such PAH bind to the DNA of prostatic epithelial cells which may result in the ultimate cellular transformation, it would be reasonable to suggest that environment and occupation could be important factors in the etiology of prostatic cancer.

Abbreviations used: AHH, aryl hydrocarbon hydroxylase; PAH, polycyclic aromatic hydrocarbons; BP, benzo(a)pyrene; 3-OHBP, 3-hydroxybenzo(a)pyrene; BA, benz(a)anthracene; DMBA, 7,12-dimethylbenz(a)anthracene; MNNG, N-methyl-N′-nitro-N-nitrosoguanidine; BPH, benign prostatic hyperplasia.

MATERIALS AND METHODS

Source of Tissue and Blood

Normal prostate of young adults was obtained from the immediate autopsy program [5] following accidental death. Blood was drawn from the same patient at the time of immediate autopsy. Tissues from BPH and prostatic carcinoma were obtained by surgery

Culture of Explant and Epithelial Cells

Tissues transported in Leibowitz medium were cut into 1mm × 1mm × 10mm strips and cultured in CMRL-1066 medium on rocker platforms [1]. For epithelial cell culture, the prostate tissue strips were minced fine and cultured in CMRL-1066 as monolayers [3].

AHH Assay

Explant cultures of prostate were treated with 10 μg BA/ml medium for 24 hours and epithelial cells were treated with BA, DMBA, or MNNG at a concentration of 5 μg/ml medium for 24 hours [3]. Tissues and cells were harvested and homogenized in 0.1 M phosphate buffer. The 600g supernatant fractions were assayed for AHH activity. AHH activity was measured by fluorometric measurement of 3-OHBP production [6,7] with an NADPH-regenerating system. One unit of AHH activity is defined as the amount of enzyme that catalyzes the formation of one nmole of phenolic product in 1 hour.

Carcinogen Binding to DNA

Monolayer culture of prostatic epithelial cells were exposed to ^{3}H-DMBA (S.A. 42 Ci/mmole) at a dose of 10 μCi/ml medium for 48 hours. Monocytes were isolated by Ficoll-Paque gradient centrifugation [8], cultured in CMRL-1066 medium for 24 hours, and exposed to ^{3}H-BP (S.A. 37 Ci/mmole) at a dose of 10 μCi/ml medium for 48 hours. Both prostatic epithelial cells and monocytes were harvested and DNA was isolated [9,10]. An aliquot of the DNA fraction was counted for radioactivity and another aliquot was assayed for DNA content(11).

RESULTS

Induction of AHH

Effect of BA treatment on AHH activity. AHH was present in all the prostate specimens studied and it was inducible by preexposure to BA (Fig. 1). In three explants of human prostate from BPH, the constitutive levels of

AHH INDUCTION

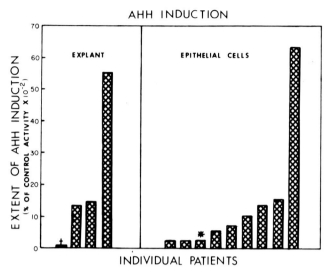

Fig. 1. AHH Induction by BA. Human prostate (BPH) was treated with BA, 10 μg/ml medium for explant cultures and 5 μg/ml medium for epithelial cell cultures for 24 hours. Extent of induction is expressed as percent of control activity. †: Carcinoma of the prostate; *: normal prostate from an accident victim obtained at immediate autopsy.

AHH ranged from 0.13–0.65 units/mg DNA. Pretreatment of these tissues with 10 μg BA/ml medium for 24 hours resulted in the increases in AHH activity by 1300–5500% of control level (left hand panel of Fig. 1).

The AHH in explant culture from carcinoma of the prostate (indicated by a cross above the bar, Fig. 1) was not induced by preexposure to BA, although the basal AHH activity was comparable to those from BPH.

Outgrowth of epithelial cells from minced tissue pieces of prostatic tissue was greater than 90% pure, as judged by light microscopy. Cells grown from one normal prostate from a 20-year-old patient (indicated by an asterisk above the bar on the right hand panel of Fig. 1) and from eight BPH specimens contained constitutive levels of AHH ranging from 0.03–0.20 units/mg protein. Exposure of cells to 5μg of BA/ml medium for 24 hours caused increases in AHH activity in all specimens resulting in the induction of 200–6300% of control activity.

The differential effect of BA and DMBA on inducing AHH was compared on the same epithelial cell preparations (Fig. 2). In all four cases studied, AHH induction by BA treatment was always higher, 1.7- to 10-fold, than those by DMBA treatment. MNNG, known to be a direct-acting carcinogen

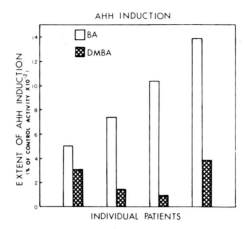

Fig. 2. AHH Induction by BA and DMBA. Outgrowth of epithelial cells from human prostate (BPH) was treated with BA or DMBA at 5 μg/ml medium for 24 hours. The extent of AHH induction is expressed as percent of control.

[12], had no inducing effect on AHH, although BA treatment caused 3- to 63-fold induction of AHH in the same epithelial cell preparations (Fig. 3).

Binding of Carcinogens to DNA

Preliminary studies on the binding of ^{3}H-DMBA to DNA of prostatic epithelial cells and the binding of ^{3}H-BP to DNA monocytes from the same patient are shown in Table I. These specimens are from normal prostates collected at immediate autopsies. The binding of ^{3}H-DMBA in three patients were 0.85, 1.50, and 1.54 pmoles of ^{3}H-DMBA/mg DNA. In the monocyte samples, two out of three showed detectable binding of ^{3}H-BP.

DISCUSSION

Human prostatic epithelium contained constitutive levels of AHH activity comparable to other human tissues [13, 14] and tissues of animal origin [6]. The variability in constitutive levels of AHH was five- to sevenfold in human prostate, which is similar to the ranges reported for human bronchus [14], and monocyte [14] and human liver [13] where approximately 10- to 20-fold variations have been recorded.

BA is a very potent inducer of AHH [15] in numerous experimental systems. Human prostate AHH was no exception in this regard. The ranges and the variabilies in AHH induction by BA were similar to those reported for other tissues [6, 16]. This interindividual variation of AHH inducibility is a genetically predetermined factor [17] which is related to individual differences in drug metabolism and carcinogen susceptibility.

AHH INDUCTION

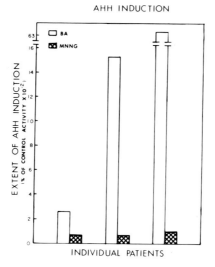

Fig. 3 AHH Induction by BA and MNNG. Outgrowth of epithelial cells from prostate (BPH) was treated with BA and MNNG at 5 μg/ml medium for 24 hours. The extent of induction is expressed as percent of control.

TABLE 1. Binding of Carcinogen to DNA*

Patient No.	Prostate[a]	Monocyte[b]
1	1.54	0.90
2	0.85	61.2
3	1.50	ND[c]

*Normal prostate tissue and monocytes were from the same patient.
[a]^{3}H-7,12-Dimethylbenz(a)anthracene, pmoles bound per mg DNA.
[b]^{3}H-Benzo(a)pyrene, fmoles bound per 10^6 cells.
[c]Not detectable.

DMBA was less effective in induction and the induction ratios for DMBA were always less than those of BA. There is no apparent correlation between the activity of a compound as an inducer and its carcinogenic potency. Since it is known that DMBA can be quite toxic to the cells [15], the dose (5 μg/ml medium) we used may have exerted toxic effects on the prostatic epithelium.

Morphological evidence of neoplastic transformation in normal human prostate by MNNG in explant culture was recently reported [2]. However, MNNG is a direct-acting carcinogen not requiring metabolic activation [12] and would not be expected to induce AHH at the dose (5 μg/ml medium) which produces morphological changes.

It might be argued that prostatic epithelial cells grown from BPH tissue might not be representative of normal tissue. However, it is known that BPH tissues behave more like normal prostatic epithelium in their metabolic behavior. BPH tissue accumulates and secretes citrate as does normal tissue; prostatic cancer cells accumulate citrate to a far lesser extent [18]. In the present study, moreover, the consititutive levels of AHH and the inducibilities were comparable to that of normal prostate collected at the immediate autopsy. In view of the great difficulties in obtaining human tissue, there seems to be no valid biochemical criterion for rejecting BPH specimens at the present time.

The covalent binding of PAH to cellular macromolecules is considered to be an essential part of their carcinogenic action [4]. The metabolism and binding of DMBA have been reported in hepatic and various extrahepatic tissues of experimental animals [19]. Intravenous injection of DMBA in castrated mice, rats, and hamsters has been shown to induce adenocarcinoma of the prostate [20]. The present report is the first in demonstrating the binding of DMBA in normal prostatic epithelium. The presence and the inducibility of AHH, together with the binding of DMBA to DNA following bioactivation via AHH, indicate that the human prostate is susceptible to environmental carcinogens and that, in addition to hormonal [21] and dietary factors [22], environmental and occupational factors might contribute to the etiology of human prostatic cancer.

The determination of the potential susceptibility of the individual and thus the evaluation of host-risk factor would be a very important approach in preventing cancer morbidity. To this end, we have an ongoing program in which the binding of carcinogen to monocytes (which would be readily available from the population for screening, if needed) are correlated with the binding of the same class of carcinogen in potential target tissues (prostate, bronchus, etc) from the same patient. The human tissues are obtained from young males at the immediate autopsy, a program in our department in which normal human tissues are obtained within 30 minutes of somatic death. The data, necessarily, are accumulating slowly and it is too early to predict what type of a correlative pattern might emerge. It is hoped that the accumulation of data in adequate amounts for statistical analysis and examination of the data in conjunction with epidemiological information would lead to means for evaluating the potential occupational or environment risk for an individual for cancer in a given tissue by the examination of readily accessible cells, ie, monocytes, from the same individual.

CONCLUSIONS

The human prostatic epithelium contained measureable constitutive levels of AHH and the enzyme was inducible by the two PAH, BA and DMBA. The extent of AHH induction by DMBA was much less than that by BA.

MNNG, a direct acting carcinogen, was not effective in inducing AHH. Significant binding of ^{3}H-DMBA to DNA in normal human prostatic epithelium was observed. These results indicate that human prostate contains the enzymatic machinery to activate carcinogenic PAH to electrophiles which bind to DNA and other informational molecules resulting in eventual cellular transformation. Thus, environmental and occupational factors might contribute to the etiology of human prostatic cancer.

ACKNOWLEDGMENTS

This work was supported in part by Public Health Service Grant CA 15798-07.

REFERENCES

1. Sanefuji H, Heatfield BM, Trump BF: Studies on carcinogenesis of human prostate. I. Technique for long-term explant culture. Tiss Cult Assoc Manual 4:855–885, 1978.
2. Sanefuji H, Heatfield BM, Trump BF: Studies on carcinogenesis of human prostate. V. Effects of the carcinogen N-methyl-N'-nitrosoguanidine (MNNG) on normal prostate during long-term explant culture. SEM/1979/part III:657–663, 1979.
3. Kahng MW, Liu W, Sanefuji H, Resau JH, Heatfield BM, Trump BF: Aryl hydrocarbon hydroxylase in human prostate. Chem-Biol Interactions 34:249–256, 1981.
4. Miller EC, Miller JA: Biochemical mechanisms of chemical carcinogenesis. In Busch H (ed): Molecular Biology of Cancer. New York: Academic Press, 1974, pp 377–402.
5. Trump BF, Valigorsky JM, Jones RT, Mergner WJ, Garcia JH, Cowley RA: The application of electron microscopy and cellular biochemistry to the autopsy: Observations on cellular changes in human shock. Hum Pathol 6:499–516, 1975.
6. Kahng MW, Jones RT, Trump BF: Induction and properties of aryl hydrocarbon hydroxylase in bovine pancreatic ducts. J Natl Cancer Inst 62:1251–1255, 1979.
7. Nebert DW, Gelboin HV: Substrate-inducible microsomal aryl hydroxylase in mammalian cell culture. I. Assay and properties of induced enzyme. J Biol Chem 243:6242–6249, 1968.
8. Bast RC Jr, Whitlock JP Jr, Miller H, Rapp HJ, Gelboin HV: Aryl hydrocarbon (benzo(a)pyrene) hydroxylase in human peripheral blood monocytes. Nature 250:664–665, 1974.
9. Belan FA, Dooley KL, Casciano DA: Rapid isolation of carcinogen bound DNA and RNA by hydroxyapatite chromatography. J Chromatogr 174:177–186, 1979.
10. Shoyab M: Binding of polycyclic aromatic hydrocarbons to DNA of cells in culture: A rapid method for its analysis using hydroxyapatite column chromatography. Chem-Biol Interactions 25:71–85, 1979.
11. Kissane JM, Robins E: Fluorometric measurement of deoxyribonucleic acid in animal tissues with special reference to the central nervous system. J Biol Chem 233:–184–188, 1979.
12. Weisburger EK: Mechanism of chemical carcinogenesis. Annu Rev Pharmacol Toxicol 18:395–415, 1978.
13. Pelkonen O: Metabolism of benzo(a)pyrene in human adult and fetal tissues. In Freudenthal RI, Jones PW (eds): Carcinogenesis. New York: Raven Press, Vol. 1, 1976, pp 9–21.
14. Kahng MW, Smith MW, Trump BF: Aryl hydrocarbon hydroxylase in human bronchial epithelium and blood monocyte. J Natl Cancer Inst 66:227–232, 1981.
15. Gelboin HV: Benzo(a)pyrene metabolism, activation and carcinogenesis: role and regulation of mixed-function oxidases and related enzymes. Physiol Rev 60:1107–1166, 1980.

16. Bast RC Jr, Okuda T, Plotkin E, Tarone R, Rapp HJ, Gelboin HV: Development of an assay for aryl hyrocarbon (benzo(a)pyrene) hydroxylase in human peripheral blood monocytes. Cancer Res 36:1967–1974, 1976.

17. Okuda T, Vesell ES, Plotkin V, Tarone R, Bast RC, Gelboin HV: Interindividual and intraindividual variations in aryl hydrocarbon hydroxylase in monocytes from monozygotic twins. Cancer Res 37:3904–3911, 1977.

18. Costello LC, Littleton GK, Franklin RB: Regulation of citrate-related metabolism in normal and neoplastic prostate. In Sharma RK, Criss WE (eds.): Endocrine Control in Neoplasia. New York: Raven Press, 1978, pp 303–312.

19. Digiovanni J, Juchau MR: Biotransformation and bioactivation of 7,12-dimethylbenz(a)anthracene. Drug Metab Rev 11:61–101, 1980.

20. Fingerhut B, Veenema RJ: An animal model for the study of prostatic adenocarcinoma. Invest Urol 15:42–48, 1977.

21. Lipsett MB: Interaction of drugs, hormones, and nutrition in the causes of cancer. Cancer 43:1967–1981, 1979.

22. Miller AB: An overview of hormone-associated cancers. Cancer Res 38:3985–3990, 1978.

The Prostatic Cell: Structure and Function
Part B, pages 191–205
© 1981 Alan R. Liss, Inc., 150 Fifth Avenue, New York, NY 10011

Induction of Cytochrome P-450 and Metabolic Activation of Mutagens in the Rat Ventral Prostate

Jan-Åke Gustafsson, Peter Söderkvist, Tapio Haaparanta, Lief Busk, Åke Pousette, Hans Glaumann, Rune Toftgård, and Bertil Högberg

INTRODUCTION

In 1951, Lasnitzki described precancerous changes induced by 3-methylcholanthrene in an organ culture of mouse prostate [1]. The changes consisted of extensive hyperplasia, squamous metaplasia, anaplasia, and in some cases invasion of the prostatic epithelium through the basement membrane. Later, similar findings have been reported by other authors using 3-methylcholanthrene-11,12-epoxide, benzo(a)pyrene, N-methyl-N-nitro-N-nitrosoguanidine, 1,2,5,6-benzathracene, and 9,10-dimethyl-1,2-benzathracene [2,3]. Horning and Dmochowski induced both sarcoma and carcinoma of the prostate by direct implantation of hydrocarbons into the prostate in vivo [4].

Cytochrome P-450-dependent activation of precarcinogens is known to play an important role in chemical carcinogenesis. Although intensive efforts have been invested to elucidate cytochrome P-450-catalyzed metabolism of xenobiotics in the liver, relatively little information is available with regard to metabolism of foreign compounds in the prostate. Ofner et al have shown that NADPH-dependent hydroxylation of steroids in the canine prostate involves a mixed function oxidase [5]. These results were later confirmed by Coffey and co-workers [6]. The presence of cytochrome P-450-dependent enzyme activities in the prostate indicates the possibility of bioactivation of exogenous chemicals in this tissue. This process is of potential importance in the etiology of prostatic carcinoma.

In a recent paper, Lee et al [7] reported that the activity of aryl hydrocarbon hydroxylase (AHH) in the rat ventral prostate increased four times after exposure to diesel emissions. Corresponding figures for the liver and the lung were 1.3 and 1.4, respectively. The same group of research workers has also briefly reported that a single intraperitoneal injection of TCDD (2,3,7,8-tetrachlorodibenzo-p-dioxin) increased the prostatic AHH-activity and the cytochrome

P-450 content 150 and 166 times, respectively [8]. These results indicate that the prostatic gland is very sensitive to certain enzyme inducers. The cytosolic receptor protein for this type of inducers is a product of the so-called Ah locus and binds TCDD with high affinity and low capacity. Poland has shown that PAHs and halogenated dioxins and dibenzofurans capable of inducing AHH bind stereospecifically to this receptor [9]. Using isoelectric focusing for measuring the ^{3}H-TCDD-receptor complex, we have shown that the TCDD-binding is competed for by 2,3,7,8-tetrachlorodibenzofuran (TCDBF), methylcholanthrene, benzo(a)pyrene and β-naphtoflavone, four inducers of AHH, but not by phenobarbital or 16α-cyanopregnenolone, inducers of other forms of cytochrome P-450 [10]. Neither was the binding competed for by dexamethasone, progesterone, estradiol, testosterone, 2-hydroxyestradiol, retinol, retinoic acid, α-tocopherol, menadione or vitamin K_1.

The present study was undertaken to investigate the inducibility of certain cytochrome P-450-related metabolic activities in the rat ventral prostate and mechanisms involved in this induction process.

MATERIALS AND METHODS
Animals

Male Sprague Dawley rats weighing 300–500 gm were obtained from Anticimex, Stockholm, Sweden. The rats were maintained on a commercial rodent diet with free access to water and were kept in a room with controlled temperature and light (10 hours dark: 14 hours light). Rats were given β-naphtoflavone (BNF), 80 mg/kg, dissolved in corn oil and phenobarbital (PB), 80 mg/kg, dissolved in 0.9% (w/v) sodium chloride intraperitoneally each day for 4 days, prior to decapitation on the fifth day, if not otherwise stated. PCB (Arochlor 1254) was given as a single dose of 500 mg/kg 5 days before decapitation. The control group received the same amount of the vehicle alone. The preparation of microsomes will be described elsewhere.

Enzyme Assays

The microsomes were assayed for 7-ethoxyresorufin-O-deethylase (7-EOD) activity at 22°C or 37°C according to the procedure described by Burke et al [11,12]. The standard incubation mixture, prepared in a fluorimeter cuvette, contained 0.25 mM NADPH, 0.5 μM 7-ethoxyresorufin dissolved in dimethylsulfoxide (DMSO), and 5–25 μl of microsomes (25 mg protein/ml). The volume was adjusted to 2 ml with 0.1 M potassium phosphate buffer, pH 7.4. The excitation wavelength was 530 nm, and the emission wavelength was 585 nm. A baseline was recorded and the reaction was started by the addition of NADPH. The concentration of DMSO was 0.5% (v/v). The reaction was unaffected by DMSO concentrations below 2.0% (v/v).

AHH-activity was determined radiometrically as described by Van Cantfort et al [13] with minor modifications. The incubation time was 30 minutes, and 1.7 mg of protein was used per incubation in case of control samples. Microsomes from the BNF-treated rats were assayed as recommended for liver (0.22 mg of protein and 10 minutes incubation time [13]). The NADPH-generating system used consisted of NADP (3.0 mM), $MnCl_2$ (30 μM), isocitrate (125 mM) and isocitrate dehydrogenase (0.36 U/ml). The incubation temperature was 37°C.

Benzo(a)pyrene (BP) metabolism was assayed by incubating 100 nmole of benzo(a)pyrene, containing 10^6 dpm ^{3}H-benzo(a)pyrene and 0.7–1.7 mg of protein in a final volume of 1 ml 0.1 M phosphate buffer, pH 7.4. The incubations were started by adding NADPH (0.5 mg/ml). The reaction was terminated after 30 minutes by adding 1 ml of acetone. Metabolites were extracted with 2×2 ml ethyl acetate containing 0.08% (w/v) butylhydroxytoluene, and the combined ethyl acetate phases were dried under nitrogen and kept in a freezer (–20°C) until analysis. Separation of the different metabolites was carried out using high performance liquid chromatography according to Holder et al [14,15]. The metabolites were identified as 9,10-,4,5-,and 7,8-dihydrodiols, quinones, phenol fraction I (mainly 9-hydroxybenzo(a)pyrene) and phenol fraction II (mainly 3-hydroxy-benzo(a)pyrene) using authentic standards.

Cytochrome P-450 was determined from the difference spectrum of dithionite reduced minus oxidized microsomes following bubbling of both cuvettes with carbon monoxide using an Aminco-Chance UV-VIS spectrophotometer. The extinction coefficient was 104 cm^{-1} mM^{-1} [16]. Protein was determined according to Lowry et al with bovine serum albumin as standard [17].

Preparation of S-5 Mix

The ventral prostate was excised and placed in ice-cold 0.17 M Tris-HC1, pH 7.3. The tissue was minced with scissors and the pieces were sedimented at 80g for 10 minutes. The pellet was suspended in medium (1 gm/2 ml) and homogenized with a Potter-Elvehjem homogenizer. The homogenate was sedimented at 300g for 10 minutes to remove cellular debris, connective tissue, muscle cells, and nuclei. The procedure was repeated once and the two supernatants were pooled and sedimented at 5000g for 7 minutes. The supernatant was designed S-5 mix.

Mutagenesis Assay

The Salmonella typhimurium histidine auxotrophs TA 98 and TA 100 were kindly provided by Professor B.N. Ames and were checked for proper genetic characteristics using the method described by Ames et al [18]. The metabolizing system (S-5 mix) contained 300 μl (PCB- or BNF-induced) or 550 μl prostate homogenate (Pb-induced or uninduced) per ml. The amount of co-factors (an

NADPH-generating system) in the S-5 mix was the same regardless of the type and volume of homogenate added. Aflatoxin B_1 (AFB_1), 2-aminofluorene (2-AF), and BP were dissolved in DMSO and added to the plates in 100 μl portions. The plates were incubated for 48 hours at 37°C and counted in a Bio Tran II automated colony counter.

Competition for ³H-TCDD-Binding to Rat Ventral Prostatic Fluid

Prostatic fluid was obtained by mincing the gland with a pair of scissors in ice-cold 50 mM Tris-HCl buffer, pH 7.4, containing 1 mM EDTA, 0.1 mM dithiothreitol (DTT), and 50 mM NaCl. The cutting resulted in release of secretory fluid from the ductules and lumina. The tissue pieces were filtered off through cheese cloth. The obtained fluid was diluted to contain 0.25 mg protein/ml. Protein concentration was measured according to Lowry et al [17] as modified by Peterson [19].

Incubations were performed in an ice bath for 2 hours and contained 200 μl diluted prostatic fluid, competitor (0.7–20 μM), ³H-TCDD (100,000 dpm, 33.0 Ci/mmole), and TCDBF (100 ng). The ³H-TCDD, TCDBF, and the different competitors were added in 1 μl dioxane. Phenobarbital was added in 1 μl water. The dioxane concentration was below 1.5% (v/v).

Separation of free ligand from ligand bound to prostatic secretion protein (PSP), also called estramustine-binding protein, was performed by isoelectric focusing in polyacrylamide gel (LKB 1804-101 Ampholine PAG-plates; LKB-Produkter AB, Bromma, Sweden) containing 2.4% (w/v) Ampholine, pH range 3.5–9.5. The focusing was carried out using an LKB 2117 Multiphor.

The plates were prefocused for 30 minutes at 50 mA, 30 W. One-hundred μl of the incubation mixture was applied to the gel, 1 cm from the cathode electrode strip, in sample frames (inner diameter 5 mm). Standard proteins (hemoglobin and ferritin) were analyzed simultaneously. The focusing was performed using 20 mA, 20 W, and 1200 V for 60 minutes. The gel was then sliced into 15 pieces and each piece was counted for radioactivity in an Intertechnique SL-4220 liquid scintillation counter (Plaisir, France) with direct calculation of dpm using the external standard technique.

RESULTS

Cytochrome P-450

Figure 1 shows the dithionite-reduced minus oxidized difference spectrum of prostatic microsomes when both cuvettes were bubbled with carbon monoxide. Following BNF treatment the cytochrome P-450 content was increased 28 times

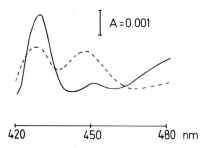

Fig. 1. The dithionite-reduced minus oxidized difference spectrum of prostatic microsomes from BNF-treated (----; 0.24 mg protein/ml) and control (——; 0.85 mg protein/ml) rats. Both cuvettes were bubbled with carbon monoxide.

from 0.002 to 0.056 nmole/mg protein. BNF treatment also caused a peak shift from 450 to 448 nm.

7-Ethoxyresorufin-O-deethylase (7-EOD) Activity

Enzymatic activities of the liver and prostatic microsomes from rats receiving BNF, PB, and corn oil are summarized in Table I. No significant differences were observed with regard to the NADPH-cytochrome c reductase activity in the prostate after either treatment, while the activity in liver microsomes showed a moderate increase after BNF treatment. On the other hand, in the prostate, BNF treatment increased the 7-EOD activity approximately 800 times when compared to control, ie, 618 as compared to 0.8 pmole/min·mg protein. The corresponding increase for liver microsomes was 108 times. Kinetic studies with prostatic and liver microsomes from BNF-treated animals showed that the substrate saturation curves for 7-EOD activity were very similar for the two tissues with the exception that the reaction velocities were about ten times higher for the liver enzyme than for the prostatic enzyme (Fig. 2). The same was true for the V_{max} values (3.11 and 0.31 nmole/min·mg protein for the liver and prostatic 7-EOD activity, respectively). The K_m values, however, were quite similar for the two tissues (0.12 and 0.077 μM for the liver and prostatic 7-EOD activity, respectively). Interestingly, both the hepatic and the prostatic 7-EOD activity displayed a pronounced substrate inhibition at higher substrate concentrations (Fig. 2).

The PB treatment increased the O-deethylase activity 6 times from 0.8 to 5.0 pmole/min·mg protein (Table I). Several experiments have shown that this difference is within the experimental variation. Consequently, PB treatment ap-

TABLE I. Effects of β-naphthoflavone and phenobarbital on drug metabolizing enzymes in microsomes from the rat liver and the rat ventral prostate

| | Enzymatic activity | | | | | |
| | Liver microsomes | | | Prostatic microsomes | | |
Treatment[a]	AHH[b]	7-ethoxyresorufin-O-deethylase[b]	NADPH-cytochrome c reductase[c]	AHH[b]	7-ethoxyresorufin-O-deethylase[b]	NADPH-cytochrome c reductase[c]
BNF	5810	7646	69.0	499 (161-1012)[d]	618 (406-1010)[d]	11.9 (4.8-23.8)[d]
PB	—	—	—	0.2	5	8.0
Corn oil	700	70.6	48.2	0.5 (0.2-8.6)[d]	0.8 (0.2-39)[d]	9.1 (2.4-46.8)[d]

[a]Rats were given β-naphthoflavone (BNF) and phenobarbital (PB), 80 mg/kg, IP, each day for 4 days. At least five animals were pooled in each group.
[b]pmole/min·mg protein. Assayed at 37°C.
[c]nmole/min·mg protein.
[d]Median values with ranges are given, n = 5. Each value represents the mean of duplicate determination.

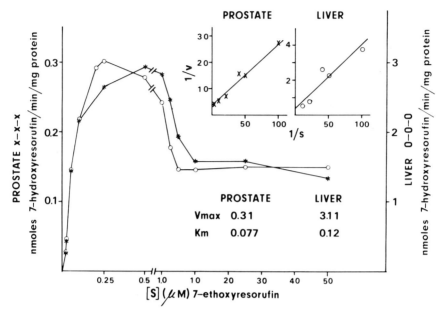

Fig. 2. Effects of varying substrate concentrations on 7-ethoxyresorufin-O-deethylase activity in liver and prostate microsomes from BNF-treated rats. The rats were given BNF, 80 mg/kg, dissolved in corn oil, intraperitoneally 24 hours prior to death. Incubations were performed at 22°C. For further details see text.

TABLE II. Metabolites isolated after incubation of benzo(a)pyrene with prostatic and liver microsomes

| Benzo(a)pyrene metabolites | Prostate | | Liver | |
	BNF-treatment[a]	Control (pmole/min, mg protein)	BNF-treatment[a]	Control
9,10-diol	4(2.2)[b]	2 (13.3)	666 (26.1)	33 (6.7)
4,5-diol	8 (4.6)	2 (13.3)[c]	104 (4.1)	28 (5.7)
7,8-diol	8 (4.6)		349 (13.7)	47 (9.6)
quinone	17 (9.7)	2 (13.3)	131 (5.1)	67 (13.6)
phenol I	28 (16.0)	3 (20.0)	198 (7.7)	71 (14.5)
phenol II	110 (62.9)	6 (40.0)	1108 (43.3)	245 (50.0)

[a]Treatment is described in Table I
[b]Values within brackets represent percentage of total metabolites.
[c]Represents the sum of 4,5- and 7,8-diol.

TABLE III. Activities of drug metabolizing enzymes in prostatic microsomes from rats of different ages

Age of rats (months)	AHH (pmole/min, mg protein)	Enzymatic activity 7-ethoxyresorufin-O-deethylase (pmole/min, mg protein)	NADPH-cytochrome c reductase (nmole/min, mg protein)
1	0.2	0.2	9.1
3	<0.1	1.0	9.8
7	<0.1	0.7	8.5

Ten prostatic glands were pooled and the values represent a mean of duplicate determinations. Assayed at 37°C.

peared to have a small or negligible effect on the 7-EOD activity in the rat ventral prostate.

Aryl Hydrocarbon Hydroxylase Activity

Following treatment with BNF, the prostatic microsomal AHH-activity increased about 1000 times from 0.5 to 499 pmole/min·mg protein. The relative increase in hepatic microsomal AHH-activity monitored in the same animals was about 8 times (Table I). Prostatic microsomes from BNF-treated rats had about the same activity as liver microsomes from control rats. No increase in AHH-activity was observed for PB-induced prostatic microsomes.

The major metabolic products found after incubation of prostatic microsomes with BP were phenols, which co-chromatographed with 9-hydroxy-(phenol I) and 3-hydroxy-benzo(a)pyrene (phenol II). They represented 60% of the total metabolites formed in case of the control and 79% in case of BNF-treated rats. As shown in Table II there was an increased formation of both dihydrodiols and phenols after BNF-treatment.

Enzymatic activities in untreated rats 1, 3, and 7 months of age are presented in Table III. No significant differences between the age groups were seen for AHH-, 7-EOD, or NADPH-cytochrome c reductase activities.

Finally, we have examined the influence of carbon monoxide (CO), NADPH, and α-naphtoflavone (α-NF) on the AHH- and 7-EOD activity (Table IV). For 7-EOD activity in prostatic microsomes from BNF-treated and control rats, a total inhibition was observed when samples were assayed without NADPH, CO-bubbled for 60 seconds or with an α-NF concentration of 70 μM. A 7-μM concentration of α-NF produced a complete inhibition of 7-EOD activity for control samples and a 98% decrease in activity with microsomes from BNF-treated rats. Complete inhibition of AHH-activity was observed in prostatic microsomes from control rats when incubated without NADPH, under a CO

TABLE IV. Influence of carbon monoxide, NADPH, and β-naphthoflavone on enzymatic activities in the rat ventral prostate of control and β-naphthoflavone-treated rats

Incubation conditions	AHH (pmole/min · mg microsomal protein)		7-Ethoxyresorufin-O-deethylase[e] (pmole/min · mg microsomal protein)	
	BNF[a]	Control[b]	BNF[c]	Control[b]
Control	410.1 (100)[d]	0.5 (100)	528 (100)	0.21 (100)
CO inhibition	5.9 (1.4)	<0.3 (<60.0)	<0.6 (<0.1)	<0.05 (<23.8)
Without NADPH	<1.2 (<0.3)	<0.3 (<60.0)	<0.6 (<0.1)	<0.05 (<23.8)
α-NF 7 μM	239.0 (58.3)	<0.3 (<60.0)	12.1 (2.3)	<0.05 (<23.8)
α-NF 70 μM	92.2 (22.5)	—	<0.6 (<0.1)	<0.05 (<23.8)

[a]The protein concentration was 0.4 mg microsomal protein/ml.
[b]The protein concentration was 5.0 mg microsomal protein/ml.
[c]The protein concentration was 0.2 mg microsomal protein/ml.
[d]Figures within brackets represent the percentage of nonmanipulated incubations.
[e]Assayed at 37°C.

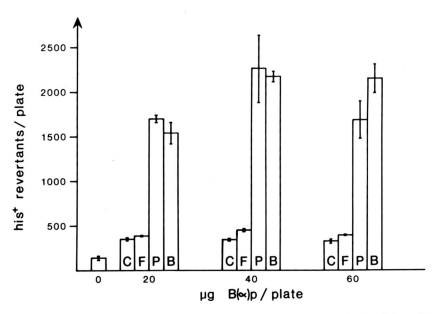

Fig. 3. Mutagenesis assay of benzo(a)pyrene (BP) according to Ames et al [18] using Salmonella typhimurium TA 100 and a fraction of rat prostatic homogenate (S-5 mix, cf text). C, control rats (untreated); F, PB-induced rats; P, PCB-induced rats; B, BNF-induced rats. For experimental details, see text.

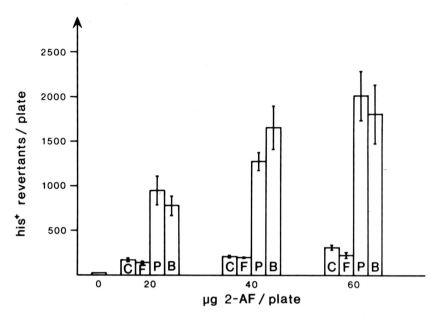

Fig. 4. Mutagenesis assay of 2-aminofluorene (2-AF) according to Ames et al [18] using Salmonella typhimurium TA 98 and a fraction of rat prostatic homogenate (S-5 mix, cf text). For explanation of symbols, see legend to Figure 3. For experimental details, see text.

atmosphere, or with an α-NF concentration of 7 μM. α-NF concentrations of 7 and 10 μM caused a 42% and 78% decrease, respectively, of AHH activity in prostatic microsomes from BNF-treated rats. NADPH-deficiency completely inhibited this reaction and incubation under a CO atmosphere resulted in a 99% inhibition. These results obtained with known inhibitors of cytochrome P-450-dependent enzymatic activities clearly indicate that the AHH- and 7-EOD activities in rat prostatic microsomes are cytochrome P-450-mediated reactions.

Metabolic Activation in Ames' Test Catalyzed by Rat Ventral Prostatic S-5 Mix

The S-5 fraction of rat prostate was capable of converting AFB_1, 2-AF, and BP to ultimate mutagenic metabolites detectable in the Ames' Salmonella test (Figs. 3–5). BP (Fig. 3) and 2-AF (Fig. 4) exhibited a stronger mutagenicity than AFB_1 (Fig. 5), but all substances showed a clear mutagenic response that was dose-dependent. The most pronounced activation was obtained with S-5 mix from BNF- and PCB-treated rats.

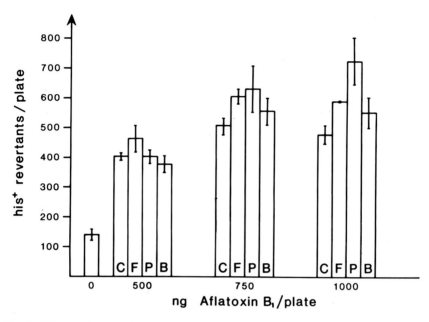

Fig. 5. Mutagenesis assay of aflatoxin B_1 (AFB$_1$) according to Ames et al [18] using Salmonella typhimurium TA 100 and a fraction of rat prostatic homogenate (S-5 mix, cf text). For explanation of symbols, see legend to Figure 3. For experimental details, see text.

Competition of TCDBF, BP, 3-MC, BNF, and LS 275 (Estramustine) for ^{3}H-TCDD-Binding to PSP

We have previously shown that the rat ventral prostate contains a major secretory protein which makes up about 20% of the total protein content in the prostate [20]. We have called this protein prostatic secretion protein (PSP) or estramustine-binding protein (EMBP) since it binds estramustine, the dephosphorylated metabolite of the drug Estracyt®, with a high affinity and a high capacity [20,21]. PSP is responsible for the selective uptake of estramustine in the ventral prostate of the rat and may possibly also play a similar role in the human [22].

When investigating the tissue distribution of the cytosolic receptor protein for TCDD, using isoelectric focusing in polyacrylamide gel, we observed the presence of a major TCDD-binding species in the rat ventral prostate [23]. The TCDD-binding protein found in the prostate did not demonstrate the characteristics of a receptor protein (high-affinity, low-capacity) and did not interact with

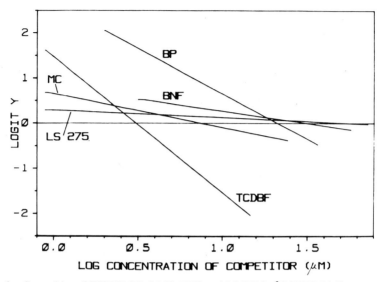

Fig. 6. Competition of TCDBF, BP, 3-MC, BNF, and LS 275 for ³H-TCDD-binding to prostatic secretion protein (PSP), also called estramustine-binding protein (EMBP). For experimental details, see text.

DNA-cellulose. This protein occurs at a much higher concentration than that of the TCDD receptor in other tissues. In addition, it has a much larger binding capacity for TCDD than the TCDD receptor. We have now identified this prostatic TCDD-binding protein as PSP. It is possible that this binder masks the occurrence of the TCDD receptor in the prostate as it focuses very closely to the receptor and occurs in such large amounts.

Figure 6 shows the relative affinities of some compounds for the ³H-TCDD-binding sites on PSP. The similar slopes of the displacing activities of TCDBF and BP may indicate that these compounds interact with the same site on PSP, whereas the mode of PSP interaction seems to be different for 3-methylchol-anthrene and BNF. LS 275 (estramustine) has a relatively weak displacing activity with respect to ³H-TCDD-binding, indicating that ³H-TCDD does not bind to the estramustine-binding site on PSP.

DISCUSSION

Our experiments give further support to the contention that the prostatic gland is very sensitive to certain enzyme inducers, since treatment with BNF resulted in a thousandfold increase in the cytochrome P-450-dependent AHH activity in the prostate, whereas the same enzyme activity increased only eight times in the liver. Furthermore, BNF-treatment resulted in an 800-fold stimulation of the cytochrome P-450-dependent 7-EOD activity in the prostate. PB treatment, however, did not affect the enzymatic activities in a significant way. PB, which is an inducer of hepatic mixed function oxidases, is reported to lack or to have a very poor inducing potency in extrahepatic tissues [24], such as lung, kidney, adrenals, testis, etc. Also in the prostate PB seems to lack inducing capacity with regard to the enzymatic activities investigated.

The reason for the higher sensitivity of the prostate to enzyme inducers of the PAH-type when compared to the liver could be related to different concentrations of the TCDD receptor in the two tissues. This, unfortunately, was difficult to assess since the electrofocusing assay of the TCDD receptor was disturbed by the great TCDD-binding capacity of PSP. However, the fact that PSP can act as a TCDD binder is very interesting in view of the 150-fold induction of AHH in the rat prostate reported by Lee et al [8]. This is a much higher level of induction than that obtained in the liver. In addition, the persistance of the AHH induction is much longer in the prostate than in the liver [8]. It cannot be excluded that the persistant high induction of AHH in the prostate following administration of TCDD may be at least partially related to a relatively high uptake of TCDD in the organ due to the presence of PSP.

The results presented in this paper indicate that PSP may also bind other inducers of cytochrome P-450, eg BNF, although with a relatively low affinity. This binding may still be of some significance in connection with the high AHH- and 7-EOD-inducing potency of BNF in the prostate in view of the large amounts in which PSP occurs. The fact that BP interacts with PSP may be of importance in chemical carcinogenesis in the prostate. Possibly, PSP may act as a trap for polycyclic aromatic hydrocarbons in the gland. Interestingly, both in the rat and the dog, methylcholanthrene is partially disposed of by secretion into the seminal fluid [25].

As is evident from Table I, there was a wide range in the control values of the enzyme activities assayed. The possibility that this was due to varying ages of the animals does not seem likely, since no significant differences in enzyme activities were observed between 1-, 3-, and 7-month-old rats (Table III). Another possible explanation is that the animals were exposed to varying concentrations of some uncontrolled inducing agent.

Treatment with BNF led to an increased formation of all BP metabolites, although the formation of phenols was stimulated most markedly. Following incubation of BP with prostatic microsomes from BNF-treated rats it was possible to quantitate the 7,8-dihydrodiol. Formation of this metabolite is important in view of its role as a precursor for the ultimate carcinogen, the 7,8-dihydrodiol-9,10-epoxide of BP [26,27].

The results obtained from the Ames' Salmonella test give further support to the contention that the prostate gland may activate BP to ultimate mutagenic metabolites. Furthermore, 2-AF and AFB_1 were also metabolically activated in this test system, indicating that the mutagen-activating capacity of the prostate is not limited to a narrow spectrum of mutagenic compounds.

The importance of xenobiotic metabolism in the prostate may be considerable. The situation in vivo is characterized by chronic exposure to small amounts of foreign compounds of environmental and occupational origin, which may be of significance although they occur at low concentrations, since the prostate seems to be very sensitive to inducing agents. Induction of cytochrome P-450-dependent enzyme systems may increase the production of reactive metabolites of precarcinogens in the prostate, a process which may be related to the etiology of prostatic carcinoma.

ACKNOWLEDGMENTS

This work was supported by grants from Forskningsrådsnämnden, the Swedish Cancer Society, and from Leo Research Foundation.

REFERENCES

1. Lasnitzki I: Precancerous changes induced by 20-methylcholanthrene in mouse prostates grown in vitro. Brit J Cancer 5: 345–352, 1951.
2. Chopra DP, Wilkoff LJ: Induction of hyperplasia and anaplasia by carcinogens in organ cultures of mouse prostate. In Vitro 13: 260–267, 1977.
3. Röller MR, Heidelberger C: Attempts to produce carcinogenesis in organ cultures of mouse prostate with polycyclic hydrocarbons. Int J Cancer 2: 509–520, 1967.
4. Horning ES, Dmochowski L: Induction of prostate tumors in mice. British J Cancer 1: 59–63, 1947.
5. Ofner P, Vena RL, Morfin RF: Acetylation and hydroxylation of 5α-androstane-3β,17β-diol by prostate and epididymis. Steroids 24: 261–279, 1974.
6. Isaacs JT, McDermott IR, Coffey DS: Characterization of two new enzymatic activities of the rat ventral prostate: 5α-androstane-3β,17β-diol 6α-hydroxylase and 5α-androstane-3β,17β-diol 7α-hydroxylase. Steroids 33: 675–692, 1979.
7. Lee IP, Suzuki K, Lee SD, Dixon RL: Aryl hydrocarbon hydroxylase induction in rat lung, liver and male reproductive organs following inhalation exposure to diesel emission. Toxicol Appl Pharmacol 52: 181–184, 1980.
8. Lee IP, Suzuki K: Differential induction of aryl hydrocarbon hydroxylase and cytochrome P-448 levels in liver, testis and prostate gland by 2,3,7,8-tetrachlorodibenzo-p-dioxin (TCDD). 7th international Congress of Pharmacology, Paris 16–21 July, 1978. Abstract 795. Paris: IUPHAR, Pergamon Press.
9. Poland A, Glover E, Kende AS: Stereospecific high affinity binding of 2,3,7,8-tetrachlorodibenzo-p-dioxin by hepatic cytosol: evidence that the binding species is receptor for induction of aryl hydrocarbon hydroxylase. J Biol Chem 251: 4936–4946, 1976.
10. Carlstedt-Duke J, Elfström G, Snochowski M, Högberg B, Gustafsson JÅ: Detection of the 2,3,7,8-tetrachlorodibenzo-p-dioxin (TCDD) receptor in rat liver by isoelectric focusing in polyacrylamide gels. Toxicology Letters 2: 365–373, 1978.
11. Burke MD, Mayer RT: Direct fluorometric assay of a microsomal O-dealkylation which is preferentially inducible by 3-methylcholanthrene. Drug Metabolism and Disposition Vol 2: p 583–588, 1974.
12. Burke MD, Prough RA, Mayer RT: Characteristics of a microsomal cytochrome P-448-mediated reaction. Ethoxyresorufin O-deethylation. Drug Metabolism and Disposition Vol 5: p 1–8, 1977.

13. Van Cantfort J, De Graeve J, Gielen JE: Radioactive assay for aryl hydrocarbon hydroxylase. Improved method and biological importance. Biochem and Biophys Res Comm 79: 505–512, 1977.

14. Holder G, Yagi H, Dansette P, Jerina DM, Lewin W, Lu AYH, Conney AH: Effects of inducers and epoxide hydrase on the metabolism of benzo(a)pyrene by liver microsomes and a reconstituted system: Analysis of high pressure liquid chromatography. Proc Natl Acad Sci 71: 4356–4360, 1974.

15. Huberman E, Sachs L, Yang SK, Gelbloin HV: Identification of mutagenic metabolites of benzo(a)pyrene in mammalian cells. Proc Natl Acad Sci 73: 607–611, 1976.

16. Matsubara T, Koike M, Touchi A, Tuchino Y, Sugeno K: Quantitative determination of cytochrome P-450 in rat liver homogenate. Anal Biochem 75: 596–603, 1976.

17. Lowry OH, Rosebrough NJ, Farr AL, Randall RJ: Protein measurement with the folin phenol reagent. J Biol Chem 193: 265–275, 1951.

18. Ames BN, McCann J, Yamasaki E: Methods for detecting carcinogens and mutagens with the Salmonella/mammalian microsome mutagenicity test. Mutation Research 31: 347–364, 1975.

19. Peterson GL: A simplification of the protein assay method of Lowry et al which is more generally applicable. Analytical Biochemistry 83: 346–356, 1977.

20. Forsgren B, Björk P, Carlström K, Gustafsson JÅ, Pousette Å, Högberg B: Purification and distribution of a major protein in rat prostate that binds estramustine, a nitrogen mustard derivative of estradiol-17β. Proc Natl Acad Sci 76: 3149–3153, 1979.

21. Forsgren B, Gustafsson JÅ, Pousette Å, Högberg B: Binding characteristics of a major protein in rat ventral prostate cytosol that interacts with estramustine, a nitrogen mustard derivative of 17β-estradiol. Cancer Research 39: 5155–5164, 1979.

22. Gustafsson JÅ, Björk P, Carlström K, Forsgren B, Hökfelt T, Pousette Å, Högberg B: On the presence of a major protein, prostatic secretion protein or estramustine-binding protein, in the rat ventral prostate and in the human prostate. In Schröder FH, de Voogt HJ (eds): Steroid receptors, metabolism and prostatic cancer, Excerpta Medica, p 86–101, 1980.

23. Carlstedt-Duke J: Tissue distribution of the receptor for 2,3,7,8-tetrachlorodibenzo-p-dioxin in the rat. Cancer Research 39: 3172–3176, 1979.

24. Burke MD, Orrenius S: Isolation and comparison of endoplasmatic reticulum membranes and their mixed function oxidase activities from mammalian extraheptic tissues. J Pharmac Ther 7: 549–599, 1979.

25. Smith ER, Hagopian M: The uptake and secretion of 3-methylcholanthrene by the prostate glands of the rat and dog. J Natl Cancer Int 59: 119–122, 1977.

26. Sims P, Groover PL: Epoxides in polycyclic aromatic hydrocarbon metabolism and carcinogenesis. Adv Cancer Res 20: 165–274, 1974.

The Prostatic Cell: Structure and Function
Part B, pages 207–228

Retinoic Acid Receptor and Surface Markers: Models for the Study of Prostatic Cancer Cells

David Brandes

INTRODUCTION

Upon withdrawal of androgen sources (orchiectomy) or administration of antiandrogenic compounds, such as stilbestrol, prostatic cells undergo atrophy and likely necrosis [3, 20, 28, 33, 34]. This has been shown to occur in the prostate of many species as well as in prostatic carcinoma in man [7]. Prostatic cells cannot sustain the integrity of their organelles after androgen deprivation or stilbestrol treatment. The mechanism of regression involves the sequestration of obsolete cellular organelles within autophagic vacuoles, where degradation is accomplished by lysosomal enzymes [3, 7, 33, 34]. Various substances, including Vitamin A compounds (retinoids) and steroid hormones [36, 37, 48], as well as x-irradiation [1, 14, 15, 32, 35] can apparently augment the intracellular release of lysosomal hydrolases and consequently may enhance the antitumor effects of conventional agents such as x-rays and chemotherapeutic drugs [2, 6, 8, 9, 16]. Retinoids and certain steroids not only are capable of labilizing the lysosomes but also appear to alter the composition and electrical charges of the cell surface [10, 22, 47]. More recently a specific binding protein for retinoic acid, cytoplasmic retinoic acid binding protein (cRABP), has been demonstrated in human and animal tissues [29, 38, 40, 41] as well as in some malignant tumors [23, 26, 30, 31, 39, 42, 45]. Generally, this protein (cRABP) is either undetectable or occurs in low concentration in the normal tissues from which the tumors originate [23, 26, 30, 31, 39, 42]. This paper discusses morphological and biochemical changes in the properties of prostatic lysosomes following orchiectomy. Studies on the distribution of cRABP in normal and malignant prostatic tissue, both in human and in the rat, and cell surface changes induced in vitro by retinoic acid and x-rays on a rat prostatic cancer cell line (PA-III) are also discussed in this presentation.

MATERIALS AND METHODS

Lysosomal Enzymes Studies

The effect of orchiectomy on prostatic lysosomes was investigated in the Carworth CFE male rats. Four days after castration, the ventral lobes of the prostate were removed, weighed, and processed for histochemistry, electron-microscopy, and biochemistry. Intact male rats of the same weights were used as controls.

For light microscopy histochemistry, 7-μm cryostat sections were incubated for acid phosphatase, β-glucuronidase and N-acetyl-β-glucosaminidase. For electron microscopy histochemistry, 36-μm cryostat sections were incubated for acid phosphatase. These sections and blocks for conventional electron microscopy were processed by standard methods.

Biochemical assays for lysosomal hydrolases. Tissues were homogenized in 0.25 M sucrose in a Potter-Elvehijem homogenizer with a teflon pestle. Whole homogenates and high speed supernatants were analyzed for β-glucuronidase, N-acetyl-β-glucosaminidase, and aryl sulfatase.

Retinoic Acid Binding Protein Studies

Human prostatic carcinoma, benign prostatic hyperplasia, and normal tissue samples were obtained from the Prostatic Tissue Collection Center, University of Miami, Florida. Normal dorsolateral and ventral prostatic lobes from the Fisher-Copenhagen F_1 rat, and four sublines of the R3327 Dunning transplantable rat prostatic carcinoma (H, hormone sensitive; HI, hormone insensitive; AT, anaplastic; ATM, anaplastic highly metastasizing) were obtained from Dr. J. Isaacs, Johns Hopkins University.

In all cases, freshly obtained tissues were rapidly frozen without cryoprotective agents and maintained at–70°C until ready to use. Control fresh frozen sections were invariably obtained to verify the histopathology of the tissues.

(³H) Retinoic acid binding assays

Human and rat prostatic tissues. Tissues were homogenized in 50 mM tris-HCl (pH 7.5) and centrifuged 1 hour at 100,000g. Aliquots of the cytosol were incubated 18 hours with (³H) retinoic acid (200 pmoles) in the presence or absence of 200-fold excess unlabelled retinoic acid. The mixture was treated with dextran-coated charcoal (100 μl) to remove free ligand. After centrifugation for 15 minutes at 1000g, 200 μl of the supernatant was layered on a 5–20% continuous sucrose gradient. Centrifugation was conducted for 2 hours at 369,400g under gradient reorienting conditions in a Sorvall TV 865 rotor. Samples (200 μl) were collected from the gradients and the amount of radioactivity was counted. The amount of radioactivity present in the 2 S region of the gradient was converted to picomoles of retinoic acid bound. Total retinoic acid bound, less that bound in the presence of 200-fold excess non-radioactive retinoic acid, provided the measure of retinoic acid specifically bound in the sample.

PA-III tumor cell lines. These cell lines [11] were propagated as mono-layers, in Eagle's minimum essential medium (MEM), with 10% fetal bovine serum, 100 μg/ml penicillin, and 100 μg/ml of streptomycin.

Cells were collected at subconfluency by scraping in phosphate buffered saline (PBS) and frozen. Procedures for assaying cRABP are similar to those described above.

Concanavalin A-horseradish peroxidase binding to the surface of PA-III cells

The cells were grown to subconfluence in 60-mm diameter tissue culture dishes according to procedures delineated above.

Retinoic acid treatment. Retinoic acid was dissolved in nitrogen gas equilibrated dimethyl sulfoxide (DMSO). After one hour incubation in the presence of 10 μg retinoic acid dissolved in 0.01 ml DMSO per 5 ml culture medium, the vitamin was removed by replacement with fresh culture medium. Controls received DMSO only. ConA-horseradish peroxidase (ConA-HRP) labelling was performed at various time points thereafter.

X-Irradiation. Cultures received 400 rads x-irradiation with a Westinghouse Quadrocondex x-ray machine, monitored with a Victoreen dosimeter (Model 555). Filters: 1.5 mm Cu, 1 mm Al; half-value thickness: 2.3 mm Cu; focus dish distance (FDD), 50 cm. Labelling with ConA was done 24 or 48 hours after x-irradiation.

Concanavalin A labelling. ConA-HRP incubation was performed on living cells prior to glutaraldehyde fixation. After washing with Ca^{++},Mg^{++}-free phosphate-buffered saline (PBS), the cultures were incubated 20 minutes in 50 μg ConA/ml in PBS, followed by 15 minutes incubation in 50 μg HRP/ml in PBS. After fixation in 4% glutaraldehyde in 0.1 M cacodylate buffer (pH 7.4), peroxidase was detected by a 15-minute treatment in 0.5 mg DAB/ml in 0.1 M Tris buffer (pH 7.4), containing 0.01% hydrogen peroxide followed by post-fixation in 1% OsO_4 in 0.1 M cacodylate buffer (pH 7.4) dehydration with a graded series of ethanol, and embedded in Araldite. After curing at 60 °C, the cultures were detached from the plastic dish and reembedded into flat blocks to obtain vertical sections. Thin sections were optionally counterstained with saturated ethanolic uranyl acetate and/or alkaline lead citrate and examined in an electron microscope.

RESULTS

Effects of Castration on Lysosomes

Four days after castration the average weight of the prostate decreased to about one-fifth of the initial values (Table I).

Light microscopy histochemistry for lysosomal enzymes reveals a redistribution from minute granules in the normal (Fig. 1) to a pattern of large conglomerates of particles in the atrophic epithelium of the castrated rats (Fig. 2). In the human prostate, a comparable shift from discrete granules in the untreated (Fig. 3) to coarser granules occurred in the prostatic cancer cells from orchiectomized patients (Fig. 4). Electron microscopy reveals gradual collapse of the endoplasmic reticulum, atrophy of the Golgi apparatus, development of acid phosphatase-rich secondary lysosomes, and sequestration of portions of endoplasmic reticulum and mitochondria within autophagic vacuoles. In later stages of development, the organelles within autophagic vacuoles appear to undergo degradation. Electron microscopical changes are illustrated in Figures 5–9.

In the castrate animals, biochemical assays of three lysosomal hydrolases, β-glucuronidase, N-acetyl-β-glucosaminidase, and aryl sulphatase, showed an increase in the specific activities of the whole homogenate (Table II) and in the percent unsedimentable absolute activities (Table III).

(^{3}H) Retinoic Acid Binding

Rat prostate tissues. In the Copenhagen-Fisher F_1 rat, cRAPB was present in the lateral lobe of the prostate, whereas the binding protein could not be detected either in the dorsal or the ventral lobes. Sucrose density gradient centrifugation of cytosol from the four sublines of the R-3327 rat prostatic carcinoma exhibited a peak of (^{3}H) retinoic acid binding in the 2S region which was

TABLE I. Average weights of prostate glands from normal and castrated rats*

Measurement	Normal prostate	Prostate from rats 4 days after castration
Number of experiments	27	20
Average weight (mg)	229.0 ± 21.2	51.8 ± 11.9
Average weight (% of normal)	100.0 ± 9.3	22.6 ± 5.2
Average pulp weight from one prostate (mg)	126.0 ± 13.3	18.0 ± 4.1

*Values are mean ± SD.

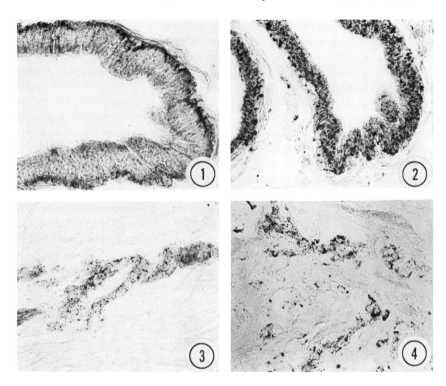

Fig. 1. Rat prostate—intact animal. Acid phosphatase-positive fine granules (secretory granules) are dispersed in the cytoplasm. Coarser granules (secondary lysosomes) are seen at the base of the epithelial cells. Acid phosphatase-lead phosphate method. × 350.

Fig. 2. Prostate from castrate rat. Acid phosphatase-positive coarse granules occupy the entire cytoplasm. These granules correspond to secondary lysosomes and autophagic vacuoles. Note atrophy of the epithelium. Acid phosphatase-lead phosphate method. × 350.

Fig. 3. Human prostatic carcinoma—untreated patient. Moderately differentiated acini show fine granular acid phosphatase-positive granules with occasional coarse granules. Acid phosphatase-lead phosphate method. × 350.

Fig. 4. Human prostatic carcinoma—orchiectomized patient. Residual groups of atrophic cells. Acid phosphatase-positive material arranged in large conglomerates (secondary lysosomes and autophagic vacuoles). × 350.

abolished by excess unlabelled ligand. A representative sample of the curves seen in the various sublines of the R-3327 tumor is shown in Figure 10. An estimate of the quantity of cRABP in the various lobes of the rat prostate and in the sublines of the Dunning R-3327 tumor is seen in Table IV.

Human prostate tissues. Sucrose density gradient centrifugation of the 100,000g cytosol extracts of human prostatic carcinoma incubated with (^{3}H)

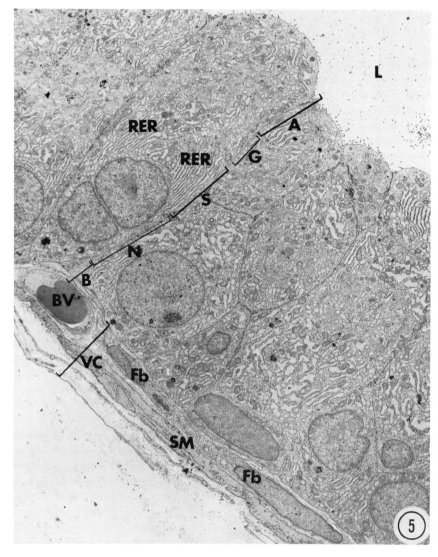

Fig. 5.   Normal rat ventral prostate.Highly differentiated cytoplasm into apical pole (A), golgi (G), supranuclear (S), and basal (B) regions. Fibrovascular compartment (VC) contains blood vessels (BV) fibroblasts (Fb), and smooth muscle fibers (SM). A markedly developed rough endoplasmic reticulum (RER) characterizes these cells. Lumen (L). × 5500.

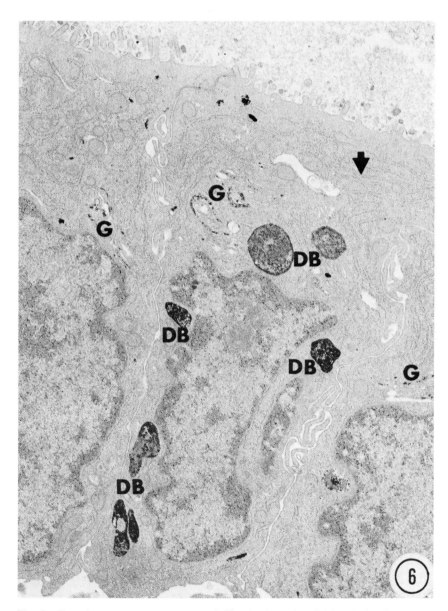

Fig. 6. Ventral prostate, post-castrate rat. Collapse and paucity of the endoplasmic reticulum (arrows); development of secondary lysosomes (DB). Appearance of a positive acid phosphatase reaction in the golgi apparatus (G) indicates activation of the lysosomal enzyme system. × 20,000.

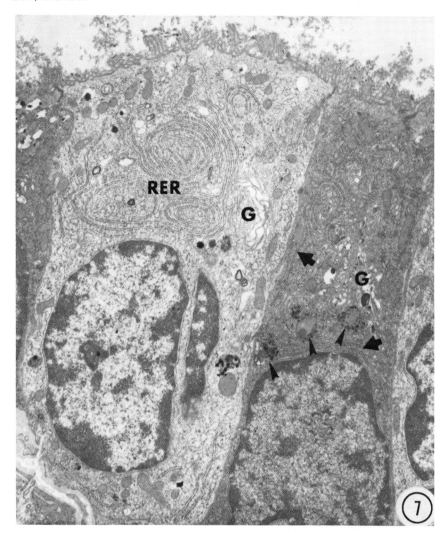

Fig. 7. Ventral prostate, post-castrate rat. Collapse (arrows) and twirling of the rough endoplasmic reticulum (RER), in preparation for sequestering within autophagic vacuoles (see Fig. 8). Golgi, G; secondary lysosomes (arrowheads). × 14,000.

retinoic acid exhibited a peak of (^{3}H) retinoic acid binding in the 2S region which was abolished by excess unlabelled retinoic acid. The assays performed on normal prostatic tissues or in prostates with benign hyperplasia (BPH) either failed to show a (^{3}H) retinoic acid binding peak in the 2S region, or showed values of cRABP far below those detected in prostatic carcinoma. Figure 11 shows a typical curve of (^{3}H) retinoic acid binding in prostatic carcinoma.

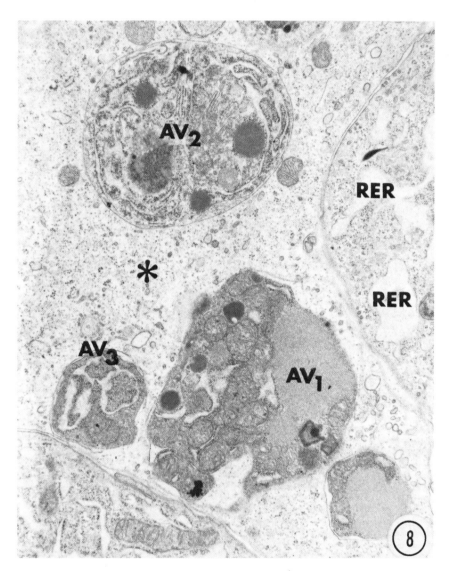

Fig. 8. Ventral prostate, post-castrate rat. Early autophagic vacuoles (AV_1, AV_2, AV_3) containing intact endoplasmic reticulum and mitochondria. Asterisk indicates paucity of unsequestered cytoplasmic organelles in these cells. An adjacent cell reveals persistent well-developed rough endoplasmic reticulum (RER), indicative of nonuniform response to hormone withdrawal. × 23,000.

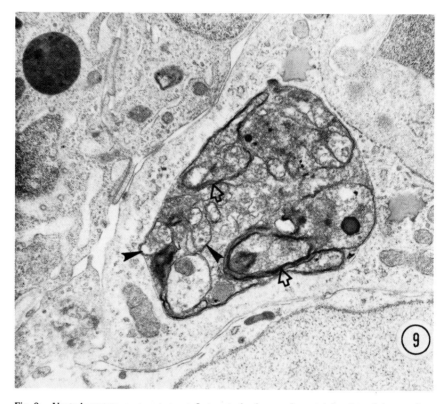

Fig. 9. Ventral prostate, post-castrate rat. Late autophagic vacuole containing degraded organelles, likely mitochondria (arrowheads). Degenerate lipoproteins evolve into lamellar bodies (open arrows). × 28,188.

PA-III Rat prostatic carcinoma cell line. Repeated assays for retinoic acid binding protein failed to detect any (^{3}H) retinoic acid binding in the 2S region.

Cell Surface Studies (PA-III Cell Line)

The general appearance of the PA-III cells growing attached to the surface of plastic culture dishes is shown in Figure 12. The cells have a tendency to pile up in multilayers giving rise to formation of scattered ridges.

In the untreated cells, Concanavalin A-Horseradish peroxidase (ConA-HRP) reaction products showed an electron-dense dispersed labelling pattern, arranged along the entire cell surface (Fig. 13). Cells treated with retinoic acid (10 μg/

TABLE II. Specific activities of acid hydrolases of whole homogenates before and after castration*

Enzyme	Normal rats	Castrated rats	Times increased	P
β-Glucuronidase	2.34	4.61	1.98	<0.01
N-Acetyl-β- glucosaminidase	20.3	47.5	2.34	<0.01
Aryl sulfatase	3.75	9.86	2.64	<0.01

*Values are enzyme units/mg protein.

TABLE III. Percent unsedimentable absolute activities of three lysosomal hydrolases in rat prostate before and after castration

Enzyme	Normal rats	Castrated rats	P*
β-Glucuronidase	52.8	74.5	<0.02
N-Acetyl-β-glucosaminidase	64.6	75.0	<0.05
Aryl sulfatase	42.6	66.7	<0.02

*P, significance of the difference between groups, as ascertained by a t test between normal and castrated rats.

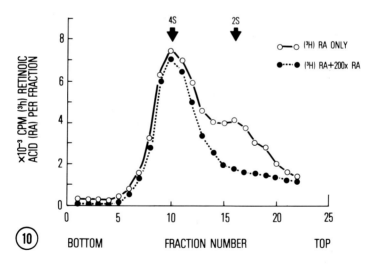

Fig. 10. Occurrence of cellular retinoic acid binding protein (cRABP) in the Dunning R-3327 anaplastic tumor. A peak of (^{3}H) retinoic acid in the 2S region, which is abolished by excess unlabelled ligand, is indicative of the presence of cRABP. Similar 2S peaks were found in the remaining sublines of the R-3327 tumor and in the normal lateral prostate. No peaks were seen in peak, or if present it was of far less magnitude than in carcinoma (see Table IVB).

TABLE IVA. ^{3}(H) Retinoic acid binding in the Copenhagen-Fisher F$_1$ prostatic lobes, and in the R-3327 rat prostatic carcinoma sublines

Tissues	^{3}(H) Retinoic acid binding/mg cytosol protein	
Normal dorsolateral prostate[a]	4100 ± 700	fmole/mg
Normal ventral prostate	0	fmole/mg
R-3327-H tumor	5100 ± 600	fmole/mg
R-3327-HI tumor	7600 ± 1700	fmole/mg
R-3327-AT tumor	5800 ± 500	fmole/mg
R-3327-MAT-LyLu tumor	8000 ± 1400	fmole/mg

TABLE IVB. ^{3}(H) Retinoic acid binding in human normal prostate, BPH, and prostatic carcinoma

Tissues	^{3}(H) Retinoic acid binding/mg cytosol protein	
Normal prostate	Usually non-detectable	
	Occasional negligible amount	
Benign prostatic hypertrophy (BPH)	3190 ± 500	fmole/mg
Prostatic carcinoma	10,620 ± 2000	fmole/mg

Binding values are presented as the mean ± SE.
[a]Separate assays for isolated dorsal and lateral lobes showed the activity to be localized exclusively in the lateral lobes.

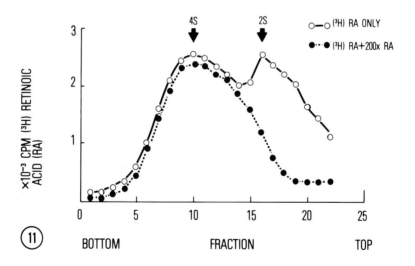

Fig. 11. cRABP in human prostatic carcinoma. (^{3}H) retinoic acid peak in the 2S region, abolished by unlabelled retinoic acid. Assays on BPH or normal prostatic tissues either failed to show a 2S peak, or if present it was of far less magnitude than in carcinoma (see Table IVB).

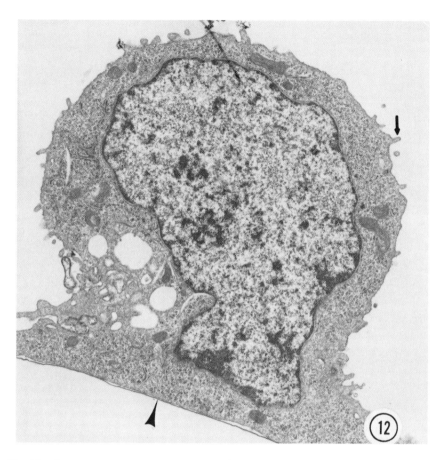

Fig. 12.   General appearance of PA-III rat prostatic carcinoma cultured cells: zone of attachment to plastic flask surface (arrowhead). Slender microprojections are seen at the free cell surface (full arrow). Free ribosomes are abundant, but rough endoplasmic reticulum is scarce. × 17,460.

ml culture medium) observed two days after treatment (Fig. 14) revealed a loss of ConA surface binding, since only occasional clusters of ConA-HRP reaction products could be seen at the cell surface. The loss of ConA-HRP binding to the cell surface became accentuated on day three after treatment (Fig. 15).

X-irradiation (400 rads) produced a similar decrease of ConA-HRP reaction products at the cell surface. This was seen in the cells examined 24 hours after irradiation and became more apparent at 48 hours (Fig. 16). Abundant secondary lysosomes became apparent after x-irradiation. Combined treatment with retinoic

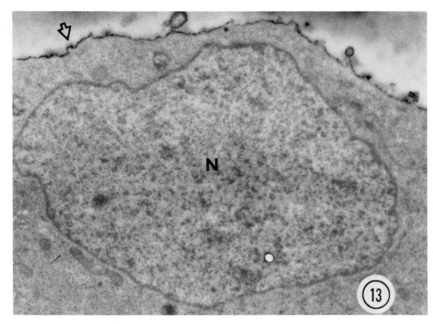

Fig. 13. PA-III cells—untreated control ConA-HRP labelling. Reaction products (open arrow) at cell surface show a dispersed labelling pattern. Nucleus, N. × 17,460.

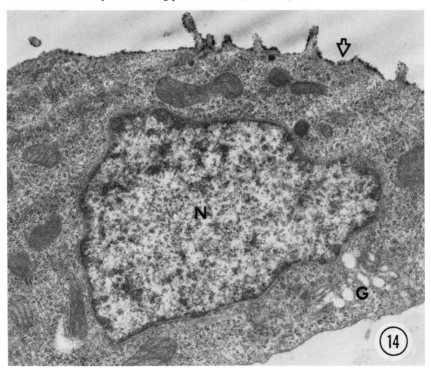

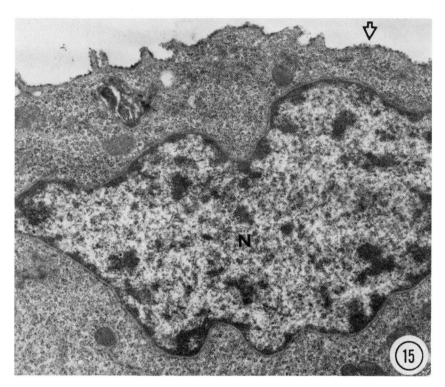

Fig. 15. PA-III cells treated with retinoic acid (10 μg/5 ml culture medium). ConA-HRP labelling performed 3 days after treatment. Loss of surface labelling (open arrow) is accentuated in comparison with day 2. Nucleus, N. × 41,680.

acid and x-irradiation, at dose levels identical to those of the separate treatments (10 μg retinoic acid; 400 rads x-irradiation), revealed the almost complete disappearance of ConA-HRP labelling indicative of an additive effect of the two agents (Fig. 17).

There was a difference in the effects of retinoic acid and x-irradiation on lectin binding sites. Whereas in the retinoic acid-treated cells, decrease in the amount of ConA-HRP reaction products could be seen if cells were fixed in glutaraldehyde immediately following ConA-HRP treatment; in the x-irradiated cells a short incubation (15–25 minutes) in PBS, prior to fixation, was required in order for the loss of lectin binding to become apparent. Forty-eight hours after treatment lysosomes and autophagic vacuoles were detected in the cells subjected to x-irradiation alone or in combination with retinoic acid, indicating damage

Fig. 14. PA-III cells treated with retinoic acid (10 μg/5 ml culture medium). ConA-HRP labelling performed 2 days after treatment. Surface labelling pattern (open arrow) shows wider unlabelled gaps than the controls. Nucleus, N; Golgi, G. × 41,680.

to cytoplasmic organelles (Figs. 16, 17). Neither secondary lysosomes nor autophagic vacuoles were detected in cells treated with retinoic acid exclusively.

DISCUSSION

Morphological and biochemical changes in lysosomes, as seen in the prostatic cells undergoing involution provoked by castration, conform to a general pattern of cell regression, both physiologic and pathologic [18, 44]. For example, a digestion of cytoplasmic organelles such as mitochondria and endoplasmic reticulum within autophagic vacuoles, and apparent translocation of hydrolases from lysosomes into the cytosol, have been observed in post-castration prostatic involution [3, 7, 28, 33, 34], in the post-lactating mammary gland [5], in postpartum uterine involution [4], and in tumor regression following x-irradiation or chemotherapeutic treatment [1, 2, 6, 8, 11, 14, 15, 32, 35]. The apparent destabilization of lysosomes in cells undergoing regressive changes has been exploited in efforts to intensify cell degradation, and possibly cell killing by the use of compounds capable of enhancing lysosomal permeability and leakage of hydrolases into the cytosol. Vitamin A compounds (retinoids) and various steroid hormones appear as the most likely candidates to fulfill this dual purpose of lysosomal labilization and hydrolase release coupled to intensification of tissue regression [2, 6, 8, 9, 15, 16, 36, 48].

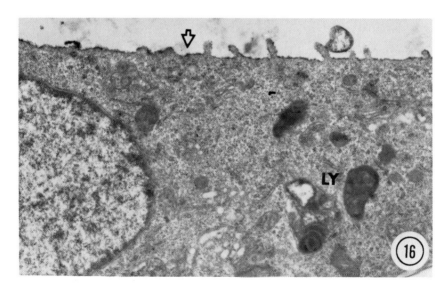

Fig. 16.   PA-III cells—x-irradiated (400 rads). ConA-HRP labelling done 3 days after treatment. Marked loss of surface labelling (open arrow). Note similarity to retinoic acid effect on day 3 (refer to Fig. 15). Secondary lysosomes are present (Ly). × 20,475.

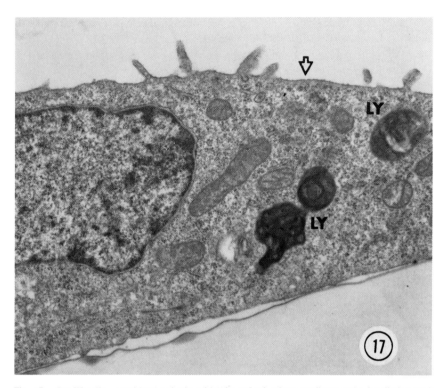

Fig. 17. PA-III cells—combined retinoic acid (10 μg/5 ml culture medium) and x-irradiation (400 rads) treatment. Surface labelling is completely lost (open arrow). Note the presence of abundant secondary lysosomes (Ly). × 41,680.

Recent studies suggest that the effects of retinoids may be mediated by other mechanisms, besides the apparent direct interaction with lysosomes, and that other cell structures may constitute targets for these compounds. A novel cytoplasmic protein, retinoic acid binding protein (cRABP), has been detected in fetal and some adult tissues, both in rats and chickens [29, 38, 40, 41]. Most pertinent to this study, cRABP has been detected in human breast and lung carcinomas, whereas in contrast, normal breast and lung tissue either do not reveal detectable levels of cRABP, or if present, the levels are far below those seen in the malignant tissues [23, 26, 30, 31, 45]. Similar findings have been reported in various animal tumors, including breast, lung, and colonic carcinoma in the rat [39, 42].

As shown in this study, cRABP is also present in human prostatic carcinoma and in the R3327 prostatic adenocarcinoma in the rat. Our results tend to indicate that a similar pattern of high levels in malignant tissues and low or undetectable levels in normal tissue, as shown with other tumors, prevails in relation to human prostatic carcinoma and the rat prostatic adenocarcinoma. Since cRABP is readily detected in fetal tissue [29, 30, 41] then tends to decrease or disappear early in the post-natal period [29] and reappears in tumors, there is good reason to consider this protein as a marker for dedifferentiation and proliferation, analogous to various other fetal proteins that are expressed in tumors [43]. By comparison, it is interesting to note that androgen receptor, which correlates positively with histologic dfifferentiation and hormone response in human prostatic carcinoma and in the R-3327 rat tumor, is not detectable in the anaplastic sublines [17, 19, 24, 25], whereas cRABP as shown here persists at high levels in the undifferentiated sublines.

There is evidence indicating that retinoids, besides their labilizing effects on lysosomes and their RABP-mediated cell growth [13, 27, 38, 40, 46, 49], can also induce alterations in cell surface components [10, 22, 49]. For example, retinoids reduce the surface binding of positively charged colloidal iron particles while enhancing the binding of negatively charged particles [10] and promote the release of sialic acid residues, possibly as a result of lysosomal neuraminidase activity [10, 22]. In the same context, retinoids affect the distribution of cell surface sugars, as evidenced by the displacement of lectin binding sites after in vitro treatment with retinol [47] or retinoic acid, as shown here in PA-III rat prostatic cancer cells. It should be mentioned that some of these cell surface effects are not mediated through a retinoid-RABP interaction mechanism, since they occur in 3T3 fibroblasts [47] and in the PA-III rat prostatic carcinoma cells, included in this study, which lack detectable levels of cRABP. The functional significance of the presence of cRABP in human prostatic carcinoma and in the various sublines of the Dunning R3327 is still uncertain. Inferences can be derived from studies with the MCF-7 human breast cancer cell line, which contains high levels of cRABP as well as several other cell systems [13, 27, 38, 40, 45, 46, 49]. From such studies, it would appear that modulation of cell growth and macromolecular synthesis could be attained through the interaction of the ligand (retinoic acid) with its specific binding protein (cRABP) including interaction at the nuclear level, in a manner similar to that of steroid hormone-receptor interaction. The presence of cRABP in human prostatic carcinoma could also be exploited in the development of combined therapeutic regimens employing retinoids as adjuvants, as shown successfully in several animal tumors and cell culture models [2, 8, 9].

CONCLUSION

Modulation of cell growth by interaction between a ligand and its specific binding protein has been demonstrated in various in vitro and in vivo systems. The best examples are represented by the well established interaction between various steroid hormones and their respective cellular receptors. Similar modulation of cell growth by ligand-receptor interaction involving retinoic acid-binding protein (RABP) has been shown by us using the MCF-7 human breast cancer cell.

The presence of RABP in human prostatic carcinoma and in various sublines of the Dunning R-3327 rat prostatic carcinoma, as shown in these studies, points to a possible endogenous modulation of prostatic cancer cell growth through ligand (retinoic acid)-receptor (RABP) interaction.

Lysosomes and cell surface componets appear as common targets for sex steroids, chemotherapeutic agents, Xrays, and retinoids. Accentuation of the release and activation of lysosomal enzymes along with alteration of cell surface composition by the concerted action of such agents may lead to a substantial enhancement of the anti-tumor effect of conventional procedures in prostatic carcinoma such as orchiectomy, estrogen therapy, and x-irradiation. The net enhancement of the anti-tumor effects of cyclophosphamide and Xrays by retinoid, attained in other animal tumor systems, substantiates these assumptions.

ACKNOWLEDGMENTS

The author would like to thank Dr. M. Pollard and Dr. S.Y. Chan for a gift of the PA-III adenocarcinoma cell line and Dr. J. T. Isaacs for sample tissues of the Dunning R-3327 tumor. Retinoids used in these studies, including ^{3}H-retinoic acid, are a generous gift from Dr. W.E. Scott of Hoffman La-Roche, Nutley, N.J.

Space and research facilities provided by the Gerontology Research Center, National Institute for Aging.

The author wishes especially to acknowledge the cooperation of the investigators that have in the past or are at present collaborating in the various studies reported here: Elsa Anton, Sandra E. Harris, Hisako Ueda, Martin J. Brandes, Mark S. Gesell, Juan C. Millan, and Joseph E. Paris.

This study was supported partly by NIH Biomedical Research Support Grant SO 7-RR-0556 and Pathology Restricted Fund (Chesapeake Physicians Professional Association).

REFERENCES

1. Aikman AA, Wills ED: Studies on lysosomes after irradiation. I. A quantitative histochemical method for the study of lysosomal permeability and acid phosphatase activity. Radiat Res 57:403, 1974.
2. Anton E, Brandes D: Lysosomes in mice mammary tumors treated with cyclophosphamide. Distribution related to course of disease. Cancer 21:483, 1968.
3. Brandes D: Hormonal regulation of fine structure. In Brandes D (ed): "Male Accessory Sex Organs: Structure and Function in Mammals." New York: Academic Press, 1974 pp 182–222.
4. Brandes D, Anton E: Lysosomes in uterine envolution: Intracytoplasmic degradation of myofilaments and collagen. J Gerontol 24:55, 1969.

5. Brandes D, Anton E, Barnard S: Lysosomes and cellular regressive changes in rat mammary gland involution. Lab Invest 20:5, 1969.

6. Brandes D, Anton E, Lam KW: Studies of the L1210 leukemia. II. Ultrastructural and cytochemical changes after treatment with cyclophosphamide (NSC-26271) and vitamin A. J Natl Cancer Inst 39:385, 1967.

7. Brandes D, Kirchheim D: Histochemistry of the prostate. In Tannenbaum M (ed): "Urologic Pathology: The Prostate." Philadelphia: Lea & Febiger, 1977, pp 99–128.

8. Brandes D, Anton E, Schofield BH, Barnard S: Role of lysosomal labilizers in treatment of mammary gland carcinomas with cyclophosphamide (NSC-26271). Preliminary report. Cancer Chemo ther Rep 50:47, 1966.

9. Brandes D, Rundell JO, Ueda H: Radiation response of L1210 leukemic cells pretreated with vitamin A alcohol. J Natl Cancer Inst 52:945–949, 1974.

10. Brandes D, Sato T, Ueda H, Rundell JO: Effect of vitamin A alcohol on the surface coat and charges of L1210 leukemic cells. Cancer Res 34:2151–2158, 1974.

11. Brandes D, Sloan KW, Anton E, Bloedorn F: The effect of x-irradiation on the lysosomes of mouse mammary gland carcinomas. Cancer Res 27:731, 1967.

12. Cham SY: Androgen and glucocorticoid receptors in the Pollard prostate adenocarcinoma cell lines. The Prostate 1:53–60, 1980.

13. Chytil L, Ong D: Mediation of retinoic acid-induced growth and anti-tumor activity. Nature 260:49–51, 1976.

14. Clarke C, Wills ED: Lysosomal enzyme activation in irradiated mammary tumours. Radiat Res 67:435, 1976.

15. Clarke C, Wills ED: The activation of lymphoid tissue lysosomal enzymes by steroid hormones. J Steroid Biochem 9:135, 1978.

16. Cohen MH, Carbone PP: Enhancement of the antitumor effect of 1,3-bis (2-choloroethyl)-1-nitrosourea and cyclophosphamide by vitamin A. J Natl Cancer Inst 48:921–926, 1972.

17. Dahlberg E, Snochowski M, Gustafsson JA: Comparison of the R-3327H rat prostatic adenocarcinoma to human benign prostatic hyperplasia and metastatic carcinoma of the prostate with regard to steroid hormone receptors. The Prostate 1:61–70, 1980.

18. DeDuve C: Lysosomes and cell injury. In Thomas LJ, Uhr JW, Grant L (eds): "International Symposium on Injury, Inflammation and Immunity." Baltimore: Williams & Wilkins, 1964 pp 283–311.

19. Geller J, Albert J, delaVega D, Loza D, Soeltzing W: Dihydrotestosterone concentration in prostate cancer tissue as a predictor of tumor differentiation and hormonal dependency. Cancer Res 38:4349–4352, 1978.

20. Groth DP, Brandes D: Correlative electronmicroscopy and biochemical studies on the effect of estradiol on the rat ventral prostate. J Ultrastruct Res 4:166, 1960.

21. Gustafsson JA, Ekman P, Snochowski M, Zetterberg A, Pousette A, Högberg B: Correlation between clinical response to hormone therapy and steroid receptor content in prostatic cancer. Cancer Res 38:4345–4348, 1978.

22. Hogan-Ryan A, Fennally JJ: Neuraminidase-like effect of vitamin A on cell surface. Eur J Cancer 14:113–116, 1978.

23. Huber PR, Geyer E, Küng W, Matter A, Torhorst J, Eppenberger U: Retinoic acid-binding protein in human breast cancer and dysplasia. J Natl Cancer Inst 61:1375–1378, 1978.

24. Isaacs JT, Heston WDW, Weissman RM, Coffey DS: Animal models of the hormone-sensitive and insensitive prostatic adenocarcinomas, Dunning 4-3327H, R-3327-HI, and R-3327-AT. Cancer Res 38:4353–4359, 1978.

25. Isaacs JT, Isaacs WB, Coffey DS: Models for development of non-receptor methods for distinguishing androgen-sensitive and insensitive prostatic tumors. Cancer Res 39:2652–2659, 1979.

26. Küng WM, Geyer E, Eppenberger U, Huber PR: Quantitative estimation of cellular retinoic acid-binding protein activity in normal, dysplastic and neoplastic human breast tissue. Cancer Res 40:4265–4269, 1980.

27. Lotan R, Nicolson GL: Inhibitory effect of retinoic acid or retinyl acetate on the growth of untransformed, transformed, and tumor cells in vitro. J Natl Cancer Inst 59:1717–1722, 1977.

28. Ofner P, Leav I, Cavazos LF: C_{19}-steroid metabolism in male sex glands. Correlation of changes in fine structure and radiometabolite patterns in the prostate of the androgen deprived dog. In Brandes D (ed): "Male Accessory Sex Organs: Structure and Function in Mammals." New York: Academic Press, 1974, pp 267–305.

29. Ong DE, Chytil F: Changes in levels of cellular retinol- and retinoic-acid-binding proteins of liver and lung during perinatal development of rat. Proc Natl Acad Sci USA 73:3976–3978, 1976.

30. Ong DE, Page DL, Chytil F: Retinoic acid-binding protein occurrence in human tumors. Science 190:60–61, 1976.

31. Palan PR, Romney SL: Cellular binding proteins for vitamin A in human carcinomas and in normal tissues. Cancer Res 40:4221–4224, 1980.

32. Paris JE, Brandes D: Effect of x-irradiation on the functional status of lysosomal enzymes of mouse mammary gland carcinomas. Cancer Res 31:392, 1971.

33. Paris JE, Brandes D: The effect of castration on histochemistry and biochemistry of acid hydrolases of rat prostatic gland. J Natl Cancer Inst 49:1685, 1972.

34. Paris JE, Brandes D: Lysosomal enzymes: Their role in secretion, involution and other processes in male sex accessory organs. In Brandes D (ed): "Male Accessory Sex Organs: Structure and Function in Mammals." New York: Academic Press, 1974, pp 223–233.

35. Reynolds C, Willis ED: The effect of irradiation on lysosomal activation in HeLa cells. Int J Radiat Biol 25:113, 1974.

36. Roels OA: The influence of vitamins A and E on lysosomes. In Dingle JT, Fell HB (eds): "Lysosomes in Biology and Pathology." Amsterdam: North-Holland Publ. Co., 1969, pp 254–275.

37. Rundell JO, Sato T, Wetzelberger E, Ueda H, Brandes D: Lysosomal enzyme release by vitamin A in L1210 leukemia cells. J Natl Cancer Inst 52:1237–1243, 1974.

38. Sani BP: Localization of retinoic acid-binding protein in nuclei. Biochem Biophys Res Commun 75:7–12, 1977.

39. Sani BP, Corbett TH: Retinoic acid-binding protein in normal tissues and experimental tumors. Cancer Res 37:209–213, 1977.

40. Sani BP, Donovan MK: Localization of retinoic acid-binding protein in nuclei and the nuclear uptake of retinoic acid. Cancer Res 39:2492–2496, 1979.

41. Sani BP, Hill DL: A retinoic acid-binding protein from chick embryo skin. Cancer Res 36:409–413, 1976.

42. Sani BP, Titus BC: Retinoic acid-binding protein in experimental tumors and in tissues with metastatic tumor foci. Cancer Res 37:4031–4034, 1977.

43. Shapira F: Isozymes and cancer. Adv Cancer Res 18:77–153, 1973.

44. Slater TF: Lysosomes and experimentally induced tissue injury. In Dingle JT, Fell HB (eds): "Lysosomes in Biology and Pathology." Amsterdam: North-Holland Publ. Co., 1969, pp 467–492.

45. Takenawa T, Ueda H, Brandes D, Millan JC: Retinoic acid-binding protein in a human cell (MCF-7) from breast carcinoma. Lab Invest 42:490–494, 1980.

46. Ueda H, Takenawa T, Millan JC, Gesell MS, Brandes D: The effects of retinoids on proliferative capacities and macromolecular synthesis in human breast cancer MCF-7 cells. Cancer 46:2203–2209, 1980.

47. Ueda H, Gesell MS, Millan JC, Harris SB, Brandes D: Effects of retinol and x-rays on con-A binding to the surface of 3T3 and SV 40-3T3 cells. J Natl Cancer Inst (submitted).

48. Weissmann G: The effects of steroids and drugs on lysosomes. In Dingle JT, Fell HB (eds): "Lysosomes in Biology and Pathology." Amsterdam: North-Holland Publ. Co., 1969, pp 276–298.

49. Wiggert B, Russell P, Lewis M, Chader G: Differential binding to soluble nuclear receptors and effects on cell viability of retinol and retinoic acid in cultured retinoblastoma cells. Biochem Biophys Res Commun 79:218–225, 1977.

50. Woessner JL Jr: The physiology of the uterus and mammary gland. In Dingle JT, Fell HB (eds): "Lysosomes in Biology and Pathology." Amsterdam: North-Holland Publ. Co., 1969, pp 299–324.

CLINICAL STUDIES

The Prostatic Cell: Structure and Function
Part B, pages 231–248
© 1981 Alan R. Liss, Inc., 150 Fifth Avenue, New York, NY 10011

The Functional Cytomorphology of Canine Prostatic Epithelium

Christoph Hohbach, Heinz Ueberberg, and Hans Deutsch

The canine prostate shows, like the human prostate, a high age-related incidence of benign prostatic hyperplasia, and among our common laboratory animals dogs have the highest frequency of spontaneously developing prostatic carcinomas [1,2]. However, both diseases show certain differences in morphology, biochemistry, hormonal regulation, or metastatic spread in the case of the carcinoma [3,4], when compared to the corresponding diseases in man. Despite these shortcomings the canine prostatic epithelium is still a suitable animal model to study basic morphological reactions of this androgen-dependent target organ, comparable to those alterations histopathologists observe in the human prostate spontaneously developed or therapeutically induced.

MATERIALS AND METHODS

For our investigations we used 24 mature Beagle dogs (CHBS-Beagle strain) divided into six groups. In comparison to the normal prostate the initial hormonal condition of the prostate was varied as follows:

1) Orchidectomy 90 days prior to the end of the experiment.
2) Application of estradiol undecylate as a single i.m. dose of 1 mg/kg body weight 14 days prior to the end of the experiment.
3) Application of the anti-androgen cyproterone acetate, 10 mg/kg body weight, orally for 21 days.

This paper is dedicated to the memory of Prof. Eberhard Altenähr, Head of the Institute of Pathology, Klinikum Steglitz, Freie Universität, Berlin.

Abbreviations –, negative; (+), questionably positive; +, weakly positive; + +, clearly positive; + + +, intensely positive; /, intermediate stage; c, control; CAS, orchidectomy; CPA, cyproterone acetate; ES, estradiol; Br, bromocriptine; PL, prolactin.

4) Ovine prolactin, 10 IU/kg body weight i.m. for 14 days.
5) Prolactin inhibition with bromocriptine, 0.3 mg/kg body weight, orally for 14 days.

In addition to the already published histological, histochemical (acid phosphatase), and ultrastructural methods [5], we studied histochemically the content and distribution of zinc in the glandular epithelium using the disulphide-method of Timm [6]. Abbreviations used for the evaluation of the histochemical reactions appear on the preceding page.

RESULTS

The Normal Prostate

Densely packed acini form approximately 40–50 lobules and are separated by a fibromuscular stroma. They are lined by a tall columnar epithelium, which is densely granulated in the apical cytoplasm. Papillary infoldings of the epithelium are protruding into the lumen of the acini (Fig. 1a).

In the same location an intense activity of acid phosphatase is to be observed. Infoldings of the epithelium simulate enzyme deposits in the glandular lumen. Basal parts of the epithelium and the nuclei show negative reactions (Fig. 2a, Table I). Zinc is also found in the apical cytoplasm as a fine dark brown granulation, ie, corresponding to the topography of acid phosphatase (Fig. 2b, Table II).

The ultrastructure of the epithelium, which has already been discussed in detail [5, 7, 8], shows the typical polar segmentation with basal nuclear region and apical accumulation of secretory organelles. The numerous electron-dense secretory granules are the outstanding ultrastructural feature. Their distribution is identical with the localization of acid phosphatase (Fig. 2a; Fig. 3). The secretory granules are secreted only by exocytosis in the area of the apical cell pole between a dense fringe of microvilli. Autophagic vacuoles and lysosomes, which we know as the actual morphological substrate of the acid phosphatase, are normally rare, mostly being involved in the degradation of secretion and not affected by exocytosis. Basal reserve cells, which represent the regenerative blastema of the epithelium, contain only a few organelles and are usually lacking secretion (Fig. 4).

The Epithelium After Prolactin and Prolactin Inhibition

After a 14-day period of prolactin and high-dose antiprolactin treatment the prostatic epithelium shows no significant qualitative deviation from its normal state with respect to the histochemistry of acid phosphatase and zinc (Tables I, II) or to ultrastructure. The cellular integrity and secretory function are well maintained. At the utmost the nuclei of basal cells seem to be occasionally more

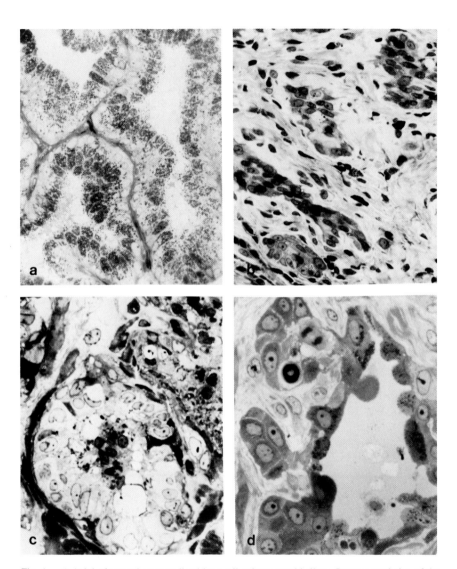

Fig. 1.   a) Acini of normal prostate lined by a tall columnar epithelium. Dense granulation of the apical cytoplasm of the secretory cells. Semithin section; × 600. b) Postcastration atrophy of the acini, fibrosis of stroma. Semithin section; × 600. c) Atrophy after cyproterone acetate with epithelial necrosis and cellular debris in the collapsed lumen. Semithin section; × 900. d) Bud-like atrophy of secretory cells and pronounced squamous cell metaplasia of proliferating basal cells after estradiol. Semithin section; × 900.

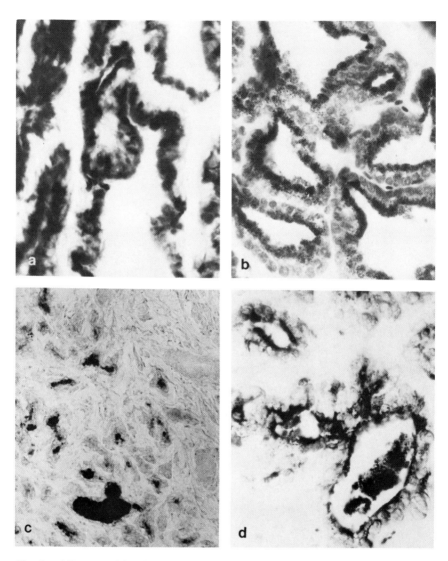

Fig. 2. a) Intense activity of acid phosphatase in the apical cytoplasm of glandular epithelium, normal prostate. × 600. b) Pronounced zinc-positive granulation of the apical portion of secretory cells, normal prostate. × 600. c) Marked loss of acid phosphatase activity after cyproterone acetate, remaining focal activity due to increased lysosomal activity and cellular debris of secretory cells. × 600. d) Reduced zinc content of secretory cells with coarse zinc-positive clusters in the lumen, corresponding to cellular debris after cyproterone acetate. × 600.

TABLE I. Activity and distribution of acid phosphatase

	Nucleus	Cytoplasm	Lumen	Stroma	Capillaries
		Glands			
C	—	+ + +	–/+	–/+	—
CAS	—	(+)/+	—	–/+	—
CPA	—	+/+ +	+/+ +	–/+	—
ES	—	+	(+)	–/+	—
BR	—	+ + +	–/+	–/+	—
PL	—	+ + +	–/+	–/+	—

TABLE II. Presence and distribution of zinc

	Nucleus	Cytoplasm	Lumen	Stroma	Capillaries
		Glands			
C	—	+ + +	–/+	—	—
CAS	—	—	—	—	—
CPA	—	+/+ +	–/+	–/+	—
ES	—	+	(+)	–/+	—
BR	—	+ + +	–/+	—	—
PL	—	+ + +	–/+	—	—

polymorphous (Fig. 5), and liposomes partly linked to autophagic vacuoles in the cytoplasm of secreting cells seem to be slightly increased after bromocriptine. However, there are no signs of functional deficiency at all.

The Epithelium After Androgen Withdrawal

Ninety days after orchidectomy the prostate is completely atrophic. Small epithelial nests line slit-like lumina and are surrounded by a broadened stroma, also with atrophic smooth muscles (Fig. 1b). Acid phosphatase has disappeared, except for almost undetectable residues, and zinc is no longer present (Tables I, II). Ultrastructurally the differentiation of the epithelium into secretory and basal reserve cells has almost completely ceased and no secretory function has been retained. Besides a few remaining secondary lysosomes, increased numbers of liposomes and glycogen deposits are present in the atrophied cytoplasm in the vicinity of the irregular nuclei (Fig. 6).

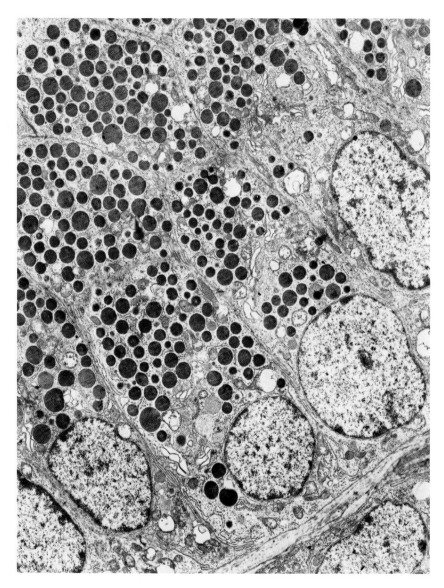

Fig. 3.   Tall columnar glandular epithelium of normal prostate, numerous electron-dense secretory granules in the apical cytoplasm. × 5400.

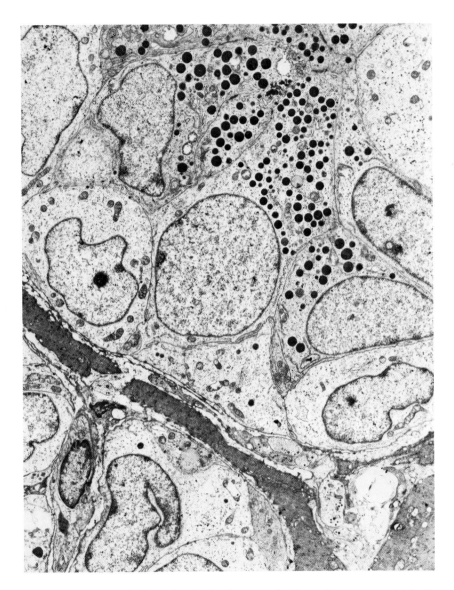

Fig. 4.   Poorly differentiated secretion-free basal reserve cells of normal prostate, granulated active superficial epithelial layer. × 6000.

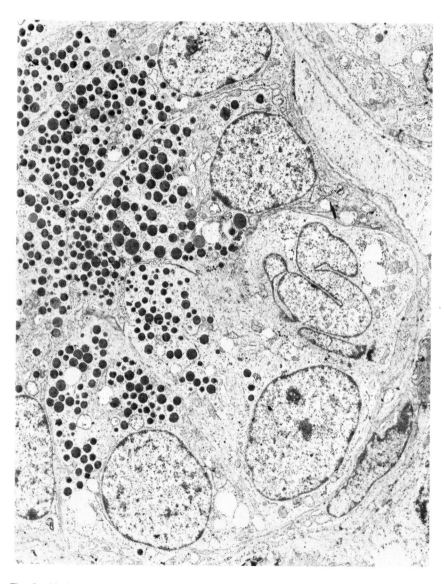

Fig. 5. Nuclear polymorphism of basal cells after bromocriptine, intact and active superficial secretory cells. × 4000.

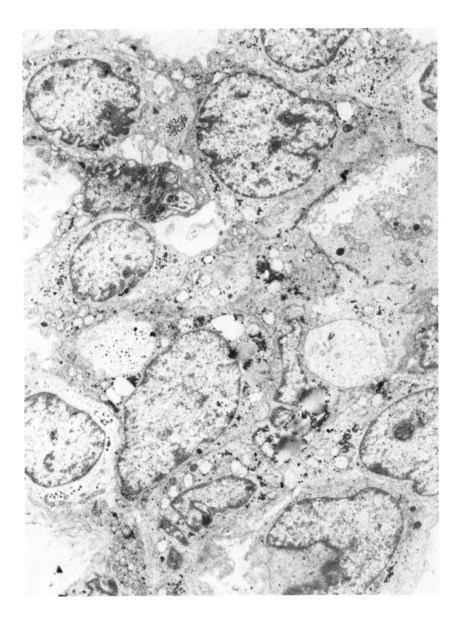

Fig. 6. Advanced atrophy of glandular epithelium after castration, loss of secretion and basal-cell-like dedifferentiation of secretory cells, paranuclear glycogen deposits and liposomes. × 4000.

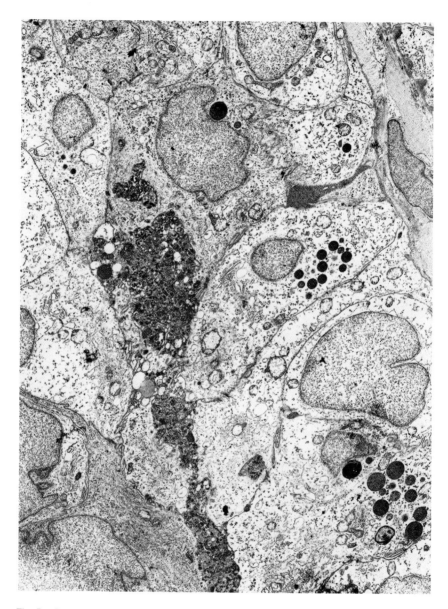

Fig. 7. Pronounced involution of glandular epithelium after cyproterone acetate, loss of secretory granules, increased number of secondary lysosomes, slit-like lumen filled with cellular debris. × 5400.

Twenty-one days after androgen receptor blocking by cyproterone acetate the glandular acini collapse. Many contain cellular debris. The cytoplasm of the epithelium is vacuolated and often contains polymorphous inclusions (Fig. 1c). Acid phosphatase is retained only as a focal coarse residual activity in the epithelium or mostly in desquamated cell clusters in the glandular lumen. The reaction of zinc is the same (Fig. 2 c,d; tables I,II). The metal is sometimes stored in macrophages of the stroma. Ultrastructurally there is a complete loss of secretory function. Instead bizarre autophagic and heterophagic vacuoles and apoptotic bodies prove the significant epithelial damage which involves basal reserve cells and secretory epithelia. Some cells even show necrosis and segregation of the basement membrane of the acini. Other regions exhibit advanced atrophy with rather decreased lysosomal activity (Figs. 7,8).

Fourteen days after a single administration of estradiol, increased mitotic activity with proliferation of basal cells which are transforming into metaplastic squamous cells is to be observed (Fig. 1d). Inclusion bodies are frequent. This is proved by the ultrastructural feature of the epithelium (Figs. 9,10). The basal cells no longer show any tendency towards secretory differentiation. Metaplastic non-cornifying squamous cells push atrophying secretory cells away from the basement membrane (Fig. 9). Secretory function ceases apart from isolated exocytosis of the few remaining granules of varying electron density. Secondary lysosomes and autophagic vacuoles indicate increased turnover and degradation of secretory granules and other organelles involved in the secretory process. Highly activated macrophages with phagocytosis of necrobiotic secretory cells prove the also augmented heterophagia (Fig. 10). Acid phosphatase shows a distinct loss of activity with a few residues in the atrophying epithelium or in macrophages migrating into the surrounding stroma. The distribution and content of zinc corresponds again to the focal residues of secretion in the involuting epithelium and in activated macrophages (tables I,II).

DISCUSSION

Prostatic Secretory Function and Its Related Histochemical Parameters

Evidently secretion is the main function of the prostatic epithelium. It is androgen-dependent and ceases rather rapidly after androgen withdrawal. Accordingly the predominating organelles of glandular epithelium are normally the numerous electron-dense secretory granules, showing species-specific differences among different animals and man [7,8]. In the dog they are secreted only via exocytosis. This mode of secretion remains unchanged in the benign prostatic hyperplasia of senile dogs [5]. In addition, our experiments with prolactin, bromocriptine, and even estradiol have shown that exocytosis is preserved in

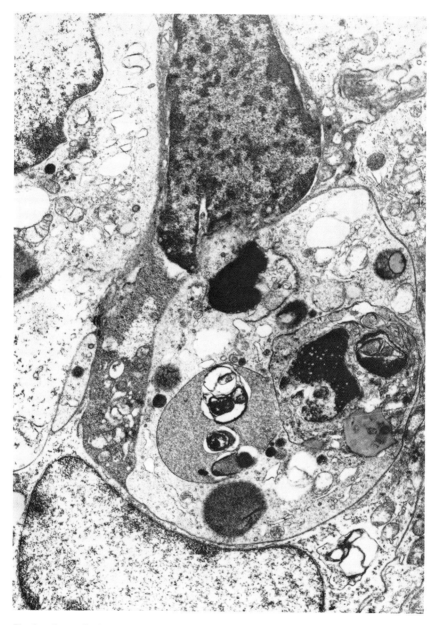

Fig. 8.   Apoptotic phagosome with condensed membrane-bound nuclear and cytoplasmic fragments in macrophage after cyproterone acetate. × 14,400.

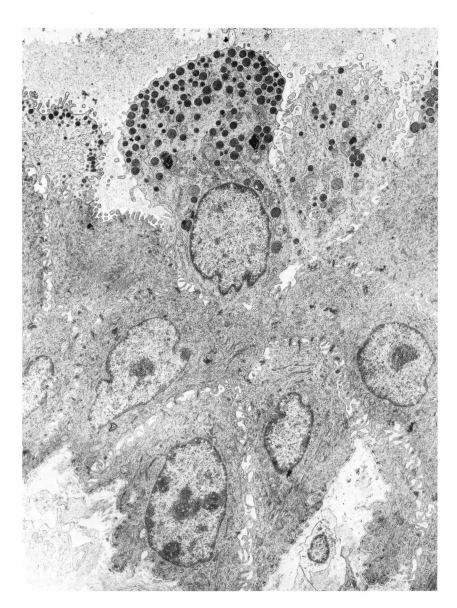

Fig. 9.   Squamous cell metaplasia of basal cells, advanced atrophy of secretory cells with distinct loss of secretory granules after estradiol. × 5400.

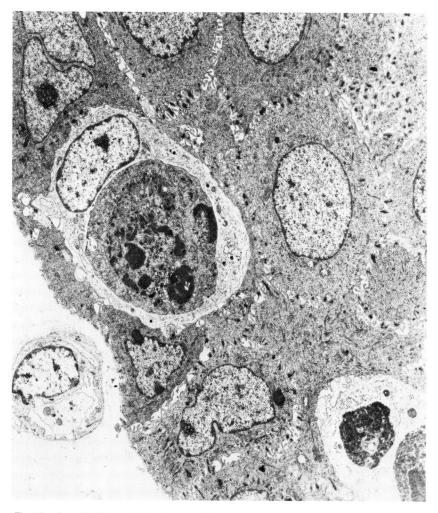

Fig. 10. Intensified heterophagia after estradiol, activated macrophages between metaplastic squamous cells containing debris of phagocytosed damaged secretory cells. × 4000.

case of deeply altered hormonal conditions of the prostate as long as the epithelium contains secretion. Yet, during maximum stimulation with intravenously applied pilocarpine, exocytosis is principally retained and only quantitatively increased [9].

Among the prostatic enzymes, acid phosphatase is of greatest importance for experimental and clinical investigations. In contrast to its rather complicated biochemistry [10,11] the enzyme has two carrier systems in the glandular epithelium easily definable by their morphological and functional properties. The quantitatively predominant part is bound to the secretory granules, whose number and distribution correspond to the enzyme activity and localization. The incorporation of acid phosphatase into the secretion is evidently androgen-dependent as it is a step in the sequence of the androgen-mediated secretory process. The quantitatively smaller part of the enzyme is integrated into the lysosomes [9,10], which are not involved in the process of exocytosis as such. However, they control a crucial point in the cycle of secretion because one of their main intracellular functions is to regulate the amount of secretion. This occurs mainly in the case of androgen deficiency when the lysosomal compartment of the atrophying epithelium is continuously activated to eliminate the excess of secretion within the bounds of the loss of secretory function [12]. The results of estradiol and anti-androgen treatment demonstrate that this elimination is done not only by increased autophagia but by intensified heterophagia as well. Both lysosomal and secretory acid phosphatase inevitably achieve the zero point in the complete atrophy 90 days after castration simply because secretory organelles, the degradation of which would require increased lysosomal activity, are no longer present.

In addition to acid phosphatase the remarkably high zinc content of glandular epithelium is another histochemical parameter of equal value for the evaluation of the functional integrity of the prostate. Concerning amount, distribution, and susceptibility to experimental manipulations of the prostate, the metal and enzyme show far-reaching analogies. As the enzyme, zinc only becomes part of the free secretion via exocytosis of the secretory granules wherein zinc is predominantly stored. From the functional morphological point of view the lysosomal system should primarily be free of zinc. With respect to our results of anti-androgen and estradiol treatment the metal is evidently incorporated into the lysosomal system only via autophagia or heterophagia of degraded secretion. Analogous to acid phosphatase, zinc metabolism of glandular epithelium is androgen dependent [13]. Androgen blocking decreases the zinc content of the prostate to a complete loss 3 months after castration. Whereas the histotopography and hormonal control of zinc can easily be studied under experimental conditions, the functional significance of the metal for male accessory sex organs remains to be established [14,15].

Atrophy of the Prostate

The importance of an intact testicular function has been known for a long time [16]. Any disorder of androgen metabolism causes atrophy of prostatic epithelium [4, 17] which is again reversible by androgens [18]. According to our results the formal pathogenesis of atrophy runs a different course. After orchidectomy secretory active epithelium and basal cells atrophy, living a vita minima until androgens will restore them functionally.

Comparable results can be achieved by the overall androgen receptor blocking with cyproterone acetate. The findings after cyproterone acetate show that initially a phase of largely increasing lysosomal activity occurs with pronounced autophagia and heterophagia which is comparatively delayed in the early postcastration phase [19–21]. The damage to cellular integrity often progresses to necrosis or to the formation of apoptotic bodies [20] causing a considerable loss of functional epithelium. Complete atrophy with expired lysosomal and secretory activity resembles the above mentioned postcastration feature. It is already present in parts of the epithelial layer and is evidently achieved more rapidly than after orchidectomy.

In addition to the very complex biochemical interactions between estradiol and androgens [4] our results suggest a direct influence of estradiol on prostatic morphology. This concerns the basal reserve cells only and is quite different to the castration or anti-androgen induced alterations. The basal cells proliferate and show squamous cell metaplasia. On the contrary the functionally specific epithelium, which is exclusively androgen-dependent, atrophies in the sense of androgen blocking. Lysosomal activity is increased as after cyproterone acetate, but is confined only to the atrophying epithelium and not to the developing metaplastic squamous cells which are evidently estrogen-dependent.

Prolactin and Prostatic Morphology

An increasing number of papers is concerned with a proliferation-enhancing synergism for the prostate between prolactin and testosterone [22,23]. This discussion has received new aspects by the development of specific prolactin inhibitors such as bromocriptine [24] and their importance to experimental investigations and possible treatment of neoplastic prostatic disease [25,26].

Morphologically comparative data of dogs were not available to us, so that our investigations still assume the character of a pilot study. To avoid a decrease of prolactin receptors in the prostate we used dogs with intact testes only [27].

However, we could neither demonstrate a typical morphological pattern of hyperprolactinemia nor of prolactin deficiency as compared to the very impressive feature of the estradiol or anti-androgen treated epithelium.

In part this negative result is surprising since suppression of prolactin with bromocriptine is said not only to lower the endogenous testosterone level, but also to hamper the in vivo uptake of testosterone into prostatic tissue as well [28]. Knowing the very sensitive reaction of prostatic glandular epithelium to androgen deficiency we expected the secretory cells at least to suffer a loss of function after bromocriptine treatment. Instead they were intact and quite active with regard to the ultrastructure and the histochemical reaction of acid phosphatase and zinc. Recently published data [29,30] which are contradictory to the current view of prolactin interactions with androgen target organs seem to support our negative findings. According to these data bromocriptine does not lower but activates the secretory function of rat ventral prostate [29] and induces dihydrotestosterone accumulation in dog prostate, whereas the content of this highly active intracellular androgen was decreased by prolactin [30]. In conclusion these results make it clear that our present knowledge concerning the prostatic effects of prolactin and bromocriptine is conflicting and incomplete and requires further investigation.

REFERENCES

1. Taylor PA: Prostatic adenocarcinoma in a dog and a summary of ten cases. Can Vet J 14: 162–166, 1973.
2. Rivenson A, Silverman J: The prostatic carcinoma in laboratory animals: A bibliographic survey from 1900 to 1977. Invest Urol 16: 468–472, 1979.
3. Walsh PC: Benign postatic hyperplasia: Etiological considerations. In Marberger H, Haschek H, Schirmer HKA, Colston JAC, Witkin E (eds): "Progress in Clinical and Biological Research." New York: Alan R. Liss, Inc., Vol 6, 1976, pp 1–7.
4. Sandberg AA: Endocrine control and physiology of the prostate. The Prostate 1: 169–184, 1980.
5. Hohbach C: Ultrastructural and histochemical studies of the prostate of dog under cyproterone acetate. Invest Urol 15: 117–123, 1977.
6. Timm F: Zur Histochemie der Schwermetalle. Das Sulfid-Silberverfahren. Dtsch Z ges gerichtl Med 46: 706–711, 1958.
7. Brandes D: The fine structure and histochemistry of prostatic glands in relation to sex hormones. Int Rev Cytol 20: 207–276, 1966.
8. Aumüller G: Prostate gland and seminal vesicles. In Oksche A, Vollrath L (eds): "Handbuch der mikroskopischen Anatomie des Menschen." Berlin, Heidelberg, New York: Springer-Verlag, 1979, Vol 7/6, pp 53–182.
9. Hohbach C: Die funktionelle Cytomorphologic des Drüenepithels—dargestellt an der Prostata des Hundes. Habilitationsschrift, Medizinische Fakultät der Universität des Saarlandes, 1979, pp 4–200.
10. Ostrowski W: Human prostatic acid phosphatase: physicochemical and catalytic properties. In Spring-Mills E, Hafez ESE (eds): "Male accessory Sex Glands." Elsevier/North-Holland Biomedical Press, 1980, pp 197–213.
11. Aumüller G, Pohl C, Seitz J: Secretory and lysosomal acid phosphatases of the male accessory sex glands. The Prostate 1: 134, 1980.
12. Bruchovsky N, Lesser B, Van Dorn E, Craven S: Hormonal effects on cell proliferation in the rat prostate. Vit Horm 33: 61–68, 1975.
13. Whithmore WF: Comments on zinc in the human and canine prostates. Natl Cancer Inst Monogr 12: 337–340, 1963.
14. Schenck B: Physiologie und Pathophysiologie der Prostata und des Prostatasekretes. In Senge T, Neumann F, Richter K (eds): "Physiologie und Pathophysiologie der Prostata." Stuttgart: Georg-Thieme-Verlag, 1975, pp 11–24.
15. Farnsworth WE: Functional biochemistry of the prostate. In Spring-Mills E, Hafez ESE (eds): "Male Accessory Sex Glands." Elsevier/North-Holland Biomedical Press, 1980, 155–182.
16. White WJ: Castration in hypertrophy of the prostate. Ann Surg 22: 1–80, 1895.
17. Tveter KJ, Dahl E, Aakvaag A: Effect of antiandrogens on the prostate gland. In Spring-Mills

E. Hafez ESE (eds): "Male Accessory Sex Glands." Elsevier/North-Holland Biomedical Press, 1980, pp 495–520.

18. Okada K, Yokoyama M, Tokue A, Takayasu H: Ultracytochemical and morphological studies of some phosphatases in the epithelial cells of the rat ventral prostate under various hormonal conditions. J Electron Microsc 23: 277–284, 1874.

19. Helminen HJ, Ericsson JLE: Ultrastructural studies on prostatic involution in the rat. Evidence for focal irreversible damage to epithelium and heterophagic digestion in macrophages. J Ultrastruct Res 39: 443–455, 1972.

20. Kerr JFR, Searle J: Deletion of cells by apoptosis during castration-induced involution of the rat prostate. Virchows Arch (Cell Pathol) 13: 87–102, 1973.

21. Dahl E, Kjaerheim A: The ultrastructure of the accessory sex organs of the male rat. II. The post-castration involution of the ventral, lateral and the dorsal prostate. Z Zellforsch 144: 167–178, 1973.

22. Farnsworth WE: Prolactin and Carcinogenesis. Prolactin and the prostate. In Boyns AR, Griffiths K (eds): Fourth Tenovus Workshop. Cardiff, Wales: Alpha Omega Alpha Publishing, 1972, pp 217–225.

23. Negro-Vilar A: Prolactin and the growth of prostate and seminal vesicles. In Spring-Mills E, Hafez ESE (eds): "Male Accessory Sex Glands." Elsevier/North-Holland Biomedical Press, 1980, pp 223–233.

24. Flückiger E:The pharmacology of bromocriptine. In Bayliss RS, Turner P, Maclay WP (eds): "Pharmacological and Clinical Aspects of Bromocriptine (Pralodel)." Turnbridge Wells Kent TN 3 ODY: MCS Consultants 1976, pp 12–26.

25. Helmerich D, Altwein JE: Effect of prolactin and the antiprolactin bromocriptine on the testosterone uptake and metabolism in androgen-sensitive and intensitive canine organs. Urol Res 4: 101–105, 1976.

26. Jacobi GH, Altwein JE: Bromocriptin, ein neues therapeutisches Prinzip beim Prostata-adenom und -carcinom. Dtsch med Wschr 103: 1–7, 1978.

27. Kledzik GS, Marshall S, Campbell GA, Gelato M, Meites J: Effects of castration, testosterone, estradiol and prolactin on specific prolactin-binding activity in ventral prostate of male rats. Endocrinology 98: 373–379, 1976.

28. Jacobi, GH, Sinterhauf K, Kurth KH, Altwein JE: Bromocriptine and prostatic carcinoma: plasmakinetics, production and tissue uptake of ^{3}H-testosterone in vivo. J Urol 119: 240–243, 1978.

29. Rohr HP, Bartsch G, Riedtmann J-J: The effect of bromocriptine on the ventral prostatic lobe of the rat. Ultr Pathol, 1980 (in press).

30. Jacobi GH: Pallivativtherapie des Prostatakarzinoms. Endokrinologische Grundlagen, klinische Situation, Prolactin—ein neues Prinzip. München: W. Zuckschwerdt Verlag, 1980, pp 29–111.

The Prostatic Cell: Structure and Function
Part B, pages 249-256
© 1981 Alan R. Liss, Inc., 150 Fifth Avenue, New York, NY 10011

Metastasis of Rat Prostate Adenocarcinoma Cells

Morris Pollard and Sham-Yuen Chan

INTRODUCTION

One of the important goals in biomedical research is the development and use of model disease systems in animals which resemble counterpart diseases in man [1, 2]. Several model tumor systems have been developed which include carcinomas of the breast, intestine, liver, and prostate [3]. In addition, model systems have been developed and used for studies on lymphatic and myelogenous leukemias, reticulum cell sarcoma, and myeloma. Some of the tumors appear "spontaneously," which means that we know neither the initiators nor the promoters of these tumors. Other model tumors develop in specific genetic strains of animals, or they result from the administration of physical, chemical, and viral oncogenic agents.

Those characteristics which are considered optimal for a model system can be listed as follows: They should be autochthonous and organ-related. They should occur in significant frequency and grow progessively. One characteristic of importance in oncology is that of metastasis, by which tumor cells spread from primary site to distant organs in which new proliferating neoplastic foci are established. It is important to know why tumor cells metastasize since this information would lead inevitably to procedures for its control: This involves promoters and antagonists of that process.

During the past six years, in the course of examining 15 aged (> 30 months) male germfree (GF) Lobund-Wistar (L-W) rats, large, grossly visible prostate adenocarcinomas (PA) were observed in 15 rats [4, 5]. Also, prostate tumors were recorded in two aged *conventional* L-W rats. In 13 of the rats with prostate tumors, metastatic lesions were observed in the lungs, and less frequently in the liver and kidneys. Microscopic evidence of PAs has been observed in additional L-W rats. The etiology or etiologies of the "spontaneous" prostate tumors are not known; however, other primary malignant carcinomas have been observed in the lung and in the livers of GF L-W male and female rats [6], which could mean that the rats had been exposed to a carcinogenic agent(s). The agent(s) responsible for the malignant neoplasms observed in GF L-W rats may be contaminants in the sterile food and bedding which they consume. It would not be appropriate to calculate the incidence of PA in L-W rats because relatively few of them are maintained into old age. However, L-W rats are uniquely susceptible to the development of metastatic PA, whatever the inducing agent may be. Other strains of GF rats (Buffalo and Sprague-Dawley), consuming the same food in the GF environment, have not developed prostate neoplasms.

Four lines of PA cells (designated PA-I, II, III, and IV) have been derived from L-W rats with "spontaneous" PA [4, 5]. The cells were cloned in vitro, and inoculated into conventional L-W rats. Each cell line manifests a defined pattern of metastasis: Three cell lines (PA-I, III, IV) spread from the subcutaneous point of implant through ipsilateral lymphatic channels to the lungs in which they establish and grow as distinct tumor foci; one cell line (PA-II) spreads through lymphatic and hematogenous routes to the lungs, liver, spleen, and bone marrow in which they develop as metastatic foci [5, 7]. The patterns of cell multiplication and spread are manifested in all L-W rats, but other lines of Wistar rats have rejected the cells.

The metastatic spread patterns of these four model PA systems are dynamic; that is they spread uniformly and spontaneously. Investigations with them may provide information which would clarify the nature of the phenomenon: Can the process of spread be accelerated or interrupted; can the organotropism be changed; and what endogenous factors are related to the process of metastasis? Does the tumor cell have a determinant role in the pattern of spread, or is this modulated by the host?

METHODS

The protocol with which the phenomenon of PA metastasis has been examined is as follows: Cells of PA-I or III were propagated as cell monolayers with medium MEM plus 10% fetal calf serum and antibiotics (penicillin and streptomycin) in a humidified atmosphere of 5% CO_2 and air at 37°C [8, 9]. When the cell cultures were confluent, they were dispersed with trypsin, counted, and 10^5 viable cells were inoculated into the footpad of the right hind foot of weaning L-W rats. Over the subsequent 4 weeks, the inoculated footpad became swollen, the popliteal and then the inguinal lymph nodes became marginally and then prominently palpable. By week 4, visible metastatic tumors had developed on and in the lungs. The rats usually survive 7–8 weeks after inoculation of tumor cells.

PA-II cells were dispersed from an enlarged lymph node, and implanted subcutaneously into the dorso-lumbar area or into a right hind footpad. Within 3 weeks bilateral peripheral lymph nodes (inguinal and axillary) were swollen, white blood cell counts were very high, and numerous PA-II cells were evident in stained blood smears. At autopsy, the lungs and bone marrow were diffusely infiltrated by tumor cells, and the liver and spleen were very large and also infiltrated by tumor cells. The rats rarely survived longer than 4 weeks after inoculation of tumor cells.

Experimental protocols were implemented to determine if the predictable patterns of metastasis could be changed by specific agents. These included administrations of sodium barbiturate, diethylstilbestrol, aspirin, indomethacin, Corynebacterium parvum, a very low density lipoprotein (VLDL), cyclophosphamide, and ICRF 159. Treatment schedules were started coincident with implantation of tumor cells or at designated periods thereafter. For assessment of results, the rats were killed for examinations when, as anticipated, the untreated controls would have developed metastases in the lungs (PA-III) or when they had died with extensive metastatic lesions in the lungs and other visceral organs (PA-II). In some experiments the rats were examined at intervals after termination of the treatment schedule.

In vitro-propagated cells, and rats with metastasizing tumors, were examined for specific enzymes which are thought to be involved in the process of metastasis. β1-4 galactosyltransferase activity was measured in the serum and in tumors from rats bearing PA-II and PA-III, and the results were compared with enzyme activities in rats bearing other transplanted and autochthonous tumors.

The isolation and purification of the plasminogen activator(s) secreted by PA-III cells were examined by the fibrin-agar plate method [10]. Urokinase served as the positive control for plasminogen activation. A chemically defined serum-free medium was developed to support the propagation of PA-III cells in order to avoid the complication of serum proteins. The cell culture medium was harvested, dialysed, and concentrated 20 × by ultrafiltration. The ultrafiltrate was examined for plasminogen activation into plasmin which was monitored by the fibrin-plate method for functional activity of plasmin and by reduced SDS polyacrylamide gel electrophoresis. Plasminogens were isolated from rat and human plasma by affinity chromatography using a lysine-Sepharose 4B column[11].

RESULTS
Modulation of Metastasis

The rate and extent of metastatic spread of PA-I and III cells were promoted by administration of sodium barbiturate (0.1%) in the drinking water [12], and the activity of PA-II cells (and not of PA-III cells) was accelerated in rats which were inoculated with diethylstilbestrol [13]. This is relevant to the demonstration of receptor sites on PA-II cells for estrogen, which could not be demonstrated on PA-III cells [14]. Tumor growth and metastasis of PA-II and PA-III cells were retarded by weekly i.p. administrations of cyclophosphamide (CPA) (50 mg/kg bodyweight); however, surviving tumor cells were reactivated following cessation of CPA treatments [15]. The immunosuppression resulting from the treatments with CPA resulted in infectious complications in some of the treated conventional rats, but not in GF counterpart rats. Intravenous inoculations of killed Corynebacterium parvum into rats retarded the rate and extent of metastatic spead to the lungs: Four weekly doses were more effective than a single dose [16]. Metastasis of PA-I and PA-III cells were retarded in rats which were administered aspirin and indomethacin, two agents which block the synthesis of prostaglandins [12].

When 10^5 PA-III cells are inoculated i.v. into L-W rats, tumor foci will develop only in the lungs. Attempts to release the tumor cells from the lungs, thereby establishing metastasis in other organs, have not been successful: Rats with PA-III lung tumors were treated with i.v. carageen, with i.m. cortisone, and with whole-body x-irradiation (450R), but the tumor foci remained only in the lungs [5]. These manipulations were administered prior to and/or subsequent to the inoculation of tumor cells.

A very low density lipoprotein-associated oncolytic factor (VLDL) was separated from the serums of rats, and the level of VLDL was significantly higher in rats which were at a late stage of pregnancy. By an in vitro tumor cell colony inhibition procedure, VLDL has demonstrated marked cytotoxicity against a number of unrelated tumor cell lines [9]. Attempts to demonstrate oncolysis by VLDL in rats with metastasizing PA-III cells have not been successful, perhaps because of (a) an inadequate supply of the lipoprotein or (b) a rapid in vivo inactivation of the agent. The VLDL was inoculated i.v. at daily intervals. There is evidence which indicates that VLDL does exert a role in metastasis: Rats which had been inoculated SC with PA-III tumor cells were administered heparin i.v. repeatedly at daily intervals, and the subsequent rate and extent of metastasis were accelerated [17]. It was demonstrated that the i.v. administration of heparin induces the production of an intravascular lipoprotein lipase which inactivated VLDL. This indirect evidence that VLDL has a role in metastasis warrants further attention.

The rate and extent of metastasis of PA-II and III cells were modified by ICRF 159 [($\pm$), 1, 2, bis (3,5-dioxopiperazin-1-γl)propane], a drug which is purported to have antimetastatic properties [18]. Groups of rats were administered ICRF 159 at daily intervals (5 days per week) starting at day 0, when the PA cells were implanted. Rats which received 60 mg ICRF 159/kg bodyweight (BW) intraperitoneally for 2 weeks were free of demonstrable PA-III tumor activity when examined at 35 days after inoculation of tumor cells. The effect of this drug on PA-III was less decisive in rats which were administered 30 mg/kg BW of the drug for 2 weeks: Some lung metastasis had appeared by day 40 after onset of the trial. When ICRF 159 treatment was delayed up to day 18, it resulted in a significant reduction of metastatic lesions compared to lesions in control rats. All of the control rats had growing tumors and metastatic lesions in the lymph nodes and lungs. In contrast to the above results, rats with PA-II cells survived during the treatment schedule with ICRF 159; however, they started to die soon after cessation of drug treatments [19]. The differences in responses of PA-II and PA-III cells to ICRF 159 were related perhaps to the rate of growth and extent of metastatic spread of the two tumors: PA-II grows rapidly and extensively, and kills the host within 4 weeks; whereas PA-III grows slower and the host will survive for weeks longer than rats with PA-II cells. It is of significance to note that ICRF 159 is relatively nontoxic at the dosages used.

Attempts to modify the organotropism of PA-II cells by sequential subcutaneous passages of cells from the bone marrow have been negative: Bone marrows to which PA-II cells had metastasized were transplanted subcutaneously through 11 passages in L-W rats, and the patterns of dissemination remained unchanged. The PA-II cells in the bone marrow produced a local tumor from which the cells spread to lymph nodes, lungs, liver, spleen, and bone marrow; and numerous PA-II cells were observed in smears prepared from the peripheral blood. There was no demonstrable change in the pattern of organotropism in the course of the entire sequence of passages [5].

Biochemical Characteristics of Metastatic PA Cells

Galactosyltransferase. βq-4 Galactosyltransferase (GalT-4) activity was measured in the serum and in tumors of rats bearing PA-II and PA-III tumors, and this was compared with enzyme activities in rats bearing other transplanted and autochthonous tumors [20]. A three- to fourfold increase in GalT-4 activity was seen in the serum of animals bearing PA-II (hematogenous metastasis) and mammary tumors (extensive tumor necrosis). A moderate increase was seen in rats bearing a transplanted lung adenocarcinoma, a transplanted IgE-producing myeloma, and autochthonous intestinal carcinomas. The latter were nonmetastasizing tumors induced in rats by 1, 2 dimethylhydrazine [21]. No increase in GalT-4 was recorded in the sera of PA-III-bearing animals, although the levels of enzyme activity demonstrable in the solid tumors of PA-II, PA-III, and mammary adenocarcinoma were comparable. This low level of activity in the serum was not attributed to an inhibitor in the serum of rats with PA-III, nor was the increase in the serum of rats with PA-II due to an activator. When the mammary adenocarcinoma was transplanted subcutaneously in the dorso-lumbar region, the level of serum GalT-4 in the rats was proportional to tumor mass.

In time-bleeding studies, the serum levels of GalT-4 activity in rats with PA-II and with mammary adenocarcinoma increased in the terminal stages of the disease. There was no significant increase of GalT-4 in serums of rats with PA-III. The increase of GalT-4 in rats with PA-II was directly related to the number of tumor cells in the blood [20].

Plasminogen activator. By means of the fibrin-agar overlay method, plasminogen-dependent, cell-associated fibrinolysis has been demonstrated in PA-II and PA-III cell lines. Since the PA cells have a high cloning efficiency (over 90%), as few as 100 cells can be plated to demonstrate fibrinolysis, which can be observed as early as 3 hours after addition of the fibrin-agar overlay. In the absence of plasminogen, no lysis of fibrin could be observed even after prolonged incubation (48 hours). By the same technique, no fibrinolysis has been observed over a 48-hour incubation period in cell lines L-929, BHK-21, Vero, and rat fibroblast line (Table I). In order to avoid the complication introduced by serum proteins, a chemically defined serum-free medium was developed [22] to support the in vitro propagation of PA-III and PA-II cells. In addition to the fibrin-agar plate method, the ^{125}I-fibrin-plate method [23] was used to demonstrate the activation of plasminogen to plasmin by the activator produced by the PA cells.

DISCUSSION

The data thus far acquired from experiments with PA-II and PA-III cells would indicate that the characteristic pattern of metastasis is an inherent quality of the tumor cell; however, treatment of the host (as with C. parvum and Na barbiturate) can modify the rate and extent of metastasis.

It is very likely that enzymological studies of the metastatic process will yield important information on this complication of cancer. It is a prerequisite to have model tumor systems with which the pattern(s) and the rates of metastasis occur spontaneously, predictably, and in high frequency. The model PA systems described here comply with these prerequisites. Extension of the experimental protocols to other organ-related tumors should reveal common or unique factors in this expression of malignancy. We can anticipate that proteolytic enzymes will be relevant to the process of metastasis. It has been postulated that tumors possessing a high level of fibrinolytic activity are more likely to metastasize than tumors showing less of this activity. Information is being sought which will confirm or deny this

TABLE I. Plasminogen-Dependent Fibrinolysis of Prostate Adenocarcinoma Cells Compared to Other Cell Lines

Cell line[a]	Fibrinolysis[b] mean diameter of zone of lysis (mm)		
	3 hr	6 hr	24 hr
PA-II	4.5	7.5	10.5
PA-III	4.0	8.0	11.0
Vero	−	−	−
L-929	−	−	−
SD (normal rat fibroblast)	−	−	−

[a]The cell density was 1000 cells per 35 mm² CoStar plate. The fibrin-agar overlay was poured 48 hours after initial cell plating.

[b]The overlay consists of fibrinogen (5 mg/ml), thrombin (5 units/ml), agarose (1.25%), and rat plasminogen (10 µg/ml). In the absence of plasminogen, no fibrinolysis could be observed in the PA cells. The fibrinogen and thrombin were depleted of plasminogen by passing through a lysine-Sepharose 4B column.

hypothesis. At this time we are examining the PA tumors for glycoprotein enzymes and for plasminogen activators, and they will be examined for collagenase, elastase, and other proteolytic enzymes. It is important to reveal what activity in the tumor cell determines if it will metastasize and, if so, through what channels and to what target organs.

ACKNOWLEDGMENTS

Supported in part by funds from USPHS grants CA 17559 and RR 00294.

REFERENCES

1. Andrews EJ, Ward BC Altman NH (eds): Spontaneous Animal Models of Human Disease." New York: Academic Press, 1979; pp 106–178.
2. Murphy GP (ed): "Models for Prostate Cancer." New York: Alan R. Liss, Inc., 1980.
3. Pollard M: Animal models for prostate cancer. The Prostate 1:207–213, 1980.
4. Pollard M: The Pollard tumors. In Murphy GP (ed): "Models for Prostate Cancer." New York: Alan R. Liss, Inc. pp 293–302, 1980.
5. Pollard M: Unpublished data. 1980.
6. Pollard M, Luckert PH: Spontaneous liver tumors in aged germfree Wistar rats. Lab Anim Sci 29:74–77, 1979.
7. Pollard M, Luckert PH: Patterns of spontaneous metastasis manifested by three rat prostate adenocarcinomas. J Surg Onco 12:371–377, 1979.
8. Chang CF, Pollard M: In vitro propagation of prostate adenocarcinoma cells from rats. Invest Urol 14:331–334, 1977.
9. Chan S-Y, Pollard M: In vitro effects of lipoprotein-associated cytotoxic factor on rat prostate adenocarcinoma cells. Cancer Res 38:2956–2962, 1978.
10. Jones PA, Benedict W, Strickland S, Reich E: Fibrin overlay methods for the detection of single transformed cells and colonies of transformed cells. Cell 5:323–329, 1975.

11. Seifring GE Jr, Castellino FJ: Metabolic turnover studies on the two major forms of rat and rabbit plasminogen. J Biol Chem 249:1434–1438, 1974.
12. Pollard M, Chang DF, Luckert PH: Investigations on prostate adenocarcinomas in rats. Oncology 34:129–132, 1977.
13. Pollard M: Prostate adenocarcinomas in Wistar rats. Rush-Presbyterian-St. Luke's Med Bull 14:17–22, 1975.
14. Chan S-Y: Androgen and glucocorticoid receptors in the Pollard prostate adenocarcinoma cell lines. The Prostate 1:53–60, 1980.
15. Pollard M, Luckert PH: Chemotherapy of metastatic prostate adenocarcinomas in germ-free rats. Cancer Treat Rep 60:619–621, 1976.
16. Pollard M, Burleson G, Luckert PH: Factors which modify the rate and extent of spontaneous metastasis of tumors in rats. In Day SB, et al (eds): "Cancer Invasion and Metastasis: Biologic Mechanisms and Therapy." New York: Raven Press, 1977, pp 349–358.
17. Chan S-Y, Pollard M: Metastasis enhancing effect of heparin and its relationship to a lipoprotein factor. J Natl Cancer Inst 64:1121–1125, 1980.
18. Hellmann K, Burrage K: Control of malignant metastasis by ICRF 159. Nature 224:273–275, 1969.
19. Pollard M, Burleson G, Luckert PH: Interference with in vivo growth and metastasis of prostate adenocarcinoma (PA-III) by ICRF 159. The Prostate 2:1–10, 1981.
20. Jenis DM, Basu S, Pollard M: Increased activity of (β1-4) galactosyltransferase in tissues of rats bearing prostate and mammary adenocarcinomas. Cancer Biochem Biophys 1981 (in press).
21. Pollard M, Luckert PH: Promotional effect of sodium barbiturate on intestinal tumors induced in rats by dimethylhydrzine. J Natl Cancer Inst 63:1089–1092, 1979.
22. Chan S-Y, Pollard M: Unpublished data, 1981.

The Prostatic Cell: Structure and Function
Part B, pages 257-267
© 1981 Alan R. Liss, Inc., 150 Fifth Avenue, New York, NY 10011

Activation of Tumoricidal Properties in Murine Macrophages by Intravenous Injection of Muramyl Dipeptide Encapsulated Within Liposomes as a Treatment for Spontaneous Metastasis

Isaiah J. Fidler and George Poste

INTRODUCTION

Recent improvements in surgical techniques and advances in general patient care have made excision of primary neoplasms a more successful cancer treatment. However, in most patients with malignant neoplasms, metastasis has already occurred at the time of diagnosis, and consequently causes most deaths from cancer (1-3). The development of metastases is dependent on an interplay between host factors and intrinsic characteristics of the malignant tumor cells (4-6). Very few tumor cells within a primary neoplasm can invade blood vessels and of those, only a few can survive in the hostile environment of the circulatory system. Similarly, not all malignant cells that survive transport can successfully be arrested in the microcirculation, undergo extravasation into the organ parenchyma, escape host defense mechanisms, and grow into metastases. Therefore, at every step of the metastatic cascade the rules of "survival of the fittest" apply to the dynamic interplay of tumor cell and host properties.

Recent studies from our laboratory suggest that metastasis is not random, but represents the selective growth of preexisting subpopulations of cells endowed with specific properties that allow them to complete the various steps

The contents of this paper do not necessarily reflect the views or policies of the Department of Health and Human Services, nor does mention of trade names, commercial products, or organizations imply endorsement by the US Government.

of the metastatic process (1, 4–6). Although cells populating metastases are metastatic (5,7) they are not necessarily uniform with regard to other biological properties, expecially if these properties are not mandatory for metastasis (5,7). For example, cells obtained from different metastases of human breast cancer exhibit variations in their estrogen receptors (8), and cells collected from different liver metastases produced by human small-cell lung cancer exhibit variations in the production of several marker enzymes (9).

There are several reasons for the failure of treatment of metastases. At the time of surgery, metastases may be too small to be detected, are often widely disseminated throughout the body, and their anatomic location(s) may be inaccessible for surgical removal. The most serious problem, however, is the emergence of metastases that are resistant to conventional therapy. Recent work suggesting that metastases may result from the proliferation of a minor subpopulation of cells within the primary tumor and that tumors are heterogeneous with regard to many phenotypic characteristics, including metastatic potential, provides a conceptual basis for explaining the emergence of such relentless tumor deposits. Phenotypic heterogeneity of this kind may also account for reports of diffferences in the response of primary and metastatic lesions to cytotoxic agents (10–12) or host effector cells (1,3,4). These findings imply that the successful approach to the eradication of metastases will be one that circumvents tumor cell heterogeneity and against which resistance is unlikely to develop.

There is considerable evidence that tumoricidal macrophages may satisfy these criteria for metastasis treatment. Unlike other host effector cells, activated macrophages can, at least in vitro, recognize and destroy tumorigenic cells and yet not harm nontumorigenic cells even in co-cultivation conditions (13–15). How tumoricidal macrophages discriminate between tumorigenic and nontumorigenic cells is not clear, but in vitro macrophage-mediated destruction of tumor cells does occur independently of such tumor cell characteristics as antigenicity, invasiveness, metastatic potential, and drug sensitivity (13–15). Although tumor cell resistance to a variety of cytotoxic drugs, antibodies, cytotoxic lymphocytes, and natural killer cells has been demonstrated, all efforts to select tumor cells that are resistant to tumoricidal macrophages have been unsuccessful (16).

A major pathway for activation of macrophages in vivo involves their interaction with microorganisms and/or their product(s) (17,18). Because such biologic agents often cause undesirable side effects, such as granuloma formation and allergic reactions (17), it is preferable to use synthetic compounds that are relatively nontoxic yet possess immune-potentiating activity to activate macrophages in vivo. N-acetylmuramyl-L-alanyl-D-isolglu-tamine (muramyl dipeptide, MDP) is the minimal structural unit (mw 492) with immune-potentiating activity that can replace mycobacteria in Freund's complete adjuvant. MDP is known to influence many macrophage functions including cytotoxic activity (19–21). It is important to note, however, that therapeutic use of water-soluble synthetic MDP is hindered by the fact that, following parenteral administration, this agent is rapidly cleared ($<$ 60 minutes) from the body and excreted in the urine (21). We have recently shown that the phagocytic uptake by macrophages of liposomes (concentric phospholipid vesicles separated by aqueous compartments containing entrapped MDP) produces highly efficient activation of rodent macrophages in vitro (22) and in vivo (23). An attractive feature of liposomes as a carrier vehicle for delivery of MDP to macrophages in situ is that the majority of liposomes injected IV are taken up by cells of the reticuloendothelial system. This "passive targeting" of liposomes to macrophages offers a means of enhancing uptake of therapeutic agents that stimulate macrophage activity.

In this report, we extend our previous observations on the use of liposome-encapsulated MDP to stimulate macrophage function in situ and examine the effectiveness of this approach for the treatment of spontaneous visceral metastases in mice.

MATERIALS AND METHODS

Animals

Specific-pathogen-free mice of the inbred strain C57BL/6N and F344 strain rats were obtained from the Frederick Cancer Research Center's Animal Production Area.

Cell Cultures

The highly invasive and metastatic B16-BL6 variant line of the B16 melanoma syngeneic to the C57BL/6 mouse was adapted to grow in vitro (24). Monolayer cultures were incubated at 37°C in a humidified atmosphere containing 5% CO_2 and were maintained in Eagle's minimal essential medium supplemented with 5% fetal bovine serum, vitamin solution, sodium pyruvate, nonessential amino acids, and L-glutamine. All cultures were free of Mycoplasma, reovirus type 3, pneumonia virus of mice, K virus, Theiler's encephalitis virus, Sendai virus, minute virus of mice, mouse adenovirus, mouse hepatitis virus, lymphocytic choriomeningitis virus, ectromelia virus, lactate dehydrogenase virus.

Preparation and Purification of Mouse Alveolar Macrophages (AM)

Mouse AM were harvested by a tracheobronchial lavage method (22,25) and 10^5 AM were plated into wells of a Microtest II plate with a surface area of 38 mm^2 (Falcon Plastics, Oxnard, CA). Nonadherent cells (fewer than 10%) were removed by washing with media 60 minutes after initial plating. At that time, more than 98% of the adherent cells had a mononuclear morphology, phagocytosed carbon particles, and opsonized sheep red blood cells (25).

MDP

MDP was purchased from Calbiochem, LaJolla, CA. The MDP did not contain endotoxins as detected with the Limulus lysate assay.

Lipids and Preparation of Liposomes

Chromatographically pure egg phosphatidylcholine (PC) and beef brain phosphatidylserine (PS) were purchased from Avanti Biochemicals, Birmingham, AL. Multilamellar vesicles (MLV) were prepared from a mixture of PC and PS (7:3 mole ratio). Encapsulation of MDP or Hanks' balanced salt solution (HBSS), or media within liposomes was achieved by methods described previously (15,23,25). We have used PS/PC-MLV as carriers for MDP because they are not toxic at the dose used here and are arrested efficiently in the lungs (and in organs of the reticuloendothelial system) when they are injected into the circulation (26).

Activation of AM Following IV Injection of Free and/or Liposome-Encapsulated MDP

Mice were injected IV with HBSS, free MDP (200 µg/ mouse) or liposomes (50 µmole MLV-phospholipids) containing either MDP (2.5 µg) or HBSS (empty liposomes). The MLV were suspended in HBSS and administered IV at a volume of 0.2 ml/mouse. Empty liposomes were suspended in HBSS containing free MDP (2.5 µg/mouse) and were injected into controls. Mice were killed at 4, 24, or 48 hours after IV injection. AM were harvested by lavage as described above (25).

Macrophage-Mediated Cytotoxicity Assay

Macrophage-mediated cytotoxicity was assessed by a radioactive release assay (25) in which 5×10^3 ^{125}I-iododeoxyuridine ([^{125}I]IUdR)-labeled melanoma cells were added to each well. Target cells alone were always plated as an additional control. Twenty-four hours after the addition of target cells, the triplicate cultures were washed and refed to remove cells that did not plate. Adherent target cells were lysed at 24 or 72 hours after incubation with 0.2 N NaOH. The lysate was adsorbed on cotton swabs which were monitored for radioactivity in a gamma counter. The percent macrophage-mediated cytotoxicity was computed with the following formula:

$$\frac{\text{cpm of target cells with} - \text{cpm of target cells with}}{\text{cpm of target cells with}} \times 100$$

$$\frac{\text{normal macrophages} \quad\; \text{activated macrophages}}{\begin{array}{c}\text{cpm of target cells with}\\ \text{normal macrophages}\end{array}} \times 100$$

The statistical significance of differences among the test groups was determined by the Student's two-tailed t-test.

Treatment of Spontaneous Metastases by Multiple IV Injections of Liposomes Containing MDP

C57BL/6 mice were injected in the footpad with 2.5×10^2 viable melanoma tumor cells. Four to five weeks later, when the tumors reached $10-15$ mm in diameter, the mice were anesthetized by methoxyflurane inhalation, and the tumor-bearing leg, including the popliteal lymph node, was amputated at midfemur. Intravenous liposome treatment began 3 days later. Each treatment consisted of an injection in the tail vein of PS/PC-MLV (5 μmoles phospholipids) suspended in 0.2 ml of HBSS. The MLV contained either MDP (2.5 μg/mouse) or HBSS (empty liposomes) suspended in HBSS containing 2.5 μg MDP/mouse. Control groups were mice that were injected IV with free MDP (200 μg/mouse) or only HBSS. Treatments were given twice weekly for 4 weeks. In some experiments, mice were killed 2 weeks after the final treatment and necropsied. The presence and number of metastases were determined with a dissecting microscope. All suspected pulmonary and extrapulmonary metastases were confirmed by microscopic examination of fixed histological sections. In a second set of survival experiments, mice were observed daily for 200 days. Dead or moribund mice were necropsied to ascertain the presence or absence of disseminated disease. Animals surviving at least 120 days after the last liposome treatment was administered were considered to be disease free (27,28).

RESULTS

Activation of Tumoricidal Properties in AM by the IV Injection of Liposomes Containing MDP

The in vitro cytotoxicity of AM harvested after IV treatment of mice was measured against the B16-BL6 tumor cells. The data are summarized in Table I. The IV injection of either 200 μg free MDP/mouse or empty liposomes suspended in 5 μg of free MDP did not render mouse AM tumoricidal. In contrast, the IV injection of MLV containing 2.5 μg MDP/mouse activated AM to become tumor cytotoxic. When harvested 4

TABLE I. Activation of tumoricidal properties in murine AM following the IV injection of free and liposome-encapsulated MDP

Treatment of AM donors[a]	Radioactivity (cpm) in live target cells[b]		
	Time of AM harvest after IV injection		
	4 hr	24 hr	48 hr
None, tumor cells alone	2206 ± 160	2100 ± 88	1890 ± 67
HBSS	2368 ± 70	2009 ± 170	1788 ± 43
Free MDP (200 μg)	2336 ± 135	2211 ± 64	1890 ± 60
Liposome-MDP (2.5 μg)[c]	1515 ± 44 (36%)[e]	1185 ± 31 (41%)[e]	1323 ± 211 (24%)[e]
"Empty" liposomes and free MDP (2.5 μg)[d]	2199 ± 33	2284 ± 67	1900 ± 161

[a]Three mice/group were injected IV with the indicated materials.
[b]10^5 AM were plated into 38-mm^2 culture wells. $5 \times 10^3 \times$ [^{125}I]IUdR-labeled B16-BL6 cells were added. Mean counts per minute $\pm$ S.D. of triplicate cultures. Cultures were terminated after 72-hour incubation.
[c]MLV, 10 μmoles total phospholipids.
[d]MLV, 10 μmoles total phospholipid containing HBSS.
[e]Percent cytotoxicity as compared with normal AM; $P < 0.005$.

hours after IV injection of liposome-encapsulated MDP, the AM were activated to lyse 36% of the target cells ($P < 0.01$). By 24 hours after IV treatment, the AM lysed 41% of the targets ($P < 0.001$) and by 48 hours after IV treatment, their cytotoxicity had diminished to 24% ($P < 0.01$).

Treatment of Spontaneous Lung and Lymph Node Metastases Following IV Injection of Liposome-Encapsulated MDP

Spontaneous pulmonary and lymph node metastases were well established in animals at the time liposome therapy was started. Melanotic metastases were visible in the inguinal and superficial iliac nodes, and parietal pulmonary metastases were visible with a dissecting microscope. Many of these pulmonary metastases contained thousands of tumor cells. Without therapy, these lesions rapidly developed into tumor foci 1–3 mm in diameter. Thus, in the first set of experiments when mice were killed 2 weeks after the last treatment with liposomes, metastases could be detected with ease. The data from these experiments are shown in Table II. The majority of mice treated with liposome-encapsulated MDP had no macroscopically or microscopically detectable metastases. Even in animals with metastatic lesions, the median number of metastases was significantly less than that found in the other treatment groups. Metastases were consistently present in a high proportion of animals in the various control groups ($P < 0.001$)

The data from the survival experiments are shown in Table III. By day 80

TABLE II. Inhibition of established B16-BL6 melanoma pulmonary metastases in C57BL/6 mice after multiple intravenous injection of liposome-encapsulated MDP

	Pulmonary metastasis		
Treatment group	Negative mice/ total	Median	Range
Control mice	4/48 (8%)	39	0–107
Free MDP (200 μg/mouse)	17/20 (15%)	51	0–98
Liposomes containing HBSS suspended in 2.5 μg MDP	3/26 (11%)	48	0–188
Liposomes containing 2.5 μg MDP	30/39 (72%)	0	0–9 <0.001

The incidence of metastasis in mice treated with liposome-encapsulated MDP was significantly decreased (P < 0.001, chi-square analysis). The data are a summary of three separate experiments.

TABLE III. Survival studies: Eradication of spontaneous metastases by the systemic administration of liposomes containing MDP

	Percentage of animals surviving by day:					
Treatment group	30	60	90	120	150	200
None, control mice	100	35	0			
Free MDP (200 μg/mouse)	100	30	0			
Liposomes containing HBSS suspended in 2.5 μg MDP	100	40	0			
Liposomes containing 2.5 μg MDP	100	68	65	65	65	65

Viable B16-BL6 cells (25,000) were implanted in the footpad of syngeneic C57BL/6 mice. Tumors (10-12 mm in diameter) were amputated 4 weeks later. Liposome therapy commenced 3 days after surgery. Each treatment consisted of IV injection of 5 μmoles lipid PS/PC MLV liposomes/mouse twice weekly for 4 weeks. These are data of two separate experiments (N = 30). The differences in median life span are highly significant (P < 0.001).

of the experiment, nearly all mice treated with MDP or control preparations had died. In contrast, 65% of mice injected IV with MLV containing MDP survived at least 120 days after the last treatment. This period exceeded by a wide margin the time (40–50 days) necessary for as few as 10 surviving tumor cells to kill their hosts (27,28). On day 200 of the experiment, all the surviving mice were killed, necropsied, and found to be disease free.

DISCUSSION

We have previously reported the feasibility of using liposome-encapsulated lymphokines to stimulate macrophage antitumor activities (30). There are, however, problems associated with the use of crude preparations of lymphokines. There is no quantitative assay for measuring activity and significant variations among different batches, and the presence of biological mediators other than macrophage-activating factors (MAF), including mitogenic, angiogenic, and vascular permeabilizing factors, must also be considered when evaluating observed host responses. It would thus be desirable, and probably mandatory for studies in man, that future efforts to stimulate macrophage function by liposome-encapsulated agents employ material(s) of defined composition and purity. For this reason, we have evaluated the efficacy of MDP encapsulated in liposomes as a potential modality for augmenting macrophage function in situ. MDP has been shown to augment the tumoricidal activity of macrophages in vitro, even when added to macrophages encapsulated within liposomes (22,23,29). As is also true of MAF encapsulated in liposomes, MDP encapsulated in liposomes is significantly more efficient in activating macrophages in vitro than the free (unencapsulated) form (22,29). In vivo, however, free MDP is cleared within 1 hour after parenteral administration (21), and even high doses of water-soluble MDP injected IV fail to elicit macrophage tumoricidal activity. Therefore, it was important to determine whether encapsulation of MDP within liposomes could circumvent the clearance problem and whether the uptake of liposomes by macrophages would enable MDP to produce a tumoricidal reponse.

The studies reported here show that the multiple IV injections of liposome-encapsulated MDP, but not free MDP or control liposome preparations, eradicated spontaneous visceral metastases in C57BL/6 mice from which a syngeneic melanoma had been surgically removed. At the start of therapy, the metastatic tumor burden in the lungs and lymph nodes may have exceeded a total body burden of 10^7 cells (23). Nonetheless, 65% of mice treated with liposome-encapsulated MDP survived at least 120 days after the final treatment. The tumor burden in these successfully treated mice was probably reduced to fewer than 10 viable cells, because they survived longer than 40–50 days, which is the median life span of mice implanted with 10 viable B16 cells (27,28). Thus, the IV injection of liposomes containing MDP, a macrophage-activating agent, brought about the complete regression of established pulmonary and lymph node metastases.

The mechanism(s) responsible for the regression of established metastases after the systemic administration of liposomes containing MDP probably involved the activation of macrophages to become tumoricidal (Table I). Evidence for the effectiveness of tumoricidal macrophages in controlling metastasis has come from adoptive transfer studies of tumoricidal macrophages into syngeneic mice bearing experimental or spontaneous metastases (31–34). For clinical therapy, however, this approach has serious limitations, such as the need to adoptively transfer many autologous or histocompatible macrophages. Because, at least in mice, macrophages from tumor-bearing animals can respond to activation stimuli and become tumoricidal (30), it is preferable to activate them in situ. Our present data indicate that the IV injection of MLV liposomes containing MDP, but not free MDP, rendered AM tumoricidal.

The ability to activate AM in situ with MDP entrapped within liposomes has several advantages. Once injected into the circulation, liposomes, like other particulate matter, are removed by cells of the reticuloendothelial system by phagocytosis. It is possible to take advantage of this physiological fact to deliver materials encapsulated within liposomes to cells of the macrophage-histiocyte series. The repeated systemic administration of specifically designed liposomes (26) is unlikely to lead to the formation of granulomas or to elicit allergic reactions associated with the systemic administration of some immune adjuvants (17,35). Finally, the encapsulation of MDP within MLV liposomes allows retention of MDP within the macrophage where it can be released over 2–3 days and can maintain the tumoricidal activities. This achieves the added advantage of a "sustained release" of the activating agent.

CONCLUSIONS

We have demonstrated that an IV injection of liposomes containing MDP can activate AM to become tumoricidal. Multiple IV injections of liposome-encapsulated MDP leads to regression of established spontaneous metastases originating from a subcutaneous murine melanoma. Although the initial results reported here are encouraging, it is unlikely that liposome-encapsulated immunomodulators could serve as a single modality in treating advanced metastatic disease. As with many other antitumor therapies, optimal application will probably require its use in combination with other antitumor agents. Therapeutic regimens designed to stimulate the antitumor properties of macrophages would probably have to follow cytoreductive treatment which would reduce tumor burden to a level low enough to allow tumoricidal macrophages to kill the remaining tumor cells that would otherwise escape destruction.

ACKNOWLEDGMENTS

We wish to thank Zoa Barnes, William Fogler, and Deborah Higdon for their excellent help.

Research was sponsored by the National Cancer Institute, DHHS, under Contract No. NO1-CO-75380 with Litton Bionetics, Inc.

REFERENCES

1. Fidler IJ, Gersten DM, Hart IR: The biology of cancer invasion and metastasis. Adv Cancer Res 28:149-250, 1978.
2. Sugarbaker EV: Cancer metastasis: A product of tumor-host interactions. Curr Prob Cancer 7:3-59, 1979.
3. Poste G, Fidler IJ: The pathogenesis of cancer metastasis. Nature 283:139-146, 1979.
4. Fidler IJ: Tumor heterogeneity and the biology of cancer invasion and metastasis. Cancer Res 37:2481-2486, 1978.
5. Fidler IJ, Cifone MA: Properties of metastatic and non-metastatic cloned subpopulations of an ultraviolet light-induced murine fibrosarcoma of recent origin. Am J Pathol 97:633−648, 1979.
6. Fidler IJ, Kripke ML: Metastasis results from preexisting variant cells within a malignant tumor. Science 197:893-895, 1977.
7. Fidler IJ, Kripke ML: Biological variability within murine neoplasms. Antibiot Chemother 28:123-129, 1980.
8. Brennan MJ, Donnegan WL, Appleby DE: The variability of estrogen receptors in metastatic breast cancer. Am J Surg 137:260-262, 1979.
9. Baylin SB, Weisburger WR, Eggleston JC, Mendelsohn GM, Beaven MA, Abeloff MD, Ettinger DS: Variable content of histaminase. L-dopa decarboxylase and calcitonin in small-cell carcinoma of the lung. Biologic and clinical implications. N Engl J Med 299:105-110, 1978.
10. Trope C: Different sensitivity to cytostatic drugs of primary tumor and metastasis of the Lewis carcinoma. Neoplasma 22:171-180, 1975.
11. Schabel FM, Jr: Concepts for systemic treatment of micrometastases. Cancer 35:15-24, 1975.
12. Heppner GH: The challenge of tumor heterogeneity. In Bulbrok RD, Taylor DJ (eds): Commentaries on Research in Breast Disease, New York: Alan R. Liss, Inc, 1979 pp 177-191.
13. Fidler IJ: Recognition and destruction of target cells by tumoricidal macrophages. Isr J Med Sci 14:177-191, 1978.
14. Fidler IJ, Darnell JH, Budmen MB: Tumoricidal properties of mouse macrophages activated with mediators from rat lymphocytes stimulated with concanavalin A. Cancer Res 36:3608-3615, 1976.
15. Poste G, Kirsh R, Fogler W, Fidler IJ. Activation of tumoricidal properties in mouse macrophages by lymphokines encapsulated in liposomes. Cancer Res 39:881-892, 1979.
16. Kerbel RS: Implications of immunological heterogeneity of tumours. Nature 280:358-360, 1979.
17. Allison AC: Mode of action of immunological adjuvants. J. Reticuloendothel Soc 26:619-630, 1979.
18. Hibbs JB Jr: Discrimination between neoplastic and non-neoplastic cells in vitro by activated macrophages. J Natl Cancer Inst 53:1487-1492, 1974.
19. Chedid L, Carelli L, Audibert F: Recent developments concerning muramyl dipeptide, a synthetic immunoregulating molecule. J Reticuloendothel Soc 26:631-641, 1979.
20. Matter A: The effects of muramyl dipeptide (MDP) in cell-mediated immunity. A comparison between in vitro and in vivo systems. Cancer Immunol Immunother 6:201-210, 1979.
21. Parant M, Parant F, Chedid L, Yapo A, Petit JF, Lederer, E: Fate of the synthetic immunoadjuvant, muramyl dipeptide (^{14}C-labelled) in the mouse. Int J Immunopharmacol 1:35-41, 1979.

22. Sone S, Fidler IJ: In vitro activation of tumoricidal properties in rat alveolar macrophages by synthetic muramyl dipeptide encapsulated in liposomes. Cell Immunol 57:42–50, 1981.
23. Fidler IJ, Sone S, Fogler WE, Barnes ZL: Eradication of spontaneous metastases and activation of alveolar macrophages by intravenous injection of liposomes containing muramyl dipeptide. Proc. Natl Acad Sci USA 78:1680–1684, 1981.
24. Hart IR: Selection and characterization of invasive varient of the B16 melanoma. Am J Pathol 97:587–600, 1979.
25. Sone S, Poste G, Fidler IJ. Rat alveolar macrophages are susceptible to activation by free and liposome-encapsulated lymphokines. J Immunol 124:2197–2202, 1980.
26. Fidler IJ, Raz A, Fogler WE, Kirsh R, Bugelski P, Poste G: The design of liposomes to improve delivery of macrophage-augmenting agents to alveolar macrophages. Cancer Res 40:4460–4466, 1980.
27. Griswold DP, Jr: Consideration of the subcutaneously implanted B16 melanoma as a screening model for potential anticancer agents. Cancer Chemother Rep 3:315–323, 1972.
28. Schabel FM Jr, Griswold DR Jr, Corbett TH, Lloyd HH: Quantitative evaluation of anticancer agent activity in experimental animals. Pharmacol Ther [A] 1:411–435, 1977.
29. Sone S, Fidler IJ. Synergistic activation by lymphokines and muramyl dipeptide of tumoricidal properties in rat alveolar macrophages. J Immunol 125:2454–2460, 1980.
30. Fidler IJ: Therapy of spontaneous metastases by intravenous injection of liposomes containing lymphokines. Science 208:1469–1471, 1980.
31. Fidler IJ: Inhibition of pulmonary metastasis by intravenous injection of sepcifically activated macrophages. Cancer Res 34:1074–1078, 1974.
32. Den Otter E, Dullens Hub FJ, Van Lovern H, Pels E: Antitumor effects of macrophages injected into animals: A review. In James K, McBride B, Stuart A (eds): The Macrophage and Cancer. Edinburgh: Econoprint, 1977, pp 119–140.
33. Liotta LA, Gattozzi C, Kleinerman J, Saidel G: Reduction of tumor cell entry into vessels by BCG-activated macrophages. Br J Cancer 36:639–641, 1977.
34. Fidler IJ, Fogler WE, Connor J: The rationale for the treatment of established experimental micrometastases with the injection of tumoricidal macrophages. In Terry W, Yamamura T. (eds): Immunobiology and Immunotherapy of Cancer, Amsterdam: Elsevier, 1979; pp 361–372.
35. Allison AC, Gregoriadis G: Liposomes as immunological adjuvants. Nature 252:252–254, 1974.

The Prostatic Cell: Structure and Function
Part B, pages 269–282
© 1981 Alan R. Liss, Inc., 150 Fifth Avenue, New York, NY 10011

Approaches to Prostatic 5α-Reductase Inhibitors

Frederick H. Batzold

INTRODUCTION

Endocrine therapy has been the most widely employed treatment for prostatic carcinoma since its inception and application by Huggins and Hodges [1] over 30 years ago. The physiologic rationale for endocrine manipulation in the management of prostatic cancer is based on the prostatic epithelium's dependence on an androgenic milieu for its growth and cellular maintenance. In an effort to deprive the prostate of the necessary androgenic stimuli a variety of approaches have been evaluated which include luteinizing hormone suppression by estrogen administration, orchiectomy, adrenalectomy, hypophysectomy, steroidogenesis blockade, and antiandrogen therapy. When compared to castration or estrogenization, the other modalities do not appear to offer any distinct long term advantages [2]. Although the aforementioned approaches to endocrine ablation for the control of prostatic growth have been widely exploited and utilized, the inhibition of Δ^4-3-ketosteroid-5α-oxidoreductase by steroid hormone analogs has not been adequately evaluated even though it has long been recognized as a potential therapeutic target. Unlike other steroid hormones, testosterone[1], in many of its target tissues such as the prostate, must be reduced to 5α-dihydrotestosterone (Fig. 1) for full androgenic expression and cellular proliferation to occur. The reduced hormone has been shown [3,4] to preferentially bind to the prostatic androgen cytosol receptor and undergo nuclear translocation which in the hormonally deprived tissue ultimately results in de novo DNA synthesis and cell proliferation. Since there appears to be a correlation between prostatic growth and the ability of various androgens to function as 5α-reductase substrates [5],

---

[1]Trivial nomenclature: testosterone, 17β-hydroxyandrost-4-en-3-one; dihydrotestosterone, 17β-hydroxy-5α-androstan-3-one; progesterone, pregn-4-en-3,20-dione; 5α-dihydroprogesterone, 5α-pregnan-3,20-dione; 17α-hydroxyprogesterone, 17α-hydroxypregn-4-en-3,20 dione; 23,24-dinorchol-4-en-22-ol-3-one, (20-R)-21-hydroxy-20-methyl-pregn-4-en-3-one; 5α-reductase, NADPH:Δ^4-3-ketosteroid-5α-oxidoreductase.

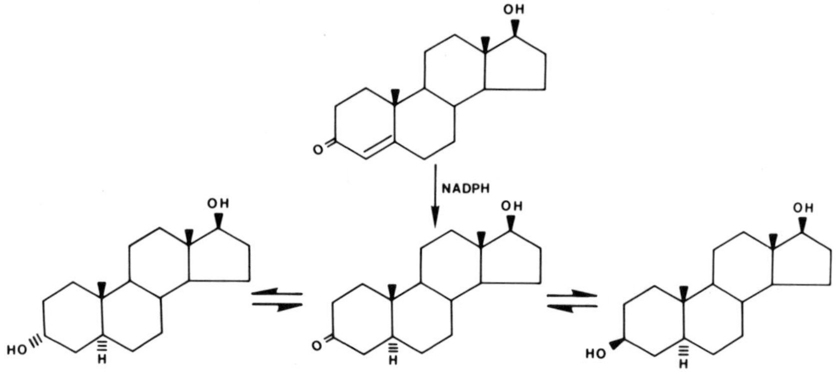

Fig. 1. Prostatic metabolism of testosterone.

it is suggested that this enzyme plays a pivotal role in regulating prostatic function and thus is an attractive target for inhibition studies.

Prostatic 5α-reductase is a membrane-bound enzyme largely associated with the nuclei and the remaining activity in the cytoplasmic particulate fraction [6]. The pH optimum for the enzyme is acidic (~6.6), and it exhibits a rigid requirement for NADPH as the reductant source [7]. Although testosterone (K_m ~1.0 μM) is accepted as the primary physiological substrate for 5α-reductase, it is capable of accepting a wide variety of Δ⁴-3-ketosteroids as substrates which are devoid of functionality at carbon center 11 of the steroid nucleus. A survey of the literature indicates that a significant number of Δ⁴-3-ketosteroids are competitive inhibitors of the 5α-reductase from diverse tissue sources. It is apparent, however, that most analogs which have been studied were modified at carbon center 17 and none has been reported to possess significant in vivo activity in suppressing prostatic growth.

Based on the possible potential of the 5α-reductase as a therapeutic target, the studies to be described herein, utilizing the rat, were undertaken to determine if appropriate steroid analogs could be realized which would provide 5α-reductase inhibitors devoid of androgenic activity for in vivo application.

MATERIALS AND METHODS

Reagents

Steroids were purchased from Sigma (St. Louis, MO) or Steraloids (Wilton, NH) and recrystallized prior to use. Other reagents were obtained from Aldrich (Milwaukee, WI) and Fisher Scientific (Fair Lawn, NJ). [1α,2α(n)-³H]-5α-dihydrotestosterone (40–60 Ci/mmol, [1α, 2α(n)-³H]-testosterone (40–60 Ci/ mmole), and [1α, 2α(n)-³H]-progesterone (40–60 Ci/mmole) were obtained from Amersham (Arlington Heights, IL). The purity of the tritiated steroids was confirmed by thin-layer chromatography.

Synthetic Steroids

Known compounds were synthesized by published procedures and conformed in all respects to the reported physical constants. 23,24-Dinorchol-4-en-22-ol-3-one was prepared by the method of Morita [8] from the corresponding aldehyde. The general procedure of Ringold [9] was used to prepare the 4-halogenated analogs with the exception of the fluorinated compounds which were kindly provided by Dr. T. Lobl of Upjohn (Kalamazoo, MI). The 2α-cyano-3-ketosteroids were generated by base treatment of the corresponding [2, 3-d]-isoxazoles [10]. The 2-methylene-Δ⁴-3-ketosteroids were prepared by the method of Manson [11].

Prostatic 5α-Reductase Assay (essentially the same as that reported in [12])

Freshly excised mature rat ventral prostate was trimmed of fat and connective tissue and thoroughly minced on ice. The tissue was suspended in phosphate buffer, pH 6.6, containing 1mM EDTA and gently homogenized at 4°C with a Brinkman Polytron. Aliquots of the homogenate (500 μl) equivalent to 50 mg tissue were incubated in 2.0 ml of buffer containing NADPH and either tritiated testosterone (0.25 μCi) or progesterone (0.25 μCi) for 1 hour at 30°C. The final NADPH concentration was 2.2×10^{-4} M, and that of the substrate was varied between 1×10^{-6} M and 5×10^{-8} M depending on the nature of the study. The synthetic analogs were added to the incubation mixture in purified methanol (50 μl) for inhibition studies. When testosterone was the substrate the incubations were terminated by extraction with ethyl acetate (3 × 5 ml) containing unlabeled carrier steroids (17β-hydroxyandrost-4-en-3-one, 17β-hydroxy-5α-androstan-3-one, 3α and 3β, 17β-dihydroxy-5α-androstane, androst-4-en-3, 17-dione, 3β, 6ξ, 17β-trihydroxy-5α-androstane, and 3β, 7ξ, 17β-trihydroxy-5α-androstane). After evaporation under nitrogen the residue was chromatographed on Merck Silica Gel 60 plates (20 × 20 cm) by a single ascent of benzene/acetone (4:1). Since progesterone yields a large number of epimeric alcohols, the incubations were extracted with methylene chloride containing pregn-4-en-3,20-dione and 5α-pregnan-3,20-dione. Prior to chromatography the residue obtained after evaporation was oxidized with chromic acid in acetone to yield essentially two products, progesterone and 5α-dihydroprogestrone which were resolved on silica gel 60 plates by a single ascent of benzene/acetone (10:1). In both cases the resolved steroids were visualized by spraying with anisaldehyde reagent and heating to 100°. The zones isopolar with the compounds of interest were transferred to vials and quantitated by liquid scintillation counting. The total 5α-reduced products generally averaged 20–30% of the total counts recovered. Activity was expressed as pmoles reduced/mg protein/hr. The initial homogenate was assayed for protein by the method of Bradford [13] with bovine serum albumin as the standard. The apparent K_I values for the various analogs were determined by the method of Dixon [14].

3α- and 3β-Hydroxysteroid Dehydrogenase Assay

The activity of the 3α- and 3β-hydroxysteroid dehydrogenases in prostatic homogenates was evaluated in a manner identical to that described for the 5α-reductase except that tritiated dihydrotestosterone (0.25 μCi) was used as the substrate. Extractions were performed with ethyl acetate containing unlabeled 17β-hydroxy-5α-androstan-3-one, 3α, 17β-dihydroxy-5α-androstane, 3β, 17β-dihydroxy-5α-androstane,3β,6ξ,17β-trihydroxy-5α-androstane, and 3β,7ξ,17β-trihydroxy-5α-androstane. Chromatographic resolution was performed on silica gel 60 by a single ascent of benzene/acetone (2:1). Quantitation was performed as described above by liquid scintillation counting.

R-3327 Adenocarcinoma

First generation (Copenhagen × Fischer, CF_1) male rats implanted with R-3327 hormone sensitive adenocarcinoma were obtained from Dr. Norman Altman, Papanicolaou Cancer Research Institute, Miami, FL. Hormone sensitivity was confirmed by the lack of tumor growth after castration. The tissue was utilized for assays when it was no larger than 1.5 cm^3 as determined by calipers. The assay of 5α-reductase activity in tumor tissue was performed as described for the rat ventral prostate.

In Vivo Evaluation of Prostatic Growth

Male Sprague Dawley rats (200–250 gm) were housed under constant conditions receiving standard rat chow and water ad libitum. Castrations were performed under ether anesthesia via the scrotal route 7 days prior to drug administration. The test substances were suspended or dissolved in propylene glycol and were administered (0.2 ml) by the intraperitoneal route daily (15 mg/day × 6). Control groups received only vehicle. On the seventh day the animals (6/group) were sacrificed by cervical dislocation and the sex accessory tissues were quickly excised and weighed. Samples of the ventral and dorsolateral prostate were retained for DNA and RNA analysis. The DNA content was determined by the method of Burton [15] and is expressed as μg DNA/mg tissue. Calf thymus DNA was used as the standard. The RNA content (μg/mg tissue) from the initial acidic hydrolsis was determined by direct reading at 260 nm with 1.0 OD unit equal to 32 μg RNA.

TABLE I. Inhibition constants of alkylated steroids for prostatic 5α-reductase

Inhibitor	Apparent K_I (μM)
6α-Methyltestosterone	2.4
6β-Methyltestosterone	4.6
4-Methyltestosterone	2.1
4-Ethyltestosterone	> 7
4-Methylprogesterone	1.2
4-Ethylprogesterone	2.5
2α-Methyltestosterone	2.8
2α-Methylprogesterone	0.8

RESULTS

In order to develop a profile as to where appropriate substituents could be introduced in the steroid nucleus A or B ring without compromising binding to the Δ^4-3-ketosteroid-5α-oxidoreductase, a series of simple alkyl derivatives was prepared and analyzed as inhibitors of the prostatic enzyme. The K_m values obtained under the conditions of our assay for testosterone and progesterone were 1.0 μM and 0.6 μM, respectively. The apparent K_I values for these competitive inhibitors as shown in Table I suggest that carbon centers C-6α, 4, and 2α were tolerant of substitution with respect to 5α-reductase binding. Positions 6β and 4, however, appeared sensitive to bulk and limits the versatility for derivatization. This was evidenced by the fact that the K_I for 4-methyltestosterone is 2.1 μM and that of the corresponding ethylated analog is greater than 7 μM. In contrast to the testosterone series, similar derivatization of progesterone did not result in a marked decrease in inhibitory activity as demonstrated by K_I values of 1.2 μM and 0.8 μM for 4-methylprogesterone and 2α-methylprogesterone, respectively.

Since numerous reports [7, 16] have indicated that a variety of C-17β side chains do not preclude enzymatic binding, functionalization of this position was sought which would possibly enhance binding, particularly when combined with appropriate A ring modification. Although many C-17 analogs of Δ^4-3-ketosteroid are acceptable, progesterone, androst-4-en-3-one-17β-carboxylic acid and 23,24-dinorchol-4-en-22-ol-3-one (21-hydroxy-20-methylpregn-4-en-3-one) were investigated based on their respective K_I values of 0.8, 1.45, and 0.44 μM. It should be noted that the carboxylic acid analogs have received little further attention due to their lack of in vivo activity.

TABLE II. Inhibition of prostatic 5α-reductase by 4-halosteroids[a]

	Molar inhibitor concentration		
	10^{-5}	10^{-6}	10^{-7}
Inhibitor		(% inhibition)	
Progesterone	64.1	48.7	21.7
4-Chloroprogesterone	50.2	45.2	32.0
4-Fluoroprogesterone	76.6	46.7	6.0
4-Chlorotestosterone	47.8	17.8	—
4-Fluorotestosterone	73.0	49.0	11.8
23,24-Dinorchol-4-en-22-ol-3-one[b]	88.4	51.2	—
4-Chloro-23,24-dinorchol-4-en-22-ol-3-one[b]	86.8	81.1	28.6

[a]Incubations were performed as described in the Methods section. [^{3}H]-testosterone = 5×10^{-8} M. Percent inhibition of reduction was calculated relative to uninhibited controls (100%).
[b][^{3}H]-testosterone = 5×10^{-7} M.

Further modification of the carbon centers associated with the Δ^4-3-ketone moiety suggested that the introduction of a halogen at carbon 4 was particularly useful and in some cases could enhance inhibitory activity. The general inhibitor profile for these derivatives is given in Table II utilizing tritiated testosterone as the substrate.

The 4-halosteroids were shown to be potent inhibitors of the 5α-reductase with 4-chloroprogesterone ($K_I = 1.25$ μM) and 4-chloro-23, 24-dinorchol-4-en-22-ol-3-one ($K_I = 0.095$ μM) being of considerable interest since the kinetic analysis of these analogs initially suggested that the inhibition was noncompetitive. However, these inhibitors are now considered to be of the mixed type since replotting the slopes from the Dixon analysis against the reciprocal substrate concentration does not go through the origin. Although this issue is not completely resolved due to the inability to purify prostatic 5α-reductase, further experiments were performed to determine if any irreversible inhibition was occurring since enzymatic reduction of the 4-chloroprogesterone unsaturation would generate an α-haloketone which could then potentially alkylate a nucleophilic residue on the enzyme resulting in inactivation. All evidence obtained, however, did not support this mechanistic possibility. When 4-chloroprogesterone (10 μM) was incubated with ventral prostatic membranes [12] and aliquots were removed over 1.5 hours, pelleted, resuspended, and assayed for 5α-reductase activity, no time-dependent inactivation was observed as compared with control incubations receiving no inhibitor. Furthermore, when [1α, 2α(n)-^{3}H]-4-chloroprogesterone (10 μM, 0.077 μCi) and NADPH (2.2×10^{-4}M) were incubated in the presence (50 mg) and absence of prostatic homogenates for one hour at 30°C, insignificant metabolic transformation of the inhibitor was observed. After extensive extraction

TABLE III. Inhibition of prostatic 5α-reductase by 2-substituted steroids

| | Molar inhibitor concentration | | |
| | 10^{-5} | 10^{-6} | 10^{-7} |
Inhibitor		(% inhibition)	
2α-Cyanotestosterone	44.0	23.8	—
2-Methylenetestosterone	42.5	28.0	—
2α-Cyanoprogesterone	42.3	18.4	—
2α-Cyano-23,24-dinorchol-4-en-22-ol-3-one	79.8	33.6	11.6
2-Methylene-23,24-dinorchol-4-en-22-ol-3-one	71.5	30.0	6.1

Incubations were performed as described in the Methods section. [^{3}H]-testosterone = 5×10^{-7} M. Percent inhibition was calculated relative to uninhibited controls (100%).

the steroidal residues were resolved by thin-layer chromatography and in incubations which had received no tissue 90% of the radioactivity was isopolar with 4-chloroprogesterone (7434 cpm) and the remainder spuriously distributed (775 cpm). In incubations which had received tissue the zone isopolar with the inhibitor contained 7431 cpm and the remainder (1341 cpm) randomly distributed.

It was concluded that a halogen substituent at the four carbon of Δ^{4}-3-ketones did not prevent binding to 5α-reductase and was effective in limiting reductive metabolism short term.

The ability of the steroid nucleus to tolerate substituents at carbon 2 was considered in view of the fact this functionization often renders androgenic compounds inactive [17]. In contrast to the four substituted analogs where binding to the 5α-reductase is not significantly diminished relative to the parent compounds, the introduction of a nitrile or methylene group at C-2 compromises binding as shown in Table III.

Thus, functionality at the two position results in a decrease in inhibitory activity. The apparent K_I for 2α-cyano-23, 24-dinorchol-4-en-22-ol-3-one was found to be 3.75 μM whereas that for the unsubstituted parent compound was 0.44 μM. In spite of this decrease in inhibitory activity, functionalization at C-2 is suggested as an important method whereby androgenic inhibitors can be rendered homonally inactive.

Having established that selected A ring substitution in Δ^{4}-3-ketosteroids was compatible with maintaining inhibitory activity toward 5α-reductase, the question of selectivity with respect to the 3α and 3β-hydroxysteroid dehydrogenases was addressed. As shown in Table IV, these analogs are modestly selective toward the prostatic 5α-reductase with the exception of the 2-methylene derivatives which do not inhibit the dehydrogenases to any significant extent.

TABLE IV. Inhibitor specificity for prostatic 5α-reductase (R) and 3ξ-hydroxysteroid dehydrogenase (HSD)

Inhibitor	% Inhibition		
	R	HSD	R/HSD
4-Chlorotestosterone	84	26	3.2/1
4-Fluorotestosterone	78	29	2.7/1
2α-Cyanotestosterone	17	10	1.7/1
2-Methylenetestosterone	35	1.0	35/1
23,24-Dinorchol-4-en-22-ol-3-one	83	36	2.3/1
4-Chloro-23,24-dinorchol-4-en-22-ol-3-one	88	21	4.2/1
2α-Cyano-23,24-dinorchol-4-en-22-ol-3-one	78	30	2.6/1
2-Methylene-23,24-dinorchol-4-en-22-ol-3-one	62	1.0	62/1
4-Chloroprogesterone	84	24	3.5/1
4-Fluoroprogesterone	83	41	2.0/1

Incubations (50 mg ventral prostatic homogenates) were carried out in a 2.5 ml system (pH 6.6) at 30°C for 1 hour containing in final concentrations NADPH (2.2×10^{-4}M), inhibitor (1 μM), and either [^{3}H]-testosterone (1 μM) or [^{3}H]-dihydrotestosterone. Percent inhibition of each substrate was based on uninhibited controls (100%) for the metabolites generated by 5α-reduction or 3-ketone reduction, respectively. The specific metabolites are given in the Methods section. The average (n = 3) percent reduction for testosterone controls was 27.5 and that for the 3-ketone of dihydrotestosterone (n = 3) 41.9%.

In order to further assess the inhibitory activity of the synthetic analogs, Δ^4-3-ketosteroid-5α-oxidoreductase from the hormone-sensitive Dunning R-3327 adenocarcinoma of prostatic origin [18] was examined. The tumor-derived enzyme had many similarities to that from ventral prostate with a pH optimum in the acidic range. The K_m values for testosterone and progesterone were 0.64 μM and 0.21 μM, respectively, as shown in Figure 2. The activity of the R-3327 5α-reductase was threefold less than that from the ventral prostate with testosterone as the substrate. Strikingly, however, no difference in activity was observed between normal and transformed tissue when progesterone was the substrate (Table V).

The R-3327 enzyme was found to be susceptible to inhibition by both C-2 and -4 substituted analogs. In general, however, the degree of inhibition was somewhat less than that observed for the ventral prostatic 5α-reductase. Representative apparent K_I values are given in Table VI.

Thus, it is suggested that the rat ventral prostate is an appropriate model for the evaluation of 5α-reductase inhibitors for studies utilizing the R-3327 tumor derived enzyme. The marked difference in the ability of tumor enzyme to me-

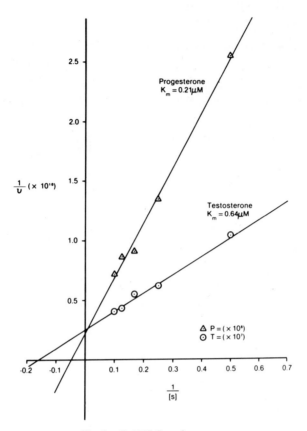

Fig. 2.   R-3327 5α-reductase.

TABLE V. Ventral prostatic and R-3327 5α-reductase activity

Substrate (5×10^{-8}M)	Pmole/ mg protein/hr
Testosterone (ventral prostate)	37.3
Progesterone (ventral prostate)	43.1
Testosterone (R-3327)	13.0
Progesterone (R-3327)	41.5

Incubations and product isolation were performed as described in the Methods section.

TABLE VI. Inhibition of R-3327 5α-reductase

Inhibitor	Apparent K_I (μM)
Progesterone	0.80 (0.80)[a]
4-Chloroprogesterone	2.86 (1.50)
2α-Cyano-17α-methyl-testosterone	18.2 (12.0)
4-Chloro-23,24-dinorchol-4-en-22-ol-3-one	0.67 (0.095)
2α-Cyano-23,24-dinorchol-4-en-22-ol-3-one	3.60 (3.75)

[a]Inhibition constants (μM) for rat ventral prostate.

TABLE VII. Effect of 5α-reductase inhibitors on the sex accessory tissues of the castrate rat

Treatment	Ventral prostate	Dorsolateral prostate	Seminal vesicles
Control (vehicle)	19 ∓ 4.2	22 ∓ 2.5	29 ∓ 2.9
4-Chloro-17α-hydroxyprogesterone	9 ∓ 1.0	15 ∓ 1.6	36 ∓ 3.0
2α-Cyano-17α-methyl testosterone	9 ∓ 1.0	26 ∓ 3.0	34 ∓ 2.0
4-Chloro- 23,24-dinorchol-4-en-22-ol-3-one	11 ∓ 1.6	19 ∓ 2.1	41 ∓ 4.0

Each value ∓ SEM (n = 6) represents tissue wet weights as mg/100gm body weight. The steroids were administered daily × 6 at a dose of 15 mg/day.

tabolize progesterone in contrast to testosterone can only be speculated on at this time.

In vivo evaluation of representative inhibitors was performed in the intact and castrate rat for effects on prostatic growth. The 4-chloro-23, 24-dinorchol-4-en-22-ol-3-one was chosen for study since it is an excellent 5α-reductase inhibitor with an apparent K_I of 0.095 μM. Although the 2α-cyano-17α-methyltestosterone was a poor inhibitor with a K_I of 12 μM, it was included for study to confirm if appropriate C-2 substituents would render active androgens hormonally inactive. The 4-chloro-17α-hydroxyprogesterone was included as a negative control since previous studies in our laboratory had shown this compound to be inactive in the intact rat in spite of being an excellent 5α-reductase inhibitor.

As shown in Table VII, none of the compounds tested exhibited any androgenic activity in stimulating prostatic growth in the castrate rat when administered daily for 6 days. This suggests that the introduction of a nitrile group at C-2 or dual modification at C-4 and C-17 results in Δ^4-3-ketosteroids which are 5α-reductase inhibitors devoid of androgenic properties.

When evaluated in the mature intact rat the 2α-cyano-17α-methyltestosterone caused a 30% (P < 0.05) suppression in the ventral prostatic weight, whereas

TABLE VIII. Effect of 5α-reductase inhibitors on the sex accessory tissues of the intact rat

Treatment	Ventral prostate	Dorsolateral prostate	Seminal vesicles
Control (vehicle)	116 ∓ 5.3	88 ∓ 4.3	132 ∓ 6.7
4-Chloro-17α-hydroxyprogesterone	111 ∓ 5.5	77 ∓ 6.0	130 ∓ 5.6
2α-Cyano-17α-methyltestosterone	80 ∓ 4.0*	67 ∓ 4.6*	113 ∓ 2.6
4-Chloro- 23,24-dinorchol-4-en-22-ol-3-one	97 ∓ 10.7	66 ∓ 4.9*	123 ∓ 6.2

Each value ∓ SEM (n = 6) represents tissue wet weights as mg/100gm body weight. The steroids were administered daily × 6 at a dose of 15 mg/day.
*$P < 0.05$.

the other analogs showed no significant effect [19]. Most interestingly, however, both the nitrile analog and the 4-chloro-23, 24-dinorchol-4-en-22-ol-3-one caused a significant decrease in the dorsolateral prostatic weights (25%, $P < 0.05$) as shown in Table VIII. Attempted correlation of the observed suppression in prostatic weights with tissue DNA and RNA was not entirely satisfactory (Table IX). The nitrile derivative which decreases ventral and dorsolateral prostate wet weights had no effect on the DNA content of the tissues. In contrast 4-chloro-23, 24-dinorchol-4-en-22-ol-3-one caused significant DNA suppression in both prostatic lobes but the wet weights were decreased in only the dorsolateral prostate. This discrepancy between wet weight data and DNA content suggests that multiple mechanisms may be operative and that they may be distinct mechanistic differences between these two active analogs requiring further study.

DISCUSSION

The necessity of an androgenic environment for prostatic growth has resulted in numerous studies aimed at depriving this tissue of the hormonal stimulus. To date estrogen administration or orchiectomy have met with the greatest success. Since testosterone must be reduced to 5α-dihydrotestosterone in the prostatic cell for full androgenic expression to occur, the studies described were performed to further evaluate the susceptibility of the Δ^4-3-ketosteroid-5α-oxidoreductase to inhibition by steroid hormone analogs. Of primary concern was defining carbon center modifications in the steroid nucleus A-ring which would not preclude analog binding to the 5α-reductase. The C-2 and C-4 positions in the A-ring can tolerate modest bulk as well as C-17 of the D-ring which is extremely versatile. Modification at C-2 did not enhance inhibitory activity, but when a nitrile substituent was introduced potent androgens became inactive. The introduction of a halogen at C-4 was particularly useful in that it appears to stabilize th Δ^4-3-ketone moiety to 5α-reduction thus prolonging the half-life of active inhibitor. When this modification was coupled with appropriate C-17 function-

TABLE IX. Effect of 5α-reductase inhibitors on the intact rat prostate DNA and RNA content

Treatment	Ventral prostate		Dorsolateral prostate	
	DNA	RNA	DNA	RNA
Control (vehicle)	2.85 ∓ 0.14	6.06 ∓ 0.41	2.06 ∓ 0.19	2.98 ∓ 0.39
4-Chloro-17α-hydroxyprogesterone	2.95 ∓ 0.33	7.58 ∓ 0.56	2.75 ∓ 0.29	3.25 ∓ 0.42
2α-Cyano-7α-methyltestosterone	2.39 ∓ 0.29	6.58 ∓ 0.37	2.17 ∓ 0.17	3.23 ∓ 0.36
4-Chloro- 23,24-dinorchol-4-en-22-ol-3-one	1.70 ∓ 0.10*	4.55 ∓ 0.50	1.07 ∓ 0.10*	2.84 ∓ 0.17

Each value ∓ SEM (n = 6) represents μg DNA or RNA/mg tissue. The steroids were administered daily × 6 at a dose of 15 mg/day.
*$P < 0.05$.

ality the inhibitory activity could be increased relative to the parent compound as demonstrated by 4-chloro-23, 24-dinorchol-4-en-22-ol-3-one which had an apparent K_I of 0.095 µM. Only the 2-methylene analogs were shown to have a high degree of specificity for inhibiting the prostatic 5α-reductase in contrast to all other analogs which to varying degrees also inhibited the 3α and 3β-hydroxysteroid dehydrogenases in prostatic homogenates.

All the analogs tested which were inhibitors of ventral prostatic 5α-reductase were also active against the R-3327 adenocarcinoma derived enzyme, although the degree of inhibition was generally less. Based on these studies, it appears that for preliminary inhibitor screening purposes the ventral prostatic enzyme is comparable to that from tumor tissue. Certain differences are apparent, however, in that the tumor enzyme was one third as active in transforming testosterone to dihydrotestosterone than ventral prostate, but no differences in activity were observed when progesterone was utilized as the substrate suggesting an iso-functional or transformed 5α-reductase may be present in the R-3327 tumor, although further studies are necessary to clarify this observation. The animal studies were particularly revealing in demonstrating that there is no correlation between in vitro 5α-reductase inhibitory activity and in vivo activity in sup-pressing prostatic growth. The nature of the C-17 side chain appeared particularly important since 4-chloro-17α-hydroxyprogesterone did not cause any reduction in dorsolateral prostatic wet weights, whereas the 4-chloro-dinorchol-4-en-22-ol-3-one did even though both are excellent 5α-reductase inhibitors. Steroid nucleus modification at carbon centers 2, 4, and 17 are compatible with in vivo activity in suppressing prostatic growth; however, the substitution pattern appears critical.

CONCLUSIONS

The results of this investigation suggest that Δ^4-3-ketosteroids can tolerate diverse substitution without significantly compromising their binding to prostatic 5α-reductase. Selected modification at C-4 and C-17 of the steroid nucleus can enhance binding to the enzyme. Halogen introduction at C-4 can limit the par-ticipation of these analogs as substrates for the 5α-reductase, whereas a nitrile substitutent at C-2 can render androgenic steroids hormonally inactive. The inhibition profile for the 5α-reductase of the R-3327 tumor parallels that for the ventral prostatic enzyme. In vitro inhibitory activity for 5α-reductase is a poor predictor of in vivo activity. However, it is concluded that appropriate steroid hormone analogs can be designed as 5α-reductase inhibitors which will be active in vivo in suppressing prostatic growth.

ACKNOWLEDGMENTS

This work was supported by US Public Health Service grant CA 23019. The technical assistance of W. Nasholds, J. Fears, and D. Moore is gratefully ac-knowledged.

REFERENCES

1. Huggins C, Hodges CV: Studies on prostatic cancer—effects of castration, of estrogens and androgen injection on serum phosphatases in metastatic carcinoma of the prostate. Cancer Res 1: 293–297, 1941.
2. Walsh PC: Physiologic basis for hormonal therapy in carcinoma of the prostate. Urol Clin N Am 2: 125–140, 1975.
3. Bruchovsky N, Wilson JD: The intranuclear binding of testosterone and 5α-androstan-17β-ol-3-one by rat prostate. J Biol Chem 243: 5953–5960, 1968.
4. Liao S, Fang S: Receptor-proteins for androgens and the mode of action of androgens on gene transcription in ventral prostate. Vit Horm 27: 17–90, 1969.
5. Bruchovsky N: Comparison of the metabolities formed in rat prostate following the in vivo administration of seven natural androgens. Endocrinology 89: 1212–1222, 1971.
6. Moore RJ, Wilson JD: Localization of the reduced nicotinamide adenine dinucleotide phosphate: Δ⁴-3-ketosteroid 5α-oxidoreductase in the nuclear membrane of the rat ventral prostate. J Biol Chem 247: 958–967, 1972.
7. Frederiksen DW, Wilson JD: Partial characterization of the nuclear reduced nictotinamide adenine dinucleotide phosphate: Δ⁴-3-ketosteroid 5α-oxidoreductase of rat prostate. J Biol Chem 246: 2584–2593, 1971.
8. Morita K: Selective oxidation of allylic alcohols with active N-halogen compounds, II. Bull Chem Soc Jpn 32: 227–232, 1959.
9. Ringold HJ, Batres E, Mancera O, Rosenkranz G: Synthesis of 4-halo hormone analogs. J Org Chem 21: 1432–1435, 1956.
10. Manson A, et al: Androstano [2, 3-d]-isoxazoles and related compounds. J Med Chem 6: 1–9, 1963.
11. Manson A, Wood D: Preparation of 2-methylene-Δ⁴-3-oxo steroids. J Org Chem 32: 3734–3737, 1967.
12. Moore RJ, Wilson JD: Reduced nicotinamide adenine dinucleotide phosphate: Δ⁴-3-ketosteroid 5α-oxido-reductase (rat ventral prostate). In O'Malley B, Hardman J (eds): "Methods in Enzymology." New York: Academic Press, 1975, Vol 36, pp 446–474. Academic Press, NY, NY.
13. Bradford M: A rapid and sensitive method for the quantitation of microgram quantities of protein utilizing the principle of protein-dye binding. Anal Biochem 72: 248–254, 1976.
14. Dixon M: The determination of enzyme inhibitor constants. Biochem J 55: 170–171, 1953.
15. Burton K: Determination of DNA concentration with diphenylamine. In Grossman L, Moldave K (eds): "Methods in Enzymology." New York: Academic Press, 1968, Vol 12B, pp 163–166.
16. Voight W, Hsia SL: Further studies on testosterone 5α-reductase of human skin. J Biol Chem 248: 4280–4285, 1973.
17. Kincl FA: Anabolic steroids. Meth Horm Res 4: 21–76, 1965.
18. Voight W, Dunning WF: In vivo metabolism of testosterone-³H in R-3327, an androgen-sensitive rat prostatic adenocarcinoma. Cancer Res 35: 1840–1846, 1975.
19. Dunnett CW: New tables for multiple comparisons with a control. Biometrics 20: 482–491, 1964.

The Prostatic Cell: Structure and Function
Part B, pages 283–297

Studies on a 5α-Reductase Inhibitor and Their Therapeutic Implications

Vladimir Petrow and Leon Lack

INTRODUCTION

Although prostatic cancer is a disease of unknown etiology, there seems little doubt that temporary remissions can be induced in many cases during the early endocrine-dependent phase, by depriving the neoplasm of endocrine support [1]. The endocrine milieu of the tumor, however, is complex and includes not only the testicular and adrenal androgens and their metabolites, but also the estrogens, corticoids, and their metabolites. An excellent review of the physiological control of prostatic growth has recently been presented by D. S. Coffey [2]. Fortunately, from among these many steroids, 17β-hydroxy-5α-androstan-3-one [dihydro-testosterone (DHT)] is generally regarded as playing a key permissive role in the oncogenic process [3–5]. It is, consequently, a legitimate target of prostatic cancer research to develop procedures which will eliminate dihydrotestosterone from the economy of the prostatic cell. Prostatic adenocarcinoma, however, is composed of a heterogeneous population of cells which differ in their requirements for androgen to perform their vital processes. It follows that inhibition of DHT-dependent growth, though palliative in the short term, cannot inhibit androgen-insensitive prostatic cells and must fail over the long term. There is thus a fatal inadequacy in the DHT approach to therapy. Until control of growth of androgen-insensitive cells is mastered, their very existence must pose a threat, like the sword of Damocles, over the head of the unfortunate sufferer. Pharmaceutical intervention of this type, however, is still justified because such intervention may well prove to be a vital part in a future complex of treatment.

Reduction of testosterone to DHT by 5α-reductase probably occurs by the concerted mechanism [6] shown in Figure 1. A therapeutically effective inhibitor of the enzyme must show marked specificity for the catalytic site of the enzyme. Moreover, as 5α-reductase is a pyridine-linked dehydrogenase, inhibition should preferably be linked to the presence of NADPH. Finally, inhibition should be irreversible in order to combat physiological dilution of the drug and to achieve prolonged inactivation.

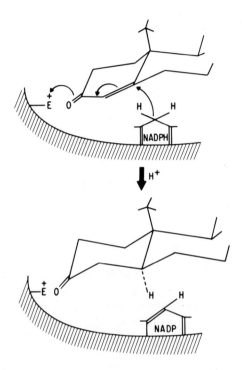

Fig. 1. Interaction of testosterone and NADPH at the active site of 5α-reductase.

Irreversible enzyme inhibitors are basically of two types. The first type, affinity-labelling reagents, resemble the substrate in structure but incorporate a chemically reactive functional group such as $-COCH_2Br$, which reacts with the enzyme when in close apposition to it with formation of a covalent bond. Such inhibitors are basically alkylating agents with limited specificity in vivo. The second group of inhibitors is known as suicide enzyme inactivators or k_{cat} inhibitors. Such inhibitors usually resemble the substrate in overall structure and possess binding affinity for the enzyme-active site. Their main characteristic lies in their possession of a latent reactive center which is activated in some manner by the catalytic action of the enzyme. When this occurs covalent binding to the enzyme takes place with its consequent inactivation [7,8]. It is to this class of inhibitors that the present work is directed.

It seems likely from Figure 1 that the driving force behind the catalytic activity of 5α-reductase resides in the polarization of the 3-keto group of testosterone. Such polarization activates C_5 which then accepts a hydride ion from the α-face of the steroid. We planned to exploit this mechanism by extending the conjugation beyond C_5 and its proximal NADPH moiety. The resulting 3-keto dienic system is known to add nucleophiles in the laboratory [9] as indicated below:

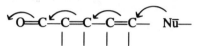

We hoped that incorporation of this system into a suitable substrate would give a steroidal inhibitor that the enzyme would mistake for testosterone. It would thus be impelled to activate the keto-diene system which, in its turn, could combine covalently with some proximal nucleophilic residue in the enzyme active site, thereby ensuring destruction of the enzyme. Such self-destruction could be regarded as "suicide."

Compounds (IV), (V), (VI), and VIII) were chosen for initial study. As (V) contains a 6-Me group, steroid (III) was included. In addition, the cross-conjugated 1,4-dien-3-one system is known to readily add nucleophiles in the laboratory [10], thereby leading to inclusion of (VII) in the study (cf Fig. 2).

Preliminary studies on these steroids showed a range of enzyme-inhibiting activites. Only steroid (VIII), however, gave promise of inhibition by a mechanism of the k_{cat} type.

MATERIALS AND METHODS

Compounds (IV) [11], (VII) [12], and (VIII) [13,14] were prepared by published methods. Compound (VI) (R5020) was from New England Nuclear and a gift from Dr. K. S. McCarty, Sr. Steroids (II), (III), and (V) were gifts from G. D. Searle and Co., The Upjohn Co., and Mead Johnson and Co., respectively. [1,2-³H] Testosterone of specific activity (50–52 Ci/mmole) was from New England Nuclear. It was purified by thin-layer chromatography (TLC) prior to use. NADPH, Tween 40, dithiothreitol, and EDTA were from Sigma Co. Chromatographic analyses utilized Polygram Sil G precoated plastic plates without gypsum and were from Brinkman Instruments Inc. Reference steroids were from Steraloids. All chemicals and solvents were of the highest purity available.

Prostatic nuclei were prepared and assayed essentially by the method of R. J. Moore and J. D. Wilson [15] employing retired male Wistar breeding rats (25–30/operation) as source of prostatic tissue. Prostatic homogenate was centrifuged at 800g and the pellet rehomogenized in 2.0 M sucrose–0.5 mM CaCl₂. Aliquots were layered over 2.2 M sucrose–0.5 mM CaCl₂ and centrifuged at 56,000g. The pellet was resuspended in 0.88 M sucrose–1.5 mM CaCl₂ and stored at −70°C.

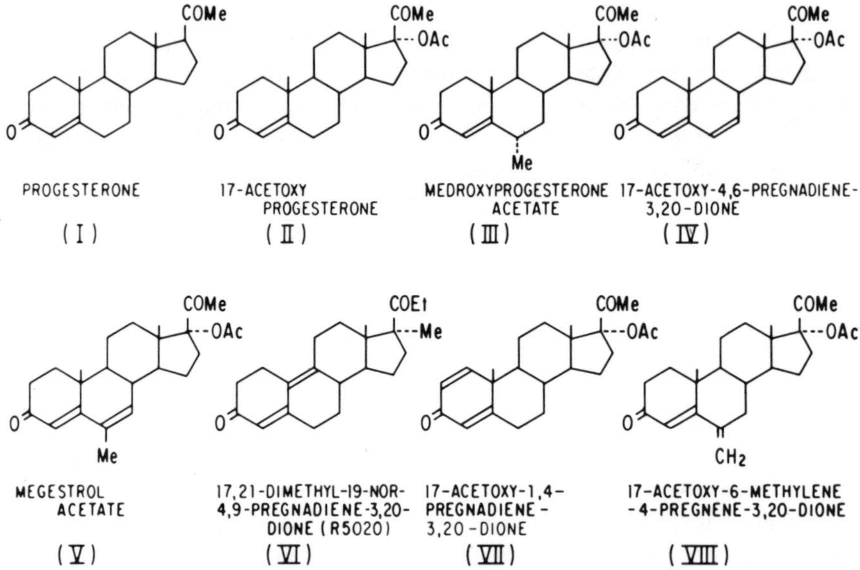

Fig. 2. Formulae of steroids examined in present study.

For assay, nuclei were suspended in 0.88 M sucrose–1.5 mM CaCl$_2$. The solution was spun at 100,000g for 30 minutes and the pellet removed and re-suspended in 0.05 M potassium phosphate buffer (pH 6.6) containing 10^{-4} M EDTA and 10 mM dithiothreitol (KED buffer) and the suspension triturated through an 18-gauge and then a 21-gauge needle. It was then centrifuged at 100,000g for 30 minutes, resuspended in KED buffer, and triturated through an 18-gauge and then a 21-gauge needle. It was then subjected to sonic disruption at 0°C. Incubations were performed on 0.8 ml or 1.0 ml final volumes unless otherwise stated. Final concentrations were 5×10^{-8} M [1,2-^{3}H]testosterone and 5×10^{-4}M NADPH in potassium phosphate-EDTA-dithiothreitol buffer. The assay mixture was incubated for the appropriate time and enzymatic reaction terminated by addition of 5 volumes of CHCl$_3$–MeOH (2:1) and processed for analysis by TLC. Reference steroids were added, the chromatograms were developed, and the spots visualized by heating with the anisaldehyde reagent [15]. The lanes were divided and cut as in the procedure of R. J. Moore and J. D. Wilson [15] and the fragments transferred to liquid scintillation vials and assayed for ^{3}H. The fraction of testosterone reduced was determined from the fraction of ^{3}H in the DHT and androstane-3β,17β-diol regions of the chromatogram to the total ^3H in the lane. Amounts of reduced testosterone were calculated from this value and the amount of testosterone originally present. Substrate blanks (incubations without enzyme) were used routinely to correct for nonenzymatic degradation and for slight impurities. These were within published limits [15].

Inhibitory activity was determined as follows: The test steroid dissolved in benzene was added to the dry incubation tubes together with 22 μg of Tween 40 dissolved in 0.2 ml benzene. Benzene was removed by a gentle stream of nitrogen and the tubes finally dried for 30 minutes in a desiccator continuously evacuated by a mechanical pump. Control tubes containing no test steroid as well as blank tubes containing the same amount of Tween 40 were treated in the same way. A portion (0.4 ml) of the substrate co-enzyme solution in KED buffer together with 0.2 ml KED buffer was added to each of these dried incubation tubes. After vortexing, the tubes were allowed to equilibrate in a 25°C waterbath and, at specified times, reactions were initiated by the addition of 0.2 ml of the enzyme preparation. After 1 hour 4 ml of $CHCl_3$–MeOH (2:1) were added and the contents of the tubes processed [15] followed by TLC. Control experiments showed that Tween 40 at twice the highest concentrations employed herein had no effect upon enzyme activity.

Preincubation studies involved exposure of the nuclear protein to the test steroid together with co-factor. The ratio of test steroid to the Tween 40 detergent was as before. All control tubes had the same amount of detergent. Preincubations were carried out for times stated in the results. Following dilution × 10, residual enzymic activity was determined as above.

RESULTS

The results of experiments assessing the potency of steroids (II) through (VIII) are given in the curves shown in Figure 3. Progesterone is included for comparison. 17-Acetoxy-6-methylene-4-pregnene-3,20-dione (VIII) [16] is clearly the most active inhibitor and equipotent with progesterone. The remaining steroids are considerably less potent. Medroxyprogesterone acetate (III) and megestrol acetate (V) are virtually inactive under the conditions of the experiment.

When the enzyme preparation was preincubated with 5×10^{-7} M of 17-acetoxy-6-methylene-4-pregnene-3,20-dione (VIII) and NADPH, then diluted × 10 and assayed for 5α-reductase activity, ca 75% of the enzymatic activity was lost (cf Table I, expts A and B). In contrast, preincubation of the steroid alone without NADPH (Table I, expt D) showed no inactivation of the enzyme. Preincubation of the enzyme with competitive inhibitors such as progesterone or testosterone under the same experimental conditions did not result in enzyme inactivation. Saturation conditions for the co-factor were optimal [16]. When the same type of preincubation studies were carried out with steroids (II) through (VII), enzyme inactivation was not observed, suggesting that any inhibition observed with these steroids (cf Fig. 2) was reversible.

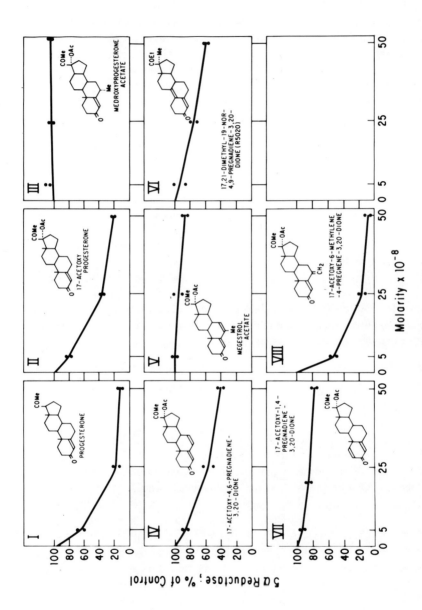

Fig. 3. Inhibition of 5α-reductase by various pregnene derivatives.

TABLE I. Effect of preincubation of enzyme with 17α-acetoxy-6-methylene-4-pregnen-3-one and NADPH on 5α-reductase activity

	Preincubation conditions (time: 15 min)		Enzymic assay conditions (time: 45 min)			Pmoles testosterone
	Inhibitor (M)	NADPH (M)	Inhibitor (M)	Testosterone (M)	NADPH (M)	reduced/mg of protein in 45 min ± SEM
A	5×10^{-7}	6×10^{-5}	5×10^{-8}	5×10^{-8}	5×10^{-4}	$0.71 \pm 0.018 n = 6$
B	0	6×10^{-5}	5×10^{-8}	5×10^{-8}	5×10^{-4}	$3.0 \pm 0.26 n = 6$
C	0	0	5×10^{-8}	5×10^{-8}	5×10^{-4}	$2.83 \pm 0.09 n = 6$
D	5×10^{-7}	0	5×10^{-8}	5×10^{-8}	5×10^{-4}	$2.63 \pm 0.18 n = 6$
E	no preincubation		0	5×10^{-8}	5×10^{-4}	$4.36 \pm 0.24 n = 4$
F	no preincubation		5×10^{-8}	5×10^{-8}	5×10^{-4}	$3.14 \pm 0.20 n = 4$

The time courses of inactivation of 5α-reductase following incubation of the enzyme with different concentrations of inhibitor (VIII) and NADPH are given in Figure 4. The assay of residual enzymic activity following incubation with the steroid employed 5×10^{-6}M testosterone.

Preincubation studies of the inhibitor with testosterone resulted in a decrease in enzymic inactivation. This is shown in Figure 6.

DISCUSSION

Comparative studies on 5α-reductase inhibition generally use progesterone (I) as standard in view of its very high potency [17]. Its rapid metabolism in the body and lack of oral activity, however, detract from its value as a therapeutic agent. By introducing a 17-acetoxy group into the molecule, 17-acetoxyprogesterone (II) is obtained, which now possesses oral activity as a progestational agent [18,19]. We have, therefore, used this basic structure (II) as far as possible in our studies. An additional attraction of this ring system is its built-in potential for anti-androgenic activity (cf for example, [20]), which property would clearly enhance its value in prostatic carcinoma.

17-Acetoxyprogesterone (II) proved to be somewhat less active than progesterone (I) as an inhibitor of 5α-reductase (Fig. 3). Introduction of a 6α-methyl group, as in medroxyprogesterone acetate (III), resulted in virtual inactivity. Extension of conjugation, as in the 4,6-diene (IV), led to significant loss in potency, which again fell to very low levels on introduction of 6-methyl as in megestrol acetate (V). The 4,9-dienic structure (IV) and the 1,4-diene (VII) were very weak inhibitors. 17-Acetoxy-6-methylene-4-pregnene-3,20-dione (VIII), in striking contrast, slightly exceeded progesterone in potency and was the most effective inhibitor of the series.

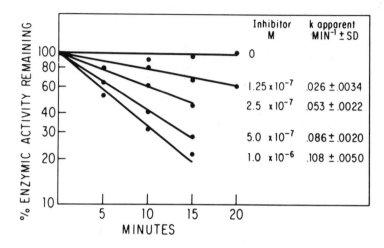

Fig. 4. Time course of inactivation of 5α-reductase following incubation of the enzyme with steroid (VIII) and NADPH. The assay of residual enzymic activity following the incubation with (VIII) utilized 5 × 10⁻⁶M testosterone. Each point is the mean of two determinations.

Mechanism of Inhibition

As outlined in the Introduction, we sought an irreversible inhibitor of the k_{cat} type which would additionally be active by the oral route. Unfortunately, the use of such standard techniques as prolonged dialysis of the enzyme-inhibitor complex to establish irreversibility is not readily applicable in this instance due to the known instability of this membrane-bound enzyme [15]. We have therefore used the "preincubation technique" to provide information on the mechanism of inhibition.

When an enzyme preparation able to reduce 4.36 pmoles testosterone /45 min/mg protein in the presence of 5×10^{-4} M of NADPH was preincubated with 5×10^{-7} M of (VIII) and NADPH for 15 minutes, diluted ×10 to bring the concentration of inhibitor to 5×10^{-8} M, and assayed in the usual way, the reducing capacity of the enzyme was found to have dropped to 0.71 pmoles testosterone /45 min/mg protein (cf Table I). NAPDH was essential during the preincubation exposure. Identical preincubation with the competitive inhibitor progesterone, in contrast, did not show a corresponding loss in activity of the enzyme. Kinetic studies were next undertaken. The enzyme was preincubated with NADPH and various concentrations of (VIII) and the residual enzymic activity assayed at specific times. As seen from Figure 4, the time course of inactivation followed pseudo-first order kinetics, which pattern of behavior is generally associated with irreversible inhibition. By plotting a reciprocal function of these rate constants as the $T_{1/2}$s against the reciprocal of the inhibitor concentrations, a straight line is obtained with a positive intercept on the y-axis (see Fig. 5), thereby indicating a saturation phenomenon. These data accord with the concept that interaction of the inhibitor (VIII) with the enzyme occurs in two steps. First there is a reversible combination of the enzyme with the inhibitor

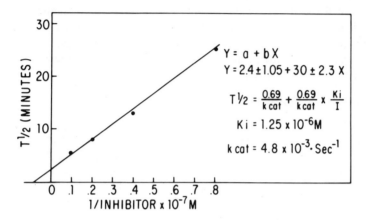

Fig. 5. The dependence of $T_{1/2}$ of the inactivation of 5α-reductase upon the reciprocal of the concentration of inhibitor (VIII).

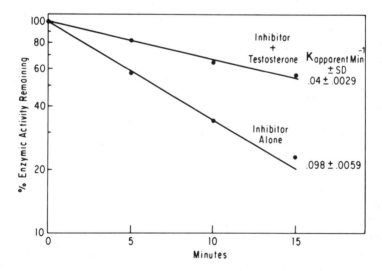

Fig. 6. Effect of testosterone upon the inactivation of 5α-reductase by inhibitor (VIII) in the presence of NADPH. Each point represents two determinations.

with a Ki of 1.25×10^{-6} M. This is followed by an irreversible step with inactivation of the enzyme. The rate constant (k_{cat}) for this step is 4.8×10^{-3}/sec. In contrast to (VIII), preincubation studies of steroids (II) through (VII) gave data compatible with only reversible inhibition.

17-Acetoxy-6-methylene-4-pregnene-3,20-dione (VIII) thus appears to fulfill the desiderata laid down in the introduction for a 5α-reductase inhibitor in that 1) it has good specificity for the enzyme site as shown by its high potency; 2) its specificity is further enhanced by the need for NADPH for the expression of inhibitory activity; and 3) it appears to be an irreversible inhibitor of the k_{cat} type. Its endocrine profile is presently under study, but it is expected that it will show activity by the oral route.

Stereochemical Aspects of Structure-Activity Relationships

Introduction of 6-ene into 17-acetoxyprogesterone (II) to give 17-acetoxy-4,6-pregnadiene-3,20-dione (IV) leads to a flattening of rings A and B (cf A in Figure 7, which shows the corresponding 6-methylated structure (V)), resulting in a significant loss in enzyme-inhibiting potency. As the diene (IV) is only a competitive inhibitor, and as such dienes readily add nucleophiles at C_7 from the α-side of the molecule [9], it seems likely that such a nucleophilic residue is not present within bonding distance of the C_7-terminal in the enzyme-active site. The 4,9-diene (VI) is likewise a weak inhibitor of the enzyme. It is true that the side chain in (VI) may play a role in reducing binding to the active side, but it seems unlikely that the decrease in activity can be explained wholly in this manner.[1] More probably, as shown in Figure 7B, the overall flattening of the rings A and B junctions is the primary factor in loss of potency. Significant loss of activity likewise follows introduction of Δ^1 into (II). Ring A in the resulting 17-acetoxy-1,4-pregnadiene-3,20-dione (VII) is flattened to give the angular structure shown in Figure 7C.

Introduction of 6α-methyl into (II) gives medroxyprogesterone acetate (III), which is now virtually inactive. As rings A and B of this steroid closely resemble (II)—which is an active inhibitor (cf Fig. 3)—its loss of activity must derive from the equatorial 6α-methyl substituent (Fig. 7D). An even greater loss of activity follows introduction of 6-methyl into the 4,6-diene (IV) to give megestrol acetate (V). As seen from Figure 7A, the methyl group in this structure is present in a pseudo-equatorial position analogous to the methyl group in medroxyprogesterone acetate, Figure 7D.

In striking contrast to the above, the introduction of the 6-methylene group into (II) gives 17-acetoxy-6-methylene-4-pregnene-3,20-dione (VIII), which is now a more potent inhibitor than progesterone and is, moreover, an apparently irreversible inhibitor under our experimental conditions. As is evident from

---

[1]Considerable variations in ring D substituents are compatible with inhibitory activity (cf [16]).

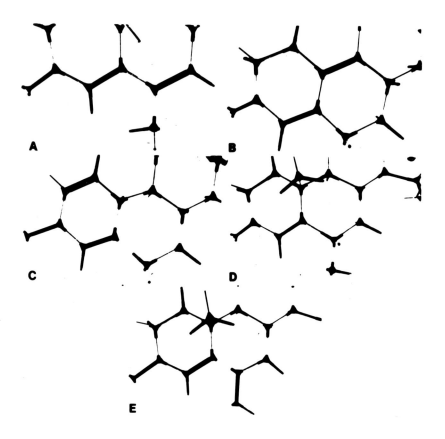

Fig. 7.   Rings A and B of Steroids (V), (VI), (VII), (III), and (VIII).

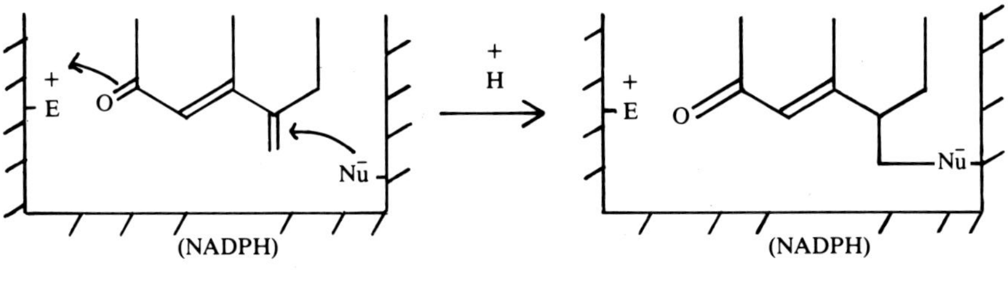

Fig. 8.   Postulated mechanism of inhibition of 5α-reductase by inhibitor (VIII).

Figure 7E, there is some flattening of rings A and B in this 6-methylenic structure. But flattening of rings A and B, as in (IV), (VI) (and (VII)), is uniformly accompanied by loss of activity, which is compounded by methyl substitution at C_6 as in (III) and (V). Based on these data, the 6-methylenic steroid (VIII) should be only weakly active. As it is the most potent inhibitor of the series and is additionally irreversible in its action, it seems likely that it can bind covalently to the enzyme-active site. As NADPH is required for the expression of such inhibitory activity, the co-enzyme must play a role in facilitating irreversible combination, for example by unmasking a nucleophilic center within bonding distance of the methylenic terminal with resulting inactivation of the enzyme as shown below. Inter alia, it may be significant that structural modification of 17-acetoxyprogesterone (II) to give (III), and (V), and (VII) results in a dramatic increase in progestational activity [21–23] which is accompanied by virtual loss of 5α-reductase-inhibiting potency.

The Case for Combination Therapy

When the preincubation experiments with steroid (VIII) were carried out in the presence of testosterone, the rates of enzymic inactivation were decreased as shown in Figure 6. This would be expected from a k_{cat} type of inhibition. It may therefore be expected that, in vivo, additional pharmacological interventions which lower testosterone levels would enhance the activity of the inhibitor. If such is indeed the case, then combination therapy of inhibitor (VIII) with, for example, a progestational agent such as megestrol acetate, which is known to lower testosterone levels by inhibiting LH, should offer therapeutic advantages over single-product therapy.

Megestrol acetate (V) was first synthesised by V. Petrow and co-workers [24,25], and shown to possess gonadotrophin-reducing, antiestrogenic and antiandrogenic properties by A. David et al [22]. Its potential value in benign prostatic hypertrophy was reported by P. E. Lebech and E. L. Nordentoft [26]. More recently, J. Geller et al [27] have reported that administration of (V) to patients with BPH leads to a significant decrease in prostatic 5α-reductase. No ^{3}H-DHT binding to a cytosol receptor protein could be demonstrated in 4/5 patients treated with the steroid. DHT levels were less than in controls and there were significantly decreased plasma levels of LH, FSH, and T at the end of the treatment period. Plasma prolactin levels were unchanged. Limited studies of the steroid in prostatic cancer [28,29] were encouraging. We were therefore surprised when megestrol acetate proved to be virtually inactive as a 5α-reductase inhibitor under our experimental conditions. Drs. A. Sandberg and N. Kadohama have kindly examined (V) and (VIII) in their tissue-culture model [30] using benign human prostatic tissue. After 1 day in the control medium, explants of tissue were maintained for 2 days in media containing 0.5 μM testosterone or

0.5 μM testosterone + 3.3–5.0 μM inhibitor, after which the tissues were exposed to ^{3}H-T for 2 hours and assayed in the usual manner. The following results were obtained:

Inhibitor	Relative inhibition
Progesterone	100
Megestrol acetate (V)	58
17-Acetoxy-6-methylene-4-pregnene-3,20-dione (VIII)	73

The simplest explanation of this in vitro data is to conclude that the inhibitory effects of (V) derive from its antiandrogenic properties [20] and, much less likely, from any possible metabolites. In vivo, however, as postulated by Geller et al [27], the antiprostatic effects of megestrol acetate (V) probably derive from LH inhibition with a consequent drop in testosterone production. In addition, the antiandrogenic effects of steroid (V) presumably lead to lower 5α-reductase levels [15]. In view of the data reported herein, there is no reason to suppose that megestrol acetate (V), per se, would exert a direct 5α-reductase-inhibiting effect in vivo by interacting with the prostatic enzyme. It seems likely that, in a clinical situation, irreversible inhibition of prostatic 5α-reductase by the 6-methylenic steroid (VIII) together with lowering of LH, T, and 5α-reductase levels by megestrol acetate (V), could well provide an advance in the therapy of prostatic cancer. The potential value of such a combination appears to warrant in vitro and in vivo studies.

CONCLUSIONS

17-Acetoxyprogesterone (II), an orally active gestagen, approaches progesterone in in vitro potency as a 5α-reductase inhibitor.

Introduction of 6α-Me and 6-Me-Δ^6 into (II) leads to virtual loss of activity. Introduction of Δ^6, Δ^9, and Δ^1 into (II) gives weak inhibitors of the enzyme.

The 6-methylene derivative (VIII), in contrast, behaves in preincubation and kinetic studies as an irreversible inhibitor of the k_{cat} type with Ki of 1.25 × 10^{-6} M and k_{cat} of 4.8 × 10^{-3} sec.

Kinetic and tissue culture studies suggest that the therapeutic effects of (VIII) in vivo would be enhanced by combination with a gonadotrophin-inhibitor such as megestrol acetate.

ACKNOWLEDGMENTS

This work was supported by research grant 1 R26 CA27374 of the National Prostatic Cancer Project (NCI). Technical assistance by Lynette Richelo, Amani Tantawi, and Douglas Rockett is gratefully acknowledged.

REFERENCES

1. Huggins C H, Hodges C V: Studies on prostatic cancer. I. The effect of castration, of estrogen and of androgen injection on serum phosphatases in metastatic carcinoma of the prostate. Cancer Res 1:293–297, 1941.
2. Coffey D S: Physiological control of prostatic growth: An overview. UICC Tech Rep Ser 48:4–23, 1979.
3. Siiteri P K, Wilson J D: Dihydrotestosterone and prostatic hypertrophy. I. The formation and content of dihydrotestosterone in the hypertrophic prostate of man. J Clin Invest 49:1737–1745, 1970.
4. Wilson J D, Loeb P M: In: "Developmental and Metabolic Control Mechanisms and Neoplasia, The University of Texas, M.D. Anderson Hospital and Tumor Institute," Baltimore: The Williams and Wilkins Co., 1965, p 375.
5. Moore R A: Benign hypertrophy and carcinoma of the prostate. In: Twombly G, Packs G (eds): "Endocrinology of Neoplastic Diseases." London, New York: Oxford Univ. Press, 1947, pp 194–212.
6. Björkhein E: Mechanism and stereochemistry of the enzymatic conversion of a Δ^4-3-oxosteroid into a 3-oxo-5α-steroid. Eur J Biochem 8:345–351, 1969; see also [15].
7. Abeles R H, Maycock A L: Suicide enzyme inactivators [review]. Accts Chem Res 9:313–319, 1976.
8. Walsh C: Recent developments in suicide substrates and other active site-directed inactivating agents of specific target enzymes [review]. Horiz Biochem Biophys 3:36–81, 1977.
9. Dodson R M, Tweit R C: 7-Acylthio-4-pregnene-3,20-diones. U.S.P. 2,904,560 (to G. D. Séarle & Co.), Sept. 15, 1959.
10. Dodson R M, Tweit R C: 1-Acylthio-4-pregnene-3,20-diones. U.S.P. 2,904,561, (to G. D. Searle & Co.), Sept. 15, 1959.
11. Sciaky R: Sintesi di analoghi di ormoni steroidi sostitui in posizione 6. Gazz Chim Ital 91:545–561, 1961.
12. Babcock J C, Pederson R L: 1-Dehydro-17-hydroxyprogesterone ester. U.S.P. 2,971,886 (to Upjohn Co.), Feb. 14, 1961.
13. Kirk D N, Petrow V: 6-Methylene steroids, B.P. 929,985 (to The British Drug Houses, Ltd.), June 26, 1963.
14. Burn D, Cooley G, Davies M T, Ducker J W, Ellis B, Feather P, Hiscock A K, Kirk D N, Leftwick A P, Petrow V, Williamson D M: Modified steroid hormones. XXXIII. Steroidal 6-formyl-3-alkoxy-3,5-dienes and some of their transformations. Tetrahedron 20:597–609, 1964.
15. Moore R J: Wilson J D: Reduced nicotinamide adenine dinucleotide phosphate: Δ^4-3-ketosteroid 5α-oxidoreductase (rat ventral prostate), Meth Enzymol 36:466–474, 1975.
16. Petrow V, Wang Y, Lack L, Sandberg A: Prostatic cancer. I. 6-Methylene-4-pregnen-3-ones as irreversible inhibitors of rat prostatic Δ^4-3-ketosteroid 5α-reductase. Submitted for publication.
17. Massa R, Martini L: Interference with the 5α-reductase system. A new approach for developing antiandrogens. Hormones and antagonists. Gynecol Invest 2:253–270, 1971/72.
18. Moffett R B, Anderson H V: Acetylation of 17α-hydroxy steroids, J Am Chem Soc 76:747–748, 1954.
19. Elton R L: Metrotropic activity of some 21-haloprogesterone derivatives. PSEBM 101:677–680, 1959; see also [21].
20. McKinney G R, Braselton J P: Antiandrogenic and antiutcrotrophic activities of three synthetic progestagens. Steroids 15:405–411, 1970.
21. Babcock J C, Gutsell E S, Herr M E, Hogg J A, Stucki J C, Barnes L E, Dulin W E: 6α-Methyl-17α-hydroxyprogesterone 17-acylates; A new class of potent progestins. J Am Chem Soc 80:2904–2905, 1958.

22. David A, Edwards K, Fellowes K P, Plummer J M: Antiovulatory and other biological properties of megestrol acetate. J Reprod Fertil 5:331–346, 1963.

23. Philibert D, Raynaud J-P: Progesterone binding in the immature mouse and rat uterus. Steroids 22:89–98, 1973.

24. Ellis B, Kirk D N, Petrow V, Waterhouse B, Williamson D M: Modified steroid hormones, Part XVII. Some 6-methyl-4,6-dien-3-ones. J Chem Soc 2828–2833, 1960.

25. Kirk D N, Petrow V, Williamson D M: Improvements in or relating to 6-methyl-3-oxo-$\Delta^{4,6}$-steroid compounds. B.P., 870,286 (to The British Drug Houses, Ltd.), June 14, 1961.

26. Lebech P E, Nordentoft E L: A study of endocrine function in the treatment of benign prostatic hypertrophy with megestrol acetate, Acta Obstet Gynecol Scand, 46 (Suppl 9):25–38, 1967.

27. Geller J, Albert J, Geller S, Lopez D, Cantor T, Yen S: Effect of megestrol acetate (Megace©) on steroid metabolism and steroid-protein binding in the human prostate. J Clin Endocrinol Metab 43:1000–1008, 1976.

28. Johnson D E, Kaesler K E, Ayala A G: Megestrol acetate for treatment of advanced carcinoma of the prostate J Surg Oncol 7:9–15, 1975.

29. Geller J, Albert J, Yen S S C: Treatment of advanced cancer of prostate with megestrol acetate. Urology 12:537–541, 1978.

30. Sandberg A: Regulation of prostate growth in organ culture. UICC Tech Rep Ser 48:165–194, 1979.

The Prostatic Cell: Structure and Function
Part B, pages 299–311

Analysis of the Androgen Receptor in Needle Biopsies From Human Prostatic Tissue

Å. Pousette, E. Borgstöm, B. Högberg, and J.-Å. Gustafsson

INTRODUCTION

Prostatic carcinoma is the most frequently occurring malignant disease in males in Sweden as well as in many other industrialized countries. Carcinoma of the prostate is almost never found in younger men, but the incidence increases rapidly in ageing males [1] and an incidence of 50% in males over 80 years of age has been reported [2]. Little is known about the etiology of prostatic carcinoma but several factors such as blood group, diet, racial origin, and socio-economic status are thought to influence prostatic tumour development [3,4]. The human prostate can be divided into separate parts with different embryological origin, hormone sensitivity, and pathogenesis [5,6]. The peripheral part is almost always the origin of prostatic carcinoma but benign prostatic hyperplasia (BPH), another prostatic disease common in senescence, always seems to develop from the periurethral parts of the gland [5,6].

The human prostate is a target tissue for androgens, and testicular activity is necessary for its normal development and function [3]. The gland atrophies after castration but it regains its normal shape, size, and secretory function after androgen therapy. The prostate is also influenced by other hormones, especially prolactin, insulin, and estrogens [7,8]. Estrogens affect the prostate probably both directly and indirectly, eg, via the testes or the central nervous system. The estrogenic action is mainly anti-androgenic.

Not only the normal prostate but often also prostatic carcinoma can be influenced by hormonal administration or withdrawal, and ever since the pioneering work of Charles Huggins in the early 1940s, endocrine manipulations have been useful tools in the treatment of prostatic carcinoma [9,10]. However, the treatment has to be individualized and several factors such as histological grading, staging, age, and general condition have to be taken into account when choosing therapy. Radical surgery can only seldom be performed and therefore endocrine treatment, chemotherapy, and irradiation are therapeutical alternatives most often used. Orchiectomy or estrogen therapy is efficient in 60–80% of patients with prostatic carcinoma but relapses occur relatively often. Moreover, estrogen therapy quite often gives rise to cardiovascular complications. Progestational anti-androgens or glucocorticoids have been beneficial in a few cases of prostatic carcinoma [11]. When attempting to select patients for endocrine therapy, cytological grading is of some help since well- and moderately well-differentiated carcinomatous tissue responds better to endocrine therapy than do malignant tissues of a low degree of differentiation. However, it would be of great clinical value if one could predict the result of endocrine treatment when choosing therapy, and therefore attempts have been made to develop predictive tests for hormonal therapy of prostatic carcinoma.

Using mainly the rat ventral prostate as a model system, the action of androgens has been at least partially clarified during the recent decade (Fig. 1). Testosterone is secreted from the testes, transported to all tissues in the body, and taken up over the cell membranes in target tissues. In the prostatic cell, testosterone is metabolized to 5α-dihydrotestosterone (DHT) which is bound to a receptor protein. The androgen-receptor complex is then translocated into the cell nucleus where it interacts with the chromatin, thereby controlling the formation of specific mRNA and thus the synthesis of specific proteins. The major protein formed, at least in the rat prostate, is prostatic secretion protein (PSP) [12,13]. A tissue is sensitive to hormonal stimulation only if a specific receptor is present in the tissue. Therefore, one can assume that a prostatic tumor containing androgen receptors is sensitive to these hormones and that the tumour will most probably regress following orchiectomy or anti-androgenic therapy. In line with these ideas, we have developed methods for quantitation of androgen receptors in prostatic carcinoma. Since fine needle aspiration biopsies are used for cytological grading in Scandinavia, a predictive test should be sensitive enough to be carried out on such material. In this report, we describe the development of a very sensitive ligand-based assay of the androgen receptor in human prostate.

MATERIALS AND METHODS

Steroids

^{3}H-Methyltrienolone (R 1881) (specific radioactivity, 80 Ci/mmole) as well as unlabelled R 1881 was purchased from New England Nuclear Chemicals, GmbH, Dreieichenhain, W. Germany. Unlabelled steroids were obtained from Sigma Chemical Co., St. Louis, MO.

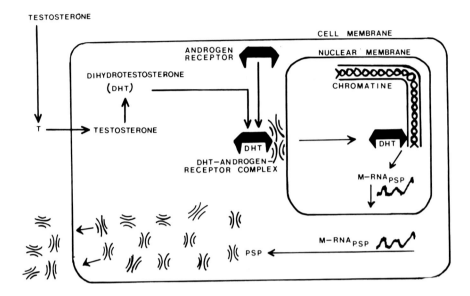

Fig. 1. Intracellular control of nuclear uptake of 5α-dihydrotestosterone receptor complex—a hypothesis. Testosterone (T) is taken up over the cell membrane in the prostatic cell and is metabolized to 5α-dihydrotestosterone (DHT). DHT is bound to the receptor and the DHT-receptor complex is translocated into the cell nucleus where, following interaction with chromatin, the synthesis of different mRNA species is stimulated. One mRNA formed is mRNA$_{PSP}$ which is translocated to the polysomes where prostatic secretion protein (PSP) is synthesized. PSP can inhibit the nuclear uptake of the DHT receptor complex [12,13].

Preparation of Cytosol

Livestock tissues collected at the slaughter house were immediately placed in a plastic bag and put in an ice-water slurry. Cytosol was prepared no later than 24 hours following removal of the tissues. Rat tissues were collected from 8-week-old Sprague-Dawley rats which were castrated 18 hours before decapitation. Human hyperplastic prostates were obtained at routine operations. Since electroresected material is unsuitable for receptor studies [14,15], only BPH tissue obtained at transvesical operations were used. "Normal" prostates were obtained in connection with cystectomy operations for bladder carcinoma, when the prostate is routinely removed. Human carcinomatous prostatic tissue was obtained using biopsies of primary tumours by the punch needle instrument designed by Veenema [16]. Cancer tissue was also obtained by fine needle aspiration biopsies. Material obtained using this technique was directly suspended in buffer. All other human tissue specimens were immediately frozen (–70°C) and later thawed on ice before being further processed. Tissues to be analyzed were homogenized in 3 volumes of ice-cold buffer A (Tris 50 mM, EDTA 1 mM, NaCl 50 mM, DTE 1 mM, pH 7.4) using an Ultra-Turrax homogenizer. The homogenate was centrifuged for 60 minutes at 105,000g. After removal of the floating lipid layer, the cytosol was decanted and the precipitate was redissolved and used for DNA determination according to Burton [17]. Protein determination was carried out according to Lowry [18]. Cytosol preparations from rat ventral prostate or human BPH tissue were divided into several equal parts and frozen at −70°C. Prior to further processing, the tubes were thawed on ice. Aliquots of cytosol were incubated with increasing amounts of ^{3}H-R 1881 in the presence or absence of a 100-fold excess of unlabelled R 1881, at 0–4°C for 16 hours.

Receptor Quantitation

In our initial experiments, receptor measurements were carried out using a dextran-coated charcoal technique [14] and B_{max} and K_d values were evaluated from Scatchard plots [19]. This technique, however, was very time-consuming, and at least 100 mg of tissue was required for analyses. A simple filter assay technique was found to be of value for measurement of androgen receptor in rat prostate [13], but this technique turned out to be unsuitable for work with human tissue. Following extensive trials, where several different quantitation methods were attempted, two techniques were found to be superior, namely isoelectric focusing in polyacrylamide gel and high-pressure liquid chromatography. When developing these methods, we used ^{3}H-R 1881-labelled cytosol prepared from BPH tissue.

Thin-Layer Polyacrylamide Gel Electrofocusing

^{3}H-R 1881-labelled cytosol (0.3 ml) containing about 5 mg of protein was saturated to 40% (w/v) with respect to ammonium sulphate by adding saturated ammonium sulphate solution prepared in buffer A. Following centrifugation at 10,000g for 10 minutes, the precipitate was resuspended in 0.3 ml of buffer A and another centrifugation was carried out before the supernatant was taken for electrofocusing. Ready-made gels from LKB Produkter AB, containing 2.4% (w/v) Ampholine, pH 3.5–9.5, were routinely used. Isoelectric focusing was performed with a Multiphor (LKB Produkter AB). Electrode strips soaked in 1 M NaOH (cathode) or 1 M sulfuric acid (anode) were added. The gel was prefocused for 15–20 minutes using a current of 15 mA.

Sample frames were used for sample application and allowed a volume of 0.3 ml. The frames were made of acrylic plastic. After the gel had been prefocused, the sample frames were placed on the gel surface 0.8–1 cm from the cathode electrode strip where the final pH was about 8–8.5. Ferritin and hemoglobin, dissolved in water, were used as standards and were focused separately. Usually eight samples were analyzed simultaneously.

Isoelectric focusing was initiated at a current of 50 mA. The voltage was increased stepwise to 1000–1200 V. When the ferritin standard was focused near the anode and the hemoglobin standard was focused in front of the sample frame (after about 1 hour), the liquid inside the sample frames was aspirated with a Pasteur pipette and the sample frames were removed. Any remaining sample solution on the gel surface was removed with a filter paper to minimize the risk of radioactive contamination.

The isoelectric focusing was continued until the current ceased to diminish. The total focusing time from the application of sample was about 1.5 hours. Effective cooling is of the utmost importance because of the rapid dissociation of the hormone-receptor complex when exposed to heat. The analysis was performed in a cold room at 2–4°C, and ice water was continuously pumped through the cooling plate of the Multiphor. pH was measured at 2–4°C with a surface pH electrode (type 403-30; Ingold, Zurich, Switzerland).

Fractionation of the Gel

The 2-mm thick gel was cut in strips, one for each sample track, and each strip was transferred to a slicing frame made of razor blades. A sheet of Parafilm (American Can Co., Greenwich, CT) was placed on the gel which was then pressed down between the razor blades with the help of a cork ring. The Parafilm was removed and each 3.3-mm broad gel slice was transferred to a plastic vial with a pair of forceps. Instagel (Packard Instrument Co., Inc., Warrenville, Downess Grove, IL), 5 ml, was added to each vial. The vials were shaken vigorously, kept at room temperature for 20 hours, and then shaken again and assayed for radioactivity in a liquid scintillation spectrometer. This incubation was sufficient to allow the ^{3}H-labelled steroid to diffuse out of the gel (data not shown).

Receptor Quantitation

The radioactivity in the vials was measured and the efficiency was calculated according to the external standard technique. The peak of radioactivity with a pI maximum between 6.8 and 7.2 represented receptor-bound ^{3}H-R 1881. For each sample a diagram was drawn and the diagrammatic baseline radioactivity was subtracted from the peak. Routinely, only a 5-cm long gel strip between pH 8 and pH 4.7 was fractionated and assayed for radioactivity.

High-Pressure Liquid Chromatography

A 30-cm SW 3000 column (Varian) was connected to a Varian isocratic model 5010 liquid chromatograph and the column eluate collected directly in 0.5-ml fractions. The system was equilibrated in buffer A and chromatography was performed at 1 ml/min using a pressure gradient starting at 25 atm. Fractions,

0.5 or 1 ml, were collected and the whole system was kept at 0–4°C. ^{3}H-Labelled cytosol from BPH tissue incubated at 0–4°C for 16 hours was used in the model experiments. No further treatment of the incubation mixture was performed prior to chromatography. Aliquots of the eluted fractions were taken for measurement of radioactivity.

Competition Experiments

The ligand specificity of the androgen binding sites was studied by adding increasing concentrations of unlabelled steroid competitors to aliquots of BPH cytosol at the same time as addition of saturating concentrations of ^{3}H-R 1881 to the incubation mixture. Following incubation, analyses were performed as described above.

RESULTS AND DISCUSSION

Endocrine therapy has been the dominating form of treatment for prostatic carcinoma for many years. However, we still do not have any reliable diagnostic aids for selecting patients for endocrine therapy. Quantitation of androgen receptors constitutes one kind of predictive test that might identify patients who will benefit from endocrine therapy. Practical application of the concept of steroid hormone receptors has already been achieved in the treatment of breast cancer. A good correlation exists between the content of estrogen receptors in the cancer tissue and the response to endocrine treatment [20,21]. We have previously investigated whether such a correlation also exists between the content of androgen receptors in prostatic cancer and response to hormonal treatment, using a dextran-coated charcoal based technique on tissue specimens obtained with Veenema biopsy [14,22]. Data from a limited number of patients suggested a relatively good correlation between the tissue content of androgen receptors and short-term response to hormonal therapy [22]. These results are encouraging and support the view that hormone receptor analysis may be a useful tool to optimize and individualize the treatment of prostatic cancer.

These results prompted us to develop a method which can be used for routine estimation of androgen receptor content in prostatic cancer tissue obtained using fine needle aspiration biopsy. Purification of the androgen receptor should make it possible to raise monoclonal antibodies against this species and develop immunoassay methods. Such a technique requires minute amounts of tissue, and adequate estimation of the receptor content may be carried out whether endogenous steroid ligands are bound to the receptor or not. Available data indicate that androgen receptor complexes in different tissues from different species have quite similar biochemical and biophysical characteristics. It may therefore be assumed that antibodies raised against the androgen receptor purified from one species will most probably crossreact with androgen receptors from other species.

Consequently, it should be possible to develop an immunoassay for quantitation of the human prostatic androgen receptor based on antibodies raised against heterologous androgen receptors. In order to identify a tissue that could serve as a suitable source for androgen receptor in purification attempts, we have screened various androgen-sensitive tissues in different species for content of cytosolic androgen receptors (Table I). Assuming that about 100 μg of receptor protein is necessary for successful raising of antibodies, no tissue was found from which it is reasonable, at the present time, to initiate purification of receptor for antibody production. In view of these considerations, we decided to try to develop ligand-based methods for androgen receptor determination in fine needle aspiration biopsies.

Initial experiments using isoelectric focusing in polyacrylamide gel of the ^{3}H-R 1881 receptor complex in human BPH cytosol were unsuccessful. The radioactivity was spread over the plate and no reproducible radioactive peak was observed. Treatment of the incubation mixture with dextran-coated charcoal or filtration through a Sephadex G-25 column to remove unbound steroid prior to electrofocusing was not successful. However, precipitation with ammonium sulphate prior to isoelectric focusing analysis was found to remove most of the unbound steroid and probably also steroid loosely attached to macromolecules. The ^{3}H-R 1881 receptor complex focused as a relatively sharp peak at pH 6.8–7.0 (Fig. 2). The peak was totally abolished when incubation was performed in the presence of a 100-fold excess of unlabelled R 1881. Using increasing concentrations of ^{3}H-R 1881 in the presence or absence of a 100-fold excess of unlabelled R 1881 and calculating specific binding as the total binding minus binding in the presence of unlabelled steroid (unspecific binding), the saturation curve in Figure 3 was obtained. The radioactive peak at pH 6.8–7.0 was always totally abolished following incubation in the presence of a 100-fold excess of unlabelled R 1881. Consequently, using saturating concentrations of ^{3}H-R 1881 only one incubation was necessary for estimation of the amount of androgen receptor. Incubations in the presence of R 2858 (11β-methoxy-17α-ethinyl-1,3,5(10)-estratriene-3,17β-diol), progesterone, triamcinolone acetonide, or dexamethasone (9α-fluoro-11β,17α,21-trihydroxy-16α-methyl-1,4-pregnadiene-3,20-dione) did not affect the radioactive peak at pH 6.8–7.0, indicating that the ^{3}H-R 1881 receptor complex represented a specific androgen receptor complex. However, progestin receptors have earlier been demonstrated in human BPH tissue and since ^{3}H-R 1881 has a certain affinity for the progestin receptor, a 100-fold excess of unlabelled triamcinolone acetonide was always routinely added to incubations with human prostatic tissue in order to saturate high-affinity, low-capacity glucocorticoid and progestin binding sites. Similarly, a 100-fold excess of R 2858 was also always routinely added in order to avoid any possible interaction between ^{3}H-R 1881 and high-affinity, low-capacity estrogen binding sites in human prostatic cytosol.

TABLE I. Cytosolic androgen receptor content in androgen-sensitive tissues which might serve as starting material for purification of androgen receptor

Tissue	Weight of tissue/animal or /operation (gm)	Total cytosolic protein (mg) prepared from one animal	Cytosolic androgen receptor fmole/mg protein	Cytosolic androgen receptor fmole/animal	μg Androgen receptor/animal assuming a receptor molecular weight of 100,000 daltons and binding ratio R 1881:receptor of 1:1	Animals needed for 100 μg of cytosolic androgen receptor
Rat prostate	0.3–0.5 (0.5)	~15	30–40 (30)	450	0.045	2220
Bull prostate	12–25 (20)	1200	7–20 (20)	24,000	2.4	42
Bull seminal vesicle	100–160 (100)	6000	8–22 (20)	120,000	12	8
Boar prostate	11–18 (15)	900	8–25 (20)	18,000	1.8	56
Boar seminal vesicle	80–120 (100)	6000	7–23 (20)	120,000	12	8
Human BPH tissue obtained from transvesical operations	20–80 (40)	3600	10–80	72,000	7.2	14

This table presents a summary of several experiments. Numbers in parentheses are values used for further calculations.

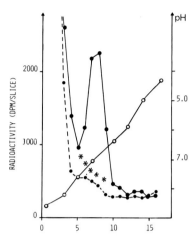

Fig. 2. Isoelectric focusing in polyacrylamide gel of cytosol prepared from BPH tissue. Cytosol was incubated with 1.5×10^6 dpm ^{3}H-R 1881 per 0.3 ml in the presence (●------●------●) or absence (●———●———●) of a 100-fold excess of unlabelled R 1881. Routine for background subtraction in case of single-point analysis: ***. pH: ○———○———○.

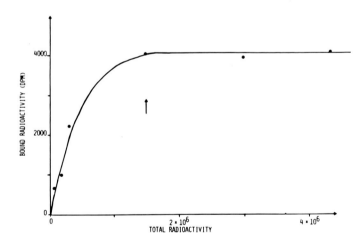

Fig. 3. Saturation curve for binding of ^{3}H-R 1881 to the high-affinity, low-capacity androgen binding sites in 0.3 ml cytosol prepared from BPH tissue using isoelectric focusing analysis in polyacrylamide gel.

Several preparations of cytosol from human BPH tissue were analyzed using isoelectric focusing (single-point assay). The interassay and intra-assay variations were about ±10%. Results obtained using the isoelectric focusing technique were in good agreement with those previously published obtained using the dextran-coated charcoal technique (Table II). Androgen receptor analyses have also been carried out on material obtained by fine needle aspiration biopsies. In some cases, the presence of an androgen receptor was observed (Fig. 4), whereas other specimens did not contain any measurable receptor. These results indicate that isoelectric focusing of the ^{3}H-R 1881 receptor complex following ammonium sulphate precipitation is a technique with high enough sensitivity to allow quantitation of androgen receptor in fine needle aspiration biopsies. Investigations are now in progress to study the reproducibility of the method and to establish the detection limit of the method with regard to the androgen receptor content in

TABLE II. Inter- and intra-assay variation of androgen-receptor content in BPH cytosol assayed using isoelectric focusing

Seven aliquots of BPH cytosol were assayed simultaneously.

fmole/mg protein
10.1
8.4
9.8
8.9
9.0
7.3
9.5
mean ± SD: 9.02 ± 0.92

Three aliquots of cytosol prepared earlier and frozen separately were thawed and analyzed 1 per week for 4 weeks.

	fmole/mg protein	mean of each assay
I	11.3	
	12.2	10.9
	9.1	
II	10.7	
	11.4	11.0
	11.0	
III	9.9	
	9.8	9.4
	8.4	
IV	10.4	
	9.6	9.4
	8.1	
	mean of assays ± SD: 10.2 ± 0.9	

We have earlier reported an androgen receptor concentration of 9–26 fmole/mg of protein in cytosol [14]. These estimations were performed using ^{3}H-R 1881 as ligand and a dextran-coated charcoal technique for separation of free and bound steroid.

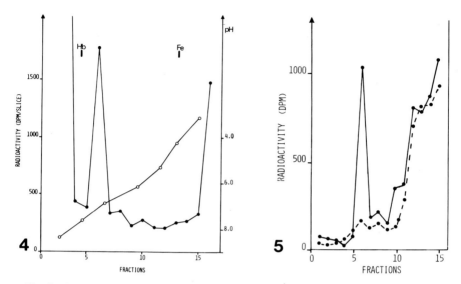

Fig. 4. Isoelectric focusing in polyacrylamide gel of ^{3}H-R 1881-labelled cytosol prepared from fine aspiration biopsies of human prostatic cancer. Cytosol, 0.3 ml, was incubated with 1.5×10^6 dpm ^{3}H-R 1881 (●———●———●). Ammonium sulphate precipitation and isoelectric focusing analyses were carried out as described in the text. pH: (○———○———○)

Fig. 5. High-pressure liquid chromatography on cytosol prepared from BPH tissue. Cytosol was incubated with 0.5×10^6 dpm ^{3}H-R 1881/0.1 ml cytosol (2.8×10^{-8} M ^{3}H-R 1881) in the absence (●———●———●) or presence (●------●------●) of a 100-fold excess of unlabelled R 1881.

relation to the amount of DNA in the specimen. Another technique which proved to be potentially useful was high-pressure liquid chromatography. The SW-3000 column separates proteins based on differing molecular weights. The ^{3}H-R 1881 receptor complex was excluded from the column and recovered in the void volume (Fig. 5). Saturation and specificity studies gave results quite similar to those obtained using isoelectric focusing. Also, high-pressure liquid chromatography was found to be sensitive enough for detection of the androgen receptor in fine needle aspiration biopsies of human prostatic tissue.

Presently, we are concentrating on the further development of the electro-focusing technique for assay of the androgen receptor in fine needle aspiration biopsies. The electrofocusing technique is less time consuming for analysis of multiple samples and therefore more suitable than the high-pressure liquid chromatography technique. In Scandinavia, fine needle aspiration biopsies are routinely used for diagnosis and follow-up of prostatic carcinoma patients. We are now attempting to develop a technique where the aspirate is suspended in buffer solution, part of which is used for cytological examination and part of which is used for receptor assay. Such a procedure will make it possible to directly correlate cytological diagnosis with androgen receptor content. The use of androgen receptor assays as predictive tests in the treatment of prostatic carcinoma may become more general and useful following development of techniques for measurement of androgen receptor in fine needle aspiration biopsies.

ACKNOWLEDGMENTS

This study was supported by grants from Riksföreningen mot Cancer and Leo Research Foundation.

REFERENCES

1. Smith DR: General Urology. Eighth ed, Lange Medical Publishing, 1975.
2. Liavåg I: Carcinoma of the Prostate. Oslo: Universitetsförl, 1966.
3. Moore RA: Benign hypertrophy and carcinoma of the prostate. Occurrence and experimental production in animals. Surgery 16:152–163, 1944.
4. Zuckerman S: The endocrine control of the prostate. Proc R Soc Med 29:1557–1568, 1936.
5. Wendel E, Brannen G, Putong P, Grayhack J: The effect of orchiectomy and estrogens on benign prostatic hyperplasia. T J Urol 108:116–119, 1972.
6. McNeal JE: Origin and development of carcinoma of the prostate. Cancer 23:24–32, 1969.
7. Jensen EV, Block BE, Smith S, Kyser K, De Sombre ER: Estrogen receptors and breast cancer response to adrenalectomy. Natl Cancer Inst Monogr 34:55–59, 1971.
8. Zachmann M, Prader A: Anabolic and androgenic effect of testosterone in sexually immature boys and its dependency on growth hormone. J Clin Endocrinol Metab 30:85–89, 1970.
9. Huggins C, Hodges CV: Studies on prostatic cancer I. The effect of castration, of estrogen and androgen injection on serum phosphatases in metastatic carcinoma of the prostate. Cancer Res 1:293–297, 1941.
10. Huggins C, Stevens RA, Hodges CV: Studies on prostatic cancer. II. Effects of castration on advanced carcinoma of the prostate gland. Arch Surg 43:209–223, 1941.
11. Mobbs BG, Johnson IE, Connolly JG: In vitro assay of androgen binding by human prostate. J Steroid Biochem 6:453–458, 1975.
12. Forsgren B, Björk P, Carlström K, Gustafsson J-Å, Pousette Å, Högberg B: Purification and distribution of a major protein in the rat prostate that binds estramustine, a nitrogen mustard derivative of estradiol-17β. Proc Natl Acad Sci USA 76:3149–3153, 1979.
13. Pousette Å, Björk P, Carlström K, Forsgren B, Högberg B, Gustafsson J-Å: Influence of prostatic secretion protein on uptake of androgen-receptor complex in prostatic cell nuclei. The Prostate, 2:23–33, 1981.
14. Snochowski M, Pousette Å, Ekman P, Bression D, Anderson L, Högberg B, Gustafsson J-Å: Characterization and measurement of the androgen receptor in human benign prostatic hyperplasia and prostatic carcinoma. J Clin Endocrinol Metab 45:920–930, 1977.
15. Gustafsson J-Å, Ekman P, Pousette Å, Snochowski M, Högberg B: Demonstration of a progestin receptor in human benign prostatic hyperplasia and prostatic carcinoma. Invest Urol 15:361–366, 1978.
16. Vecnema RK. A simplified prostatic perineal biopsy punch. J Urol 69:320–322, 1953.
17. Burton K: Determination of DNA concentration with diphenylamine. Meth Enzymol 12B:163–166, 1968.

18. Lowry OH, Rosebrough NJ, Farr AL, Randall RJ: Protein measurement with the Folin phenol reagent. J Biol Chem 193:265–275, 1951.

19. Scatchard G: The attraction of proteins for small molecules and ions. Ann NY Acad Sci 51:660–672, 1949.

20. Jensen EV, Jacobson HI: Biological Activities of Steroids in Relation to Cancer. New York: Academic Press, 1960.

21. McGuire WL, Carbone PP, Sears ME, Escher GC: Estrogen Receptors in Human Breast Cancer. New York: Raven Press, 1975.

22. Gustafsson J-Å, Ekman P, Snochowski M, Zetterberg A, Pousette Å, Högberg B: Correlation between clinical response to hormone therapy and steroid receptor content in prostatic cancer. Cancer Res 38:4345–4348, 1978.

The Prostatic Cell: Structure and Function
Part B, pages 313–327
© 1981 Alan R. Liss, Inc., 150 Fifth Avenue, New York, NY 10011

The Development of Gamma-Emitting Hormone Analogs as Imaging Agents for Receptor-Positive Tumors

John A. Katzenellenbogen

Receptors for hormones and drugs are proteins that demonstrate high affinity binding, specific for their cognate ligands; they are also usually found in highest concentrations in target tissues for the particular hormone or drug. Thus, through this combination of selective distribution and specific, high affinity binding, receptors provide an opportunity for the selective localization of chemical agents within an organism in vivo. In an effort to utilize receptors as a localizing mechanism, a number of groups have been developing "receptor binding radio-pharmaceuticals," [1] that is, agents that contain a gamma-emitting radionuclide and have a high affinity for a certain receptor. In most cases, the intended use of the radiopharmaceutical is for diagnostic purposes, to provide an "image" of a target tissue or of a tumor derived from that tissue. Some receptors that are being considered in these terms are muscarinic, cholinergic, and β-adrenergic receptors in the myocardium, estrogen receptors in breast tumors, dopamine and opiate receptors in the brain, and glycoprotein receptors in the liver [1].

In this report we will review efforts that we have made towards the development of gamma-emitting estrogen analogs as imaging agents for human breast tumors. In addition, we will cover the characteristics needed for successful development and optimization of receptor-binding radiopharmaceuticals in general, and we will discuss the prospects of this approach to study the prostate and prostatic cancer.

ESTROGEN RECEPTORS IN BREAST CANCER

Estrogen receptors can be detected in ca. 60% of primary human breast tumors [2–4], and in most cases receptor levels in tumors exceed those in normal breast tissue. The assay of the estrogen receptor content of breast tumor biopsy samples now forms the most reliable basis for the selection of alternative therapies for the management of the breast cancer [5,6]. Since estrogens administered at physiological doses are known to be concentrated in target tissues [7,8], including human breast tumors [9–12], through their interaction with estrogen receptors, a suitable gamma-emitting estrogen should act as a breast tumor-imaging agent. Such an agent might be useful in many respects: Through selective accumulation in receptor-positive tumors, it might permit a more refined or sensitive delineation of the primary tumor and might assist in locating metastatic tumors. It might also provide a means of assessing the degree of lymph node involvement non-invasively. Since its uptake would be based on binding to the estrogen receptor, such an agent would provide, noninvasively, an assay of receptor that would reveal not only the presence of receptor but would display the full dynamics of estrogen-receptor interaction in vivo. It is possible that this more complete elucidation of the kinetics of estrogen binding by the tumor might help to distinguish between receptor-positive tumors that will respond to hormone therapy and those that will not respond [2,5].

FACTORS THAT DETERMINE THE UPTAKE CHARACTERISTICS OF IMAGING AGENTS BY BREAST TUMORS

While the presence of a high affinity binding protein in a specific tissue or tumor provides a theoretical basis for the selective localization of a radiopharmaceutical agent, it is essential to determine whether sufficient uptake can be achieved and whether the uptake ratio between target and nontarget sites will be adequate for imaging purposes. The uptake of an estrogen by a receptor-positive tumor will depend upon the receptor concentration, the fractional saturation of receptor that is attainable, and the specific activity of the radiopharmaceutical. It is known that receptor-positive tumors contain levels of receptor in the range of 0.1–10 nM [5]. Taking 1 nM as a typical concentration and assuming a fractional saturation of 0.1 would be attainable, we can calculate that a radiopharmaceutical would need to have a specific activity of 1,000 Ci/mmole in order for a 1-cm^3 tumor to accumulate 0.1 μCi, which is generally considered to be the lower level of detectability of conventional imaging equipment. These specific activities can be obtained with current radiosynthetic methodology.

The second factor that limits the effectiveness of an estrogen receptor-based imaging agent is binding selectivity. Estrogens are lipophilic molecules and they interact with hydrophobic binding sites on nonreceptor molecules (nonspecific binding). Since this nonreceptor binding is not localized to target tissues, it forms a background upon which receptor-mediated uptake must be observed. This means that a breast tumor-imaging agent must have not only a high affinity for the estrogen receptor, but a low affinity for nonreceptor proteins, ie, a good binding selectivity. Our initial studies on estrogen radiopharmaceuticals [13] convinced us that binding selectivity was going to prove to be a crucial issue in the design of breast tumor imaging agents.

BINDING SELECTIVITY AND THE BINDING SELECTIVITY INDEX

By binding selectivity, we mean the characteristic distribution that a potential radiopharmaceutical agent displays between the desired target-binding sites and other nontarget (background) binding sites [14]. With a breast tumor imaging agent, the desired binding is, of course, to the estrogen receptor. Background binding, or binding to nonreceptor proteins, is of two types, high affinity and low affinity. Examples of the former type are the serum proteins, sex-steroid binding protein, found in humans [15], and α-fetoprotein, found in rodents [16]. These serum-binding proteins display a narrow structure and stereospecificity that is distinctly different from that of the receptor [14]. Thus, one can "design away" from them, without compromising binding to receptor.

The second component of nonreceptor binding is of low affinity and does not display the marked structural and stereospecificity of the high affinity binding. Thus, it is not possible to "design away" from these sites. Low affinity, nonreceptor binding is generally referred to as "nonspecific binding" and is comprised of interactions with albumin, hydrophobic sites on other proteins, and interaction with lipoidal and membranous phases [14]. This type of binding is found to be dependent mainly upon lipophilicity.

In order to compare the binding selectivity of different estrogen analogs as candidate breast tumor imaging agents, we have found it convenient to devise a quantitative expression for binding selectivity. For this purpose, we have proposed the use of the ratio of receptor binding affinity to nonspecific binding affinity, which we term the "binding selectivity index" (BSI) [14].

$$\text{Binding selectivity index (BSI)} = \frac{\text{Receptor binding affinity}}{\text{Nonspecific binding affinity}} \qquad (1)$$

We have simplified the definition of the binding selectivity index further by normalizing receptor and nonspecific binding to that of estradiol, ie, as RAC over NSB: RAC or the "ratio of association constants" is a standard

$$\text{BSI} = \frac{\text{RAC}}{\text{NSB}} \frac{(100 \text{ for estradiol})}{(1 \text{ for estradiol})} \qquad (2)$$

measure of the affinity of a compound for the estrogen receptor, relative to that of estradiol (which is 100 by definition), and NSB or "nonspecific binding" is the ratio of the binding index (site concentration times affinity) that the agent has for the low affinity, nonreceptor sites relative to that of estradiol.

The binding selectivity index is clearly a simplistic expression of the true binding distribution in vivo, but it is an expression that is easily evaluated by simple in vitro binding measurements (see below), and while it does not consider such factors as blood flow and the kinetics of ligand association and dissociation, it does embody both receptor and nonreceptor binding, and thus proves to be superior to the consideration of receptor binding affinity alone.

EVALUATION OF THE BINDING SELECTIVITY INDEX OF RECEPTOR-BASED RADIOPHARMACEUTICALS: IN VITRO BINDING STUDIES

The binding affinity of an estrogen analog for the estrogen receptor is easily determined by a competitive binding assay. The analog need not be available in radiolabeled form, since its affinity is determined relative to that of a tracer ligand (typically ^{3}H-estradiol) by its effectiveness in displacing the tracer from the receptor binding site. Results are obtained as the ratio of association constants or RAC. The nonspecific binding encountered by estrogens and other steroid derivatives is of too low an affinity to be measured by competitive binding assays. However, nonspecific binding depends to a major extent on compound hydrophobicity [17–19], and within a series of related compounds it can be predicted on the basis of alcohol-water partition coefficients. In fact, we have measured the binding indices of a group of radiolabeled estrogen analogs with uterine cytosol by equilibrium dialysis, under conditions where only low affinity binding was being measured, and we have found that these could be related directly to the octanol-water partition coefficients calculated by the fragment method of Rekker [20] (see equation 3).

$$\log nk = 0.447 \log P_{calc} - 2.08 \tag{3}$$

Thus, we can evaluate the binding selectivity index for any new estrogen derivative simply by determining its affinity for receptor relative to that of estradiol by a competitive binding assay (RAC) and by calculating its nonspecific binding (NSB), using our empirically derived expression relating nonspecific binding to calculated octanol-water partition coefficients (equation 4) [14].

$$\log NSB = 0.447 (\log P_{calc} - 4.63) \tag{4}$$

RECEPTOR AFFINITY, NONSPECIFIC BINDING, AND BINDING SELECTIVITY INDICES OF HALOGENATED ESTROGENS

We have prepared a number of steroidal and nonsteroidal estrogen derivatives bearing halogen substituents at aromatic and aliphatic positions [21,22], and we have measured the receptor affinity and calculated the nonspecific binding and the binding selectivity indices of these compounds [14]. These data are summarized in Tables I–III.

There are a number of patterns evident in the binding characteristics of these compounds. First of all, with the aromatic substituted compounds, only substi-

TABLE I. Receptor binding affinity (RAC), calculated partition coefficients (P_{calc}), nonspecific binding (NSB), and binding selectivity indices (BSI) of aromatic halogenated estrogen derivatives

	X	Y	RAC[a] × 100%	log P_{calc}[b]	NSB[c]	BSI[d]
ESTRADIOLS						
	H	H	100	(4.63)	1.00	100
	F	H	101	(4.84)	1.24	81
	H	F	128	(4.84)	1.24	103
	Br	H	1.2	(5.60)	2.71	0.44
	H	Br	10	(5.60)	2.71	3.7
	I	H	<0.1[e]	(5.89)	3.66	<0.03
	H	I	<0.1[f]	(5.89)	3.66	<0.03
HEXESTROLS						
	H	H	300	(5.66)	2.89	104
	F	H	240	(5.79)	3.30	73
	Br	H	19	(6.55)	7.21	2.6
	I	H	14[g]	(6.84)	9.72	1.4
	H	F	180	(5.79)	3.30	55
	H	I	29	(6.84)	9.72	3.0

[a]Various concentrations of unlabeled compounds (10^{-4}–10^{-10} M) were incubated with 10^{-8} M [^{3}H]-estradiol and lamb uterine cytosol (ca. 2.5 nM receptor site concentration) for 16 hours at 0°C. Free ligands were removed by a brief treatment with dextran-coated charcoal. For details see [23]. The affinity relative to that of estradiol is expressed by RAC × 100%, which is the ratio of association constants ($K_a^{compd}/K_a^{estradiol}$) × 100%.
[b]log P_{calc} is the octanol-water partition coefficient calculated by the fragment method of Rekker [20].
[c]NSB is the nonspecific binding, calculated by equation 4.
[d]BSI is the binding selectivity index calculated by equation 2.
[e]Data taken from [24–26].
[f]The receptor binding affinity of 4-iodoestradiol is reported to be somewhat less than that of 2-iodoestradiol, although data were not presented in quantitative form [27].
[g]Datum is from [13].

tution with fluorine results in compounds with affinities comparable to that of estradiol; a bromine or iodine at positions 2 or 4 in estradiol reduces affinity 10- to 100-fold; the same is true in the hexestrol series. Also, aromatic halogen substituents are quite lipophilizing; thus the compounds substituted with the larger halogens have not only low receptor affinity but high nonspecific binding as well. Therefore, their binding selectivity indices are very low compared to the parent compounds and to the fluorine-substituted analogs.

With the hexestrol derivatives bearing halogen in the side chain (Table II), the trends are quite different. In the hexestrol series, the fluoro compound again has the highest affinity. Though its receptor binding is lower than that of *ortho-*

fluorohexestrol, its nonspecific binding is also lower, since halogen at an aliphatic position is less lipophilizing than at an aromatic position. Thus, its binding selectivity is close to 100. While substitution with a larger halogen at an aromatic position caused a major decrease in binding (cf. Table I), a bromine or iodine substituent at the end of the hexane chain was tolerated reasonably well; again, because of the lower lipophilizing effect of an aliphatic vs aromatic halogen, these derivatives have binding selectivity indices that are nearly tenfold greater than those of the aromatic halogenated compounds.

In the norhexestrol series (Table II), the bromo and iodo derivatives, which are nearly isosteric with hexestrol, have an affinity close to that of hexestrol. However, because they have one fewer methylene unit, these derivatives have lower nonspecific binding than do the corresponding bromo and iodohexestrols, and their binding selectivity indices of ca. 100 are among the highest of the bromo and iodo compounds we have prepared to date. The fluoro norhexestrol has a somewhat lower affinity, comparable to that of norhexestrol itself, but because of its low nonspecific binding, it has the highest binding selectivity index of any compound we have prepared.

The binding characteristics of some estradiol derivatives bearing halogens at C-16 are shown in Table III. The chloro, bromo, and iodo groups are well tolerated at this position when they are oriented α, which suggests that the receptor must have a room for hydrophobic groups of considerable size at this site. Again, since halogens at aliphatic positions cause relatively little increase in the predicted nonspecific binding, these compounds have binding selectivity indices that are nearly as high as that of estradiol.

UPTAKE SELECTIVITY IN VIVO

We have prepared a number of these halogenated estrogens in radiolabeled form in order to study the selectivity of their uptake in vivo [30,31]. In some cases, the derivatives have been labeled with tritium, and in one case with a radiohalogen (16α-[^{77}Br]-bromoestradiol-17β). These radiolabeled derivatives have been injected intravenously into immature female rats, and after 1 hour their tissue distribution was determined. These data are summarized in Figure 1. In these studies it has proved most convenient to express uptake selectivities in terms of target tissue uptake relative to the average level of nontarget tissue uptake.*

---

*Tissue uptake is generally expressed as the ratio of tissue uptake/gm to blood activity/gm. With the tritium-labeled compounds (estradiol, o-fluorohexestrol, and 1-fluoro-, 1-bromo-, and 1-iodo-hexestrol), however, accurate blood activities were difficult to obtain due to extensive color quenching. Therefore, for each compound we have expressed tissue uptakes relative to the average uptake observed in four nontarget tissues: esophagus, muscle, lung, and spleen.

TABLE II. Receptor binding affinity (RAC), calculated partition coefficients (P_{calc}), nonspecific binding (NSB), and binding selectivity indices (BSI) of hexestrol derivatives halogenated on the side chain

	H	RAC[a] × 100%	log P_{calc}[a]	NSB[a]	BSI[a]
HEXESTROLS					
	H	300	(5.66)	2.98	104
	F	127	(4.98)	1.43	89
	Br	65	(5.73)	3.10	21
	I	60	(5.08)	4.45	12
NORHEXESTROLS					
	H	133	(5.13)	1.67	80
	F	135	(4.45)	0.83	163
	Br	200	(5.20)	1.80	110
	I	172	(5.55)	2.58	67

[a]See Table I, footnotes a–d.

TABLE III. Receptor binding affinity (RAC), calculated partition coefficients (P_{calc}), nonspecific binding (NSB), and binding selectivity indices (BSI) of estrogen derivatives bearing halogen at C-16

	X	RAC[a] × 100%	log P_{calc}[a]	NSB[a]	BSI[a]
	H	(estradiol) 100	(4.63)	1.00	100
	(α)Cl	100	(4.86)	1.27	79
	(α)Br	139	(5.04)	1.52	91
	(β)Br	4.7	(5.04)	1.52	3.1
	(α)I	78[b]	(5.39)	2.19	36
	(β)I	57[c]	(5.39)	2.19	26

[a]See footnotes a–d, Table I.
[b]RAC × 100% of ca. 100 is reported by Hochberg [28] and Hochberg and Rosner [29].
[c]Datum is from Arunchalam [24].

There are a number of striking features about these data. First of all, as expected for a receptor-mediated process, the uptake by a target tissue such as the uterus is much more pronounced than that of the nontarget tissues: esophagus, muscle, lung, spleen, and stomach. Some of the compounds show substantial levels in tissues involved in hormone metabolism (liver) and/or excretion (kidney), but material which is extracted from these tissues consists almost exclusively of metabolites, while that from the uterus is essentially unmetabolized. The intestinal contents have very high activity, all of which is due to polar metabolites or conjugates (data not shown).

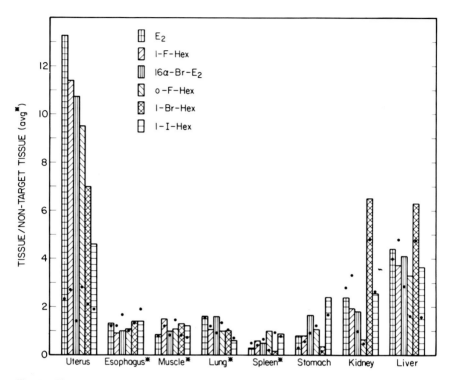

Fig. 1. Tissue uptake selectivity of radiolabeled halogenated estrogen derivatives. Immature (day 25) female Holtzmann rats were injected intravenously (tail vein) with 2–20 μCi of the indicated compounds in the absence (vertical bars) or presence (dots) of an excess (13 μg) of unlabeled estradiol (to determine nonspecific uptake). Uptake levels, determined after 1 hour, are expressed as the uptake per gm relative to the average uptake in the nontarget tissues: esophagus, muscle, lung, spleen (see text).

In order to ascertain whether the uptake by the target tissue was due to the receptor binding, parallel experiments were conducted in which uptake was determined in rats that were treated simultaneously with an amount of unlabeled estradiol sufficient to occupy estrogen receptors fully. In this case (indicated by the dots), the uptake into nontarget tissues was essentially the same as before, while the uptake by the uterus was depressed nearly to the level seen in the nontarget tissues.

We have attempted to compare in a quantitative fashion how well the uptake selectivity of these compounds observed in vivo correlates with their binding selectivity index, and how well it correlates with their receptor binding affinity alone. To do this, we have defined another index, the target tissue uptake selectivity index (TSI), that expresses the selectivity of target tissue uptake observed in vivo:

Target tissue uptake selectivity index (TSI) =

$$\frac{\text{Target tissue uptake} - \text{nontarget tissue uptake (avg)}}{\text{Nontarget tissue uptake (avg)}}$$

This index is simply the receptor-mediated binding in the target tissue (that is, the target tissue uptake in the absence of excess unlabeled ligand, minus the average uptake in the nontarget tissues), divided by the average uptake in the nontarget tissues. In the case of the halogenated estrogens, receptor-mediated uptake is determined in the uterus in the absence of unlabeled estradiol, and the nontarget tissues are esophagus, lung, muscle, and spleen.

The correlations between the log of the target tissue uptake selectivity index and the log of the receptor binding affinity or the binding selectivity index are shown in Figure 2. In this figure, the scales on the abscissa have been adjusted so that the correlation lines superimpose; thus, the goodness of fit is apparently simply from the spread of points about the line (and from the correlation coefficients).

The relationship between target tissue uptake selectivity and the binding selectivity index is very good (r = 0.97). In each case, a decrease in the value of the binding selectivity index is reflected by a decreased target tissue selective uptake. On the other hand, the receptor affinity (RAC) alone is a very poor predictor of target tissue uptake selectivity (r = 0.62). In fact, for the first four compounds, estradiol, 1-fluorohexestrol, 16α-bromoestradiol, and *ortho*-fluorohexestrol, target tissue uptake selectivity decreases, while receptor affinity actually increases. In contrast, the binding selectivity index does register the fact that although the receptor affinity of these compounds is increasing, their nonspecific binding is increasing to a greater extent, so it correctly predicts that their selectivity of uptake in vivo should decrease. Thus, simplistic though it may be, the binding selectivity index is clearly a much more successful predictor of the in vivo uptake selectivity of these halogenated estrogen derivatives than is their receptor binding affinity alone.

MAMMARY TUMOR UPTAKE AND IMAGING IN RATS

Using 16α-bromoestradiol labeled with the gamma-emitter bromine-77, we have studied uptake by dimethylbenz(a)anthracene-induced mammary tumors in adult rats [31]. These tumors have relatively high levels of estrogen receptor, and over 90% of them are hormone responsive [32,33]. In these animals we have seen tumor-to-blood ratios ranging from 4–22. In general, higher uptake ratios were evident in the tumors that were small and well vascularized. We have also been able to image mammary tumors in rats using this gamma-emitting estrogen [31]. A scintigram of a tumor-bearing rat is shown in Figure 3. The left panel shows the neck region of the rat, with a tumor evident as an area of greatly increased activity. The right panel illustrates an area of increased uptake in the

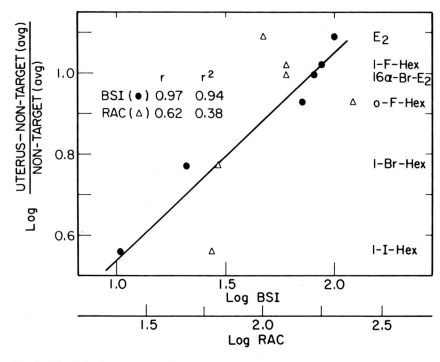

Fig. 2. Correlation between target tissue uptake selectivity index and binding selectivity index and receptor affinity. The tissue uptake data in Figure 1 were recalculated in terms of the target tissue uptake selectivity index (see text). The $\log_{10}$ of these indices were correlated with the $\log_{10}$ of the binding selectivity indices (BSI) and the receptor affinities (RAC) of the individual compounds. The scales on the abscissa were adjusted so that the two correlation lines coincide. The structures of the compounds are evident from the abbreviations.

abdomen of the rat; two adjacent tumors were found in this region upon sacrificing the rat.

PROSPECTS FOR THE DEVELOPMENT OF GAMMA-EMITTING IMAGING AGENTS FOR THE PROSTATE

The possibilities for developing gamma-emitting steroid analogs that may accumulate selectively in the prostate, on the basis of selective uptake by specific binding proteins in the prostate, appear to be as good, and perhaps even better, than those for the development of breast tumor-imaging agents [14]. Such agents might be useful in the diagnosis of prostatic disorders and cancer, and in the assessment of the dissemination of disease and the efficacy of treatment.

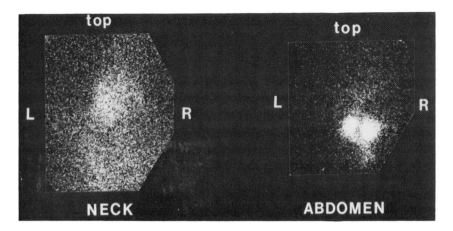

Fig. 3. Scintigraphic images of mammary tumors in a rat. A Sprague-Dawley female rat was injected on day 50 with 5 mg of 7,12-dimethylbenz(a)-anthracene, and mammary tumors were allowed to develop for 60–90 days. The animal was injected intravenously via the femoral vein with 150 μCi of $16\alpha[^{77}Br]$-bromoestradiol and imaged using a gamma camera and a pinhole collimator 1 hour postinjection. The panel on the left shows a tumor as an area of enhanced uptake in the neck region, and the image at the right shows an area of increased uptake in the abdomen where two adjacent tumors were located.

There have been many studies in which the concentration of steroid receptors in the human prostate has been determined [34], and in many cases there appear to be receptors for androgens, estrogens, progestins, and glucocorticoids. Selected data on the concentration of androgen receptors, taken from recent work of Mobbs, Johnson, and Connolly [35], are presented in Table IV. The levels of androgen receptor in the prostate are significant and are comparable to the levels of estrogen receptor in mammary tumors (which have proved to be sufficient for imaging purposes). The amount of androgen receptor that is measured depends upon whether free or total sites are assayed, total site concentration often being several-fold higher than the free. The occupation of androgen receptors by endogenous ligands may vary, depending upon alterations in the concentration of circulating androgens and differences in androgen metabolism in localized regions of the prostate. The highest levels of free sites are found with estrogen treatment; this is probably the result of suppression of gonadal androgen production. It is under these conditions that the prostate would appear to be in the most suitable state for imaging, using agents whose uptake is based upon binding to the androgen receptor. By utilizing an approach analogous to the one we have followed with the estrogen receptor, it should be possible to develop a gamma-emitting androgen with high affinity for the androgen receptor

TABLE IV. Androgen receptor in human prostatic tissue[a]

Tissue (treatment)	Androgen receptor concentration pmoles/ gm tissue average (range)			
	Free		Total	
Muscle	0		0.2	
Nonprostatic cancer (orchiectomy)	0.3		1.5	
Prostate (none)	0.5	(0.2–0.9)	2.0	(0.8–3.9)
(orchiectomy or E)	0.6	(0.3–0.9)	1.0	(0.4, 1.5)
Benign prostatic hypertrophy	0.3	(0–1.2)	2.9	(0.5–4.3)
Prostatic carcinoma (none)	1.2	(0–9.1)	3.4	(0.4–10.2)
(orchiectomy)	0.7	(0.2–2.1)	1.7	(0.9–4.2)
(E)	3.2	(0.7–9.9)	6.0	(1.4–12.6)
(orchiectomy + E)	3.1	(0.3–6.3)	3.2	(0.3, 6.1)

[a]From [35]. Determined by preparation of tissue cytosols in the presence of [^{3}H]-5α-dihydrotestosterone and incubating for 1 hour at 0°C (to determine free sites) and for 16 hours at 25°C (to determine total sites). Measurement of bound steroid was done by protamine precipitation.

of the prostate, and low affinity for nonreceptor proteins. The androgen receptor-mediated uptake of such an agent by the prostate should be adequate and sufficiently selective for imaging purposes.

But the prostate holds additional prospects for the development of imaging agents. In a series of studies on the anticancer agent estramustine, Forsgren has found that in rat prostate there is a protein that binds this agent and appears to be responsible for its selective accumulation in the prostate [36]. The binding protein is very different from the androgen receptor: It is a secreted, rather than an intracellular protein; and its affinity for the ligand is ca. 100-fold less than that of the steroid receptors for their ligands, but its concentration in the rat prostate is many thousand-fold greater than that of receptors. This protein also appears to be present in high concentrations only in prostatic tissue [37]. Only limited studies on structure binding affinity relationships have been done, but it appears that this protein requires the presence of the aromatic bis-chloroethylcarbamate unit, as well as a relatively unperturbed estrogen structure. So far, the function of this protein has only been the subject of speculation [36]; it may be the same as certain prostatic proteins that have been studied by others [38,39].

Estramustine

Although it is tempting to speculate that the efficacy of estramustine in the treatment of human prostatic cancer is the result of an estramustine-binding protein in the human prostate, the presence of such a binder in humans is, as yet, not certain. If such a protein is present in human prostate, and is there in sufficient concentration, then it would be a very attractive target upon which to base the design of selective agents for imaging the human prostate.

CONCLUSION

In our studies on the development of gamma-emitting estrogen analogs as receptor-based agents for imaging breast tumors, we have tried to develop a rational approach to the design of agents that will be optimal in their selectivity and thus most ideally suited for use in humans. We have considered binding selectivity to be the key factor in determining the success of these agents, and we have formulated the binding selectivity index as a simple means for quantitating the binding selectivity of candidate compounds and as a guide for the development of new agents. So far, this index has proved to be a remarkably good predictor of in vivo uptake selectivity.

The approach we have taken in the development of imaging agents for breast tumors should be adaptable to the development of imaging agents based on specific, high affinity binding proteins present in other tissues. In this regard, the androgen receptor, and possibly also an estramustine-binding protein, could form the basis for the development of agents for imaging the human prostate.

ACKNOWLEDGMENTS

Support for our work on the development of breast tumor-imaging agents has come from the National Institutes of Health (PHS HHS CA 25836) and from the American Cancer Society (BC-223). I am grateful for the efforts of my colleagues: D. F. Heiman, K. E. Carlson, S. G. Senderoff, R. Goswami, S. W. Landvatter, J. Ng, and J. E. Lloyd. The work on 16α-[^{77}Br]-bromoestradiol was done in collaboration with Drs. K. D. McElvany and M. J. Welsh of the Washington University School of Medicine, St. Louis, and utilized bromine-77 produced by the Los Alamos National Laboratories Medical Radioisotope Group.

REFERENCES

1. Eckelman W C (ed): "Receptor Binding Radiotracers." Vol X in the Uniscience Series "Radiotracers in Biology and Medicine." (L. G. Colombetti, series editor) Boca Raton: CRC Press, 1981.
2. McGuire W D, Carbone P P, Vollmer E P: "Estrogen Receptors in Human Breast Cancer." New York: Raven Press, 1975.
3. McGuire W L, Horwitz K B, Pearson O H, Segaloff A: Current status of estrogen and progesterone receptors in breast cancer. Cancer 39: 2934–2947, 1977.
4. McGuire W L, Chamness G C, Horwitz K B, Zava D J: Hormones and their receptors in breast cancer. In O'Malley B W, Birnbaumer L (eds): "Receptors and Hormone Action II." New York: Academic Press, 1978, pp 401–441.

5. Allegra J C, Lippman M E, Thompson E B, Simorn R, Barlock A, Green L, Huff K K, Do H M T, Aitken S: Distribution, frequency, and quantitative analysis of estrogen, progesterone, androgen, and glucocorticoid receptors in human breast cancer. Cancer Res 39: 1447–1454, 1979.

6. Thompson E B, Lippman M E (eds): "Steroid Receptors and the Management of Cancer." Boca Raton: CRC Press, Vol 1, 1979.

7. Jensen E V, Jacobson H I: Basic guides to the mechanism of estrogen action. Rec Prog Horm Res 18: 387–414, 1962.

8. Glascock R F, Hoekstra W G: Selective accumulation of tritium-labeled hexestrol by reproductive organs of immature female goats and sheep. Biochem J, 72: 673–782, 1959.

9. Folca P J, Glascock R F, Irvine W T: Studies with tritium-labeled hexestrol in advanced breast cancer. Lancet 796–798, 1961.

10. Desphande N, Jensen V, Bulbrook R D, Berne T, Ellis F: Accumulation of tritiated oestradiol by human breast tissue. Steroids 10: 219–232, 1967.

11. Pearlman W H, DeHertogh R, Lauman K R, Pearlman M R J: Metabolism and tissue uptake of estrogen in women with advanced carcinoma of the breast. J Clin Endocrinol 29: 707–720, 1969.

12. James F, James V H T, Carter A E, Irvine W T: A comparison of in vivo and in vitro uptake of estradiol by human breast tumors and the relationship to steroid excretion. Cancer Res 31: 1268–1272, 1971.

13. Katzenellenbogen J A, Hsiung H M, Carlson K E, McGuire W L, Kraay R J, Katzenellenbogen B S: Iodohexestrols II. Characterization of the binding and estrogenic activity of iodinated hexestrol derivatives in vitro and in vivo. Biochemistry 14: 1742–1750, 1975.

14. Katzenellenbogen J A, Heiman D F, Carlson K E, Lloyd J E: In vitro and in vivo steroid receptor assays in the design of estrogen radiopharmaceuticals. In Eckelman W C (ed): "Receptor Binding Radiotracers." Boca Raton: CRC Press, Vol 10, 1981.

15. Petra P H: The serum sex steroid-binding protein. Purification, characterization and immunological properties of the human and rabbit proteins. J Steroid Biochem 11: 245–252, 1979.

16. Nunez E, Valette G, Benassayag C, Jayle M-F: Comparative study on the binding of estrogens by human and rat serum proteins in development. Biochem Biophys Res Commun 57: 126–133, 1974.

17. Hansch C, Kiehs K, Lawrence G L: The role of substituents in the hydrophobic bonding of phenols by serum and mitochondrial protein. J Am Chem Soc 87: 5770–5773, 1965.

18. Helmer F, Kiehs K, Hansch C: The linear free-energy relationship between partition coefficients and the binding and conformational perturbation of macromolecules by small organic compounds. Biochemistry 7: 2858–2863, 1969.

19. Scholtan W: Bestimmungsmethoden und Gesetzmässigkeiten der Serum-protein-binding von Arzneimitteln. Arzneim.-forsch 28: 1037–1047, 1978.

20. Rekker R F: The Hydrophobic Fragmental Constant. New York: Elsevier North Holland, 1978.

21. Heiman D F, Senderoff S G, Katzenellenbogen J A, Neeley R J: Estrogen receptor based imaging agents. 1. Synthesis and receptor binding affinity of some aromatic and D-ring halogenated estrogens. J Med Chem 23: 994–1002, 1980.

22. Goswami R, Harsy S G, Heiman D F, Katzenellenbogen J A: Estrogen receptor based imaging agents. 2. Synthesis and receptor binding affinity of side-chain halogenated hexestrol derivatives. J Med Chem 23: 1002–1008, 1980.

23. Katzenellenbogen, J A, Johnson H J, Jr, Myers H N: Photoaffinity labels for estrogen binding proteins of rat uterus. Biochemistry 12: 4085–4092, 1973.

24. Arunachalam T, Longcope C, Caspi E: Iodoestrogens, synthesis, and interaction with uterine receptors. J Biol Chem 254: 5900–5905, 1979.

25. Komai T, Eckelman W C, Johnsonbaugh R E, Mazaitis A, Kubota H, Reba R C: Estrogen

derivatives for the external localization of estrogen-dependent malignancy. J Nucl Med 18: 360–366, 1977.

26. Mazaitis J K, Gibson R E, Komai T, Eckelman W C, Francis B, Reba R C: Radioiodinated estrogen derivatives. J Nucl Med 21: 142–146, 1980.

27. Maysinger D: Ph.D. Thesis. Univ. Southern California, 1976.

28. Hochberg R B: Iodine-125-labelled estradiol: A gamma-emitting analog of estradiol that binds to the estrogen receptor. Science 205: 1138–1140, 1979.

29. Hochberg R B, Rosner W: Interaction of $16\alpha[^{125}I]$ iodo-estradiol with estrogen receptor and other steroid binding proteins. Proc Natl Acad Sci USA 77: 328–332, 1980.

30. Katzenellenbogen J A, Carlson K E, Heiman D F, Goswami R: Receptor-binding radiopharmaceuticals for imaging breast tumors: Estrogen receptor interactions and selectivity of tissue uptake of halogenated estrogen analogs. J Nucl Med 21: 550–558, 1980.

31. Katzenellenbogen J A, Senderoff S G, McElvany K D, O'Brien H A, Welch M J: $[^{77}Br]$-16α-Bromoestradiol-17β: A high specific activity gamma-emitting estrogen that shows selective, receptor-mediated uptake by uterus and DMBA-induced mammary tumors in rats. J Nucl Med 22: 42–47, 1981.

32. Tsai T L, Katzenellenbogen B S: Antagonism of development and growth of 7,12-dimethylbenz(a)anthracene-induced rat mammary tumors by the antiestrogen U23,469 and effects on estrogen and progesterone receptors. Cancer Res 37: 1537–1543, 1977.

33. Tsai T L-S, Rutledge S, Katzenellenbogen B S: Antiestrogen modulation of the growth and properties of ovarian-autonomous and ovarian-dependent mammary tumors in rats. Cancer Res 39: 5043–5050, 1979.

34. Karr J P, Sandberg A A: Steroid receptors in prostatic cancer. In Murphy G P (ed): "Prostatic Cancer." Littleton: PSG Publishing, 1979, pp 49–74.

35. Mobbs B G, Johnson I E, Connolly J G: The effect of therapy on the concentration and occupancy of androgen receptors in human prostatic cytosol. The Prostate 1: 37–51, 1980.

36. Forsgren B, Gustafsson J-Å, Pousette Å, Högberg B: Binding characteristics of a major protein in rat ventral prostate cytosol that interacts with estramustine, a nitrogen mustard derivative of 17β-estradiol. Cancer Res 39: 5155–5164, 1979.

37. Forsgren B, Bjork P, Carlstrom K, Gustafsson J-Å, Pousette Å, Högberg B: Purification and distribution of a major protein in rat prostate that binds estramustine, a nitrogen mustard derivative of estradiol-17β. Proc Natl Acad Sci USA 76: 3149–3153, 1979.

38. Chen C, Hipakka R A, Liao S: Prostate α-protein: Subunit structure polyamine binding, and inhibition of nuclear chromatin binding of androgen-receptor complex. J Steroid Biochem 11: 401–405, 1979.

39. Heyns W, Mous P J, Rombauts W, DeMoor P: Androgen-dependent synthesis of a prostatic binding protein by rat prostate. J Steroid Biochem 11: 209–213, 1979.

The Prostatic Cell: Structure and Function
Part B, pages 329-334
© 1981 Alan R. Liss, Inc., 150 Fifth Avenue, New York, NY 10011

Mitochondrial Damage Produced by Estradiol Valerate in the Dunning (R3327H) Rat Prostatic Adenocarcinoma: A Preliminary Report

John A. Arcadi and S. Poolsawat

INTRODUCTION

Huggins and his associates [1, 2, 3] in 1941 showed that the epithelial cells of the prostate of the dog and man are dependent on testicular androgen (or parenteral testosterone propionate) for their growth and metabolism. That the prostatic epithelial growth was decreased or inhibited by orchiectomy or estrogen administration had been demonstrated previously in 1935 by Moore [4]. With both of these observations clearly demonstrated, Huggins utilized orchiectomy and stilbestrol to treat humans with metastatic prostatic carcinoma. The results proved excellent for at least a year in which 80% of the patients responded—but then relapsed.

The concept, proposed by Huggins, in which diminished testosterone or added estrogen therapy resulted in the decrease of prostatic epithelial growth has been further explored in the use of "anti-androgens" and various female hormones.

That there are estrogen (and particularly estradiol) receptors in the prostate has been demonstrated by several workers [5]. The use of estradiol with an attached nitrogen mustard has been used to selectively affect the prostatic epithelium [6].

Lehninger describes β-oxidation in the metabolism of fatty acids as a process that occurs exclusively inside the mitochondria [7]. Since this is so, the longer chain fatty acid (valeric) attached to estradiol would be held in the prostatic cell mitochondria for a much longer time than estradiol or its salt. (β-oxidation is such that the "fatty acids are degraded into two-carbon units that can enter the Krebs . . . cycle" [7].)

One of us (JAA) postulated from the above findings that estradiol attached to a fatty acid would necessitate the longer action of estradiol in the mitochondria, theoretically producing more destruction of the cell. Estradiol valerate is estradiol attached to a 5-carbon fatty acid.

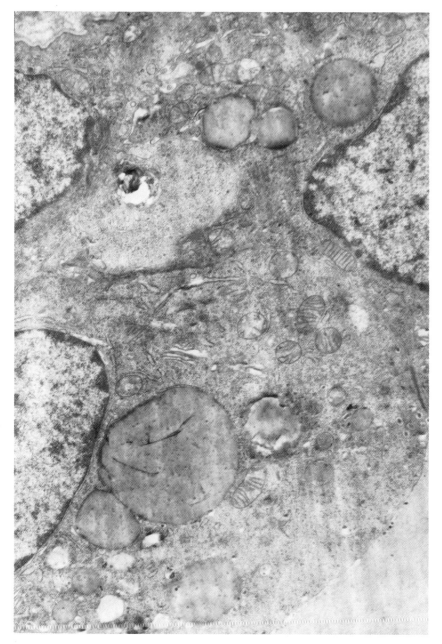

Fig. 1.   The untreated R3372H rat prostatic carcinoma. Mitochondria are seen with normal cristae. There are large lipid granules previously described [9] with a peroxidase membrane. The intensity of the nuclear membrane, dense nucleoli, and the endoplasmic reticulum are finely developed, with ribosomes clearly seen.   × 13,600.

With these observations in mind it was hypothesized that estradiol valerate might have a direct destructive effect on prostatic epithelium—perhaps even more so in prostatic cancer since there are more lipid droplets (into which the fatty acids with estradiol will dissolve) and an increasing number of mitochondria [8, p 113] with denser cristae, which should accept more estradiol valerate—to destroy the cell and slow the growth or destroy prostatic carcinoma.

MATERIALS AND METHODS

Male hybrids from the mating of a Copenhagen male and a Fischer female, provided by the Papanicolou Laboratory, Miami, FL, through the National Prostatic Cancer Project and Dr. N. Altman, were used throughout this study. The rats were either used to carry, or were carrying, the R3327H Dunning prostatic tumor subcutaneously or were used as controls for their own prostates. Tumor tissue was obtained from either The Johns Hopkins Hospital, Baltimore, MD, or from the Papanicolou Institute.

Animals bearing the subcutaneously implanted tumors were sent to our laboratory. These animals were cared for until palpable tumors were felt. These tumors were surgically biopsied under moderately sterile conditions using ether anesthesia. The normal ultrastructural morphology was recently published in detail by Arcadi [9], and a histochemical study is in preparation.

The tumor-bearing rats were treated either by 1) orchiectomy; 2) implantation of 500 mg/kg rat of estradiol valerate; 3) implantation of 500 mg/kg of stilbestrol; or 4) a rebiopsy of the untreated tumor-bearing rat. The estradiol and stilbestrol were implanted subcutaneously as powder without a solvent.

RESULTS

In the untreated tumor the mitochondria were very slightly increased in number (Fig. 1) with slight increase of the cristae of these structures. Larger lipid globules previously shown to be surrounded by a peroxidase membrane were seen [9].

The tumor-bearing rat, orchiectomized 10 days prior to the second biopsy, showed some changes in the nuclei with nuclear membrane irregularity and thinning. The endoplasmic reticulum appeared almost normal. The mitochondria were normal in some areas, but showed changes usually described by minimal testosterone deficiency.

Stilbestrol therapy (a single dose of 500 mg/kg) produced some degenerative changes as seen in the orchiectomized group (Fig. 2).

In those rats bearing tumors that 10 days previously were given subcutaneously 500 mg/kg of estradiol valerate, there are striking changes in the intramitochondrial structures (Fig. 3). There was breakdown of the cristae with disarray, hyaline body formation, and general dissolution and distortion of the mitochondria, the most significant energy source of the cell. Since the source of ATP energy bonds are principally in mitochondria, the problem arises as to how this cell can function, grow, or replicate.

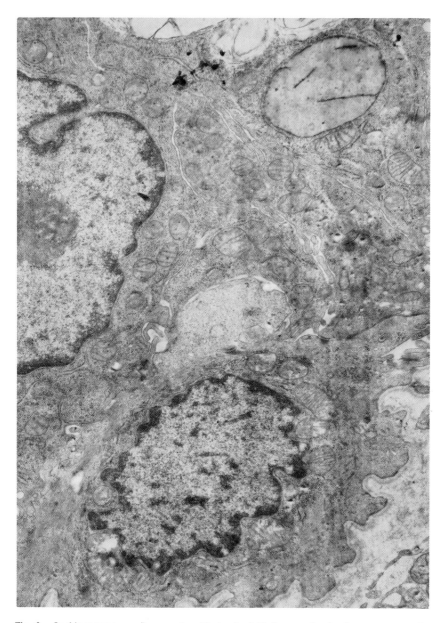

Fig. 2.   In this tumor tissue from a rat orchiectomized 10 days previously, there are some mitochondria undergoing alterations with destruction of parts of the cell. The nuclear membranes are thinning and the intranuclear structure has become disarranged. The mitochondrial structure is basically intact.   × 13,600.

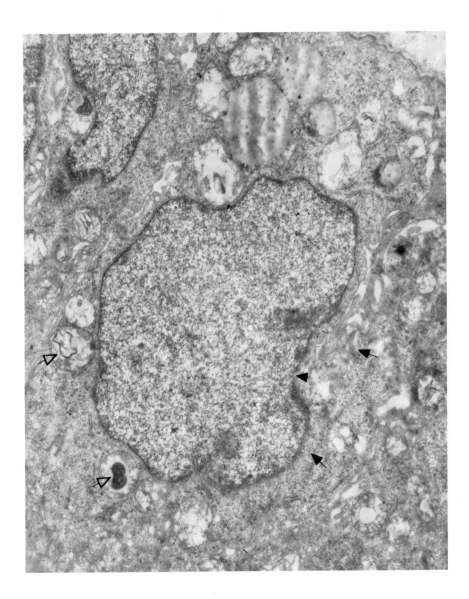

Fig. 3. There is an obvious destruction of the mitochondria. "Hyaline bodies" (open arrows) are seen in many of the mitochondria. Solid arrows indicate general cellular and membrane destruction. This is as prominent a change as has been seen by the authors. × 20,700.

The answer, then, is that since other energy sources cannot sustain the cell, it will die. The tumor cell, as noted above, is rich in these mitochondrial structures. Thus, if "familiarity breeds contempt," we suggest that the mitochondrion and its ATP will leave the cell in a dying state.

Significant studies presented at this seminar suggest that the nuclear matrix is of great importance in the growth of the prostatic cancer cell. This is only partially true. The competence of the cytoplasmic structures such as mitochondria, Golgi structure, and endoplasmic reticulum cannot be ignored in prostatic cell function.

ACKNOWLEDGMENTS

This study was supported by the Whittier College Cancer Research Fund and its generous contributors.

REFERENCES

1. Huggins C, Hodges CV: Studies on prostatic cancer. I. The effect of castration, of estrogen, and of androgen injection on serum phosphatases in metabolic carcinoma of the prostate. Cancer Res 1:293–297, 1941.
2. Huggins C, Stevens RE, Hodges CV: Studies on prostatic cancer. II. The effects of castration on advanced carcinoma of the prostate gland. Arch Surg 43:209–223, 1941.
3. Huggins C, Scott WW, Hodges CV: Studies on prostatic cancer. III. The effects of fever, of desoxycorticosterone and of estrogen on clinical patients with metastatic carcinoma of the prostate. J Urol 46:997–1006, 1941.
4. Moore RA: The evolution and involution of the prostate gland. Am J. Pathol 12:559–624, 1956.
5. Markland FS, Chopp RT, Cosgrove MD, Howard EB: Characterization of the steroid hormone receptors in the Dunning R3327 rat prostatic adenocarcinoma. Cancer Res 38:2818–2826, 1978.
6. Kirdani, RY, Muntzing J, Varkarakis MJ, Murphy GP, Sandberg AA: Studies on the antiprostatic action of Estracyt, a nitrogen mustard of estradiol. Cancer Res 34:1031–1037, 1974.
7. Lehninger AL: Biochemistry Work Publishers, 1970.
8. Tannenbaum M (ed) "Urologic Pathology: The Prostate." Philadelphia: Lea and Febiger, 1977.
9. Arcadi JA: Cytochemical localization of lipid, peroxidase, and carbohydrate substances in the Dunning prostatic adenocarcinoma R3327H. An ultastructural analysis. J Surg. Oncol 15:287–296, 1980.

The Prostatic Cell: Structure and Function
Part B, pages 335–339
© 1981 Alan R. Liss, Inc., 150 Fifth Avenue, New York, NY 10011

Critical Issues in Prostatic Cancer: The Clinical Trial in Localized Disease

Frank M. Torti

At every stage of prostatic carcinoma, from A1 to D2, the appropriate therapy is disputed. Although disagreement about cancer management is not unique to prostatic cancer, the range of approaches, from therapeutic nihilism to aggressive intervention, is not encountered in most solid tumor research. This is most evident in the apparently localized, palpable prostatic nodule, where radical prostatectomy, external beam irradiation, radioactive implants, endocrine therapy, and even no initial therapy have been advocated and are currently practiced.

Physicians can find excellent clinical studies to support any of these views. The reason that controversy persists is not due to insufficient investigations, but is based on at least two more fundamental factors: 1) statistical considerations in the design and interpretation of studies of localized disease, and 2) the current technology available to stage patients with presumed localized disease.

STAGING

In order to compare local therapies of prostatic carcinoma effectively, staging must be sufficiently accurate to select a group of patients who are unlikely to have occult metastatic disease. Only in the group of patients who have tumor confined to the prostate can surgery, irradiation, or any other local modality be tested. The higher the fraction of patients with unrecognized metastatic disease, the more futile attempts at curative local treatment become.

The current staging tools for prostatic cancer are, at best, modestly effective in identifying patients with regionally and distantly metastatic disease. The current staging procedures which have been utilized and evaluated are the acid phosphatase, bone scan, lymphagiogram, and staging lymphadenectomy. Pelvic ultrasound and CT scans may play an important role in the future, but have not been prospectively utilized in large series. Acid phosphatase determined by enzymatic methods, even in the face of overt metastatic disease, is negative in up to 40% of cases [1]. Thus, although when elevated acid phosphatase can be useful in following the course of metastatic disease, as a staging tool it is of very modest utility. Bone scan is a considerably more sensitive test than bone x-rays for the identification of metastatic disease [2, 3], and has improved the staging of patients wth prostatic cancer. However, a significant number of patients with negative bone scans will fail. For example, for all patients with B lesions, distant metastases occurred in approximately 20% in the Stanford series [4].

Staging lymphadenectomy or, to a lesser extent, lymphangiogram defines a group of patients who have regionally metastatic disease. Patients with positive nodes do poorly; most will not be cured. Positive nodes cannot adequately be predicted from examination of the prostate; 21.2% of patients with "B" nodules in the Stanford series have tumor found in the regional nodes at lymphadenectomy [5]. Thus lymphadenectomy or the evaluation of regional adenopathy by lymphangiogram [6] is an important staging tool. Although up to 25% of patients with negative lymph nodes will develop metastatic disease [7], only in the group with negative nodes can the efficacy of local therapy be reasonably tested.

Progress has been made in the detection of occult metastases, but current staging may still be inadequate. In the Jewett series of B1 nodules [8, 9], 37% of patients died of prostatic carcinoma. Presumably, this number would have been smaller if bone scans and lymphangiograms were available. In the Stanford series reported by Bagshaw in 1977, 86.5% of patients with negative staging lymphadenectomy and bone scan were free of disease, with a median follow-up of 22 months [5]. Follow-up is not long enough to know what the eventual relapse rate will be. With longer follow-up, this and other surgically staged series will define a group of patients who probably had micrometastases at diagnosis undetected by bone scan, acid phosphatase, and lymphadenectomy. This group is not amenable to cure with local treatment.

Staging techniques for localized prostatic carcinoma have improved but have not yet been refined to where a group of patients can be selected with localized cancer. This hinders the ability to test and evaluate local therapy, which is being applied to patients with occult metastatic disease, the progression of whose disease will be independent of the efficacy of local treatments.

As will be discussed below, once a group unlikely to have occult metastatic disease is defined by adequate staging, it is this group in which the efficacy of local therapy can be tested. However, such a group may have a low biological potential for metastases. The results of ongoing studies such as that of the Veterans Administration Cooperative Urological Research Group, which have a no-treatment arm, will be important in our final decisions on how to manage these tumors [10].

STATISTICAL CONSIDERATIONS: THE IMPACT OF NATURAL HISTORY

Prostatic carcinoma is a complex disease with a variable natural history. Figure 1 illustrates one way of expressing the variablility in the biologic behavior of the disease. At its inception, the disease is occult. Some patients will never have the disease diagnosed antemortem. Others will have disease diagnosed incidentally at a TURBT for presumed benign disease; the heterogeneity of the biologic behavior of these stage "A" tumors is well known. Other patients will go on to develop clinically evident disease. What is important to note on Figure 1 is that even in the subset of patients with clinical disease, there is a competition among the forces of mortality: that due to prostatic cancer and those due to intercurrent disease. This is due to the age of the patient as well as the variability in the natural history of the disease.

At age 63 the 10-year survival of the normal population, derived from life standard tables, is approximately 64%. Thus, patients at this age are high risk of death from intercurrent illness. Although death from intercurrent illness would not introduce bias into a randomized study of local treatment methods, it does cause a dilutional effect on the overall survival [11]. That is, many patients in both arms of the study die of unrelated diseases. Considerably more patients are, therefore, required to demonstrate a difference between therapeutic interventions.

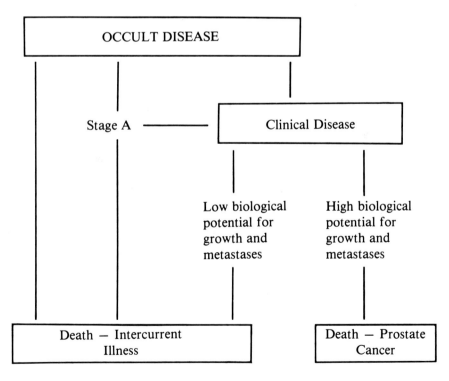

Fig. 1.   Natural history of prostatic cancers.

Compounding this problem is the data from the Veterans Administration Cooperative Urological Research Group on the natural history of low grade, low stage prostatic carcinoma. In Gleason categories 3–8, only about one in ten patients died of prostatic carinoma [12]. Tumors in these patients have a low biologic potential for metastases (Fig. 1). Again, although one can compare two local treatments in this population, it dramatically increases the number of cases required to evaluate the impact of local therapy. If 90% of the patients will die of unrelated causes even though they have histologically documented cancer, even dramatic differences in cancer-related deaths will go unnoticed. Using overall survival as an end point, the futility of attempting to evaluate a local treatment in prostatic carcinoma becomes evident.

There is no curative salvage therapy for disseminated prostatic carcinoma. Thus failure of local treatment will eventually be translated into death from prostatic cancer unless death from intercurrent illness supervenes. For studies of the efficacy of local therapy for localized disease, relapse-free survival should be the end point. A patient treated for local disease is a failure of local therapy (or staging) if either local recurrence or a bony metastasis occurs, regardless of whether the patient eventually dies of cardiac disease or prostate cancer. Reporting relapse-free survival would circumvent many of the difficulties created by the large number of deaths due to intercurrent illness. Studies of therapy for localized disease must report relapse-free as well as overall survival if any critical judgement of the effectiveness of that particular therapy is to be made.

Relapse-free survival is critically dependent on the frequency and uniformity of the diagnostic tests. For example, if bone scans are done only when pain occurs in one study and routinely every 6 months in another study, the former study will appear to have a much improved disease-free survival simply as an artifact of more frequent ascertainment. Further, for localized disease, reporting must differentiate between clinical progression and biopsy-only evidence of persistent disease.

Standard criteria of progression, with diagnostic tests done at uniform intervals, would aid significantly in the resolution of the controversies in localized prostatic carcinoma.

REFERENCES

1. Schaffer DL, Pendergrass HP: Comparison of enzyme, clinical, radiographic, and radionuclide methods of detecting bone metastases from carcinoma of the prostate. Radiology 121:431–434, 1976.
2. Pistenma DA, McDougall IR, Kriss JP: Screening for bone metastases. Are only scans necessary? JAMA 231(1):46–50, 1975.
3. Shafer RB, Reinke DB: Contribution of the bone scan, serum acid and alkaline phosphatase, and the radiographic bone survey to the management of newly diagnosed carcinoma of the prostate. Clin Nuclear Med 2(6):200–203, 1977.

4. Bagshaw M: Personal communication.

5. Bagshaw MA, Pistenma DA, Ray GR, Freiha FS, Kempson RL: Evaluation of extended-field radiotherapy for prostatic neoplasm: 1976 progress report. Cancer Treat Rep 61(2):297–306, 1977.

6. Spellman MC, Castellino RA, Ray GR, et al: An evaluation of lymphography in localized carcinoma of the prostate. Radiology 125:637–644, 1977.

7. Hilaris BS, Whitmore WF, Batata M, Barzell W: Behavioral patterns of prostate adenocarcinoma following an ^{125}I implant and pelvic node dissection. Int J Radiat Oncol Biol Phys 2:631–637, 1977.

8. Jewett HJ: The case for radical perineal prostatectomy. J Urol 103:195–199, 1970.

9. Jewett HJ: The present status of radical prostatectomy for stages A and B prostatic cancer. Urol Clin N Amer 2(1):105–124, 1975.

10. Madsen PO: Radical prostatectomy for carcinoma of the prostate: stage I + II. "Proceedings of the International Symposium on Therapy of Cancer of the Prostate." Rost A, Fielder U, (eds). Berlin: Urologische Klinik, Klinikum Steglitz, Freie University, 1978, p 46.

11. Torti FM, Carter SK: The chemotherapy of prostatic adenocarcinoma. Ann Intern Med 92(5):681–689, 1980.

12. Byar DP: VACURG studies on prostatic carcinoma. In: Tannenbaum M (ed): "Urologic Pathology: The Prostate." Philadelphia: Lea and Febiger, 1977, p 241.

The Prostatic Cell: Structure and Function
Part B, pages 341–346
© 1981 Alan R. Liss, Inc., 150 Fifth Avenue, New York, NY 10011

Cooperative Clinical Trials in Prostate Cancer

Gerald P. Murphy and Nelson H. Slack

Cooperative efforts to study treatment modalities for prostate cancer on a prospective basis appear to have been first undertaken in the 50s by the Cooperative Study Group in Prostatic Cancer headed by Dr. H. Brendler of New York University. This group completed its first trial in 1960, comparing a placebo with stilphostrol in orchiectomy failures, but failed to demonstrate any treatment difference [1].

Shortly thereafter the Veterans Administration Cooperative Urological Research Group (VACURG) was organized. In 1960 the first of three well-known cooperative trials of hormone therapies for prostate cancer was started that contrasted diethylstilbestrol (DES), orchiectomy or placebo singly and/or in combinations [2]. No appreciable treatment differences were observed in any of the 14 relatively large groups, totaling over 2,300 patients in the first study, but DES at 5 mg/day was found to be associated with cardiovascular toxicity [2]. The second study compared three different doses of DES and a placebo in 12 groups, totaling 561 patients. This group found 1.0 mg/day to be as effective as 5 mg/day without the associated toxicity [2]. The third study consisted of 12 groups totaling 1,112 patients and contrasted a placebo and DES (1.0 mg/day) with Premarin (a conjugated natural estrogen) or Provera (a progestational agent), neither of which were found to be any better than treatment with DES [3].

Nonhormonal chemotherapy in a trial specifically for prostate cancer was not studied on a cooperative basis until the National Prostatic Cancer Project (NPCP) instituted its first study in July, 1973 [5]. Such agents had been studied in small uncontrolled series. One such early study reported in 1947 found that nitrogen mustard had a beneficial effect in patients with hormone refractory disease [6,7]. It has been pointed out by Schmidt that to adequately study the effects of these agents it is essential to have as homogeneous a population as possible, as accomplished by rigid entry criteria, but also to acquire a relatively large sample size [7]. Only through prospectively randomized cooperative trials is it possible to accomplish both in a reasonable time span [4]. The only other cooperative effort for some time, however, was the Eastern Cooperative Oncology Group

(ECOG), who started a clinical trial in prostate cancer to compare adriamycin and 5-FU after the NPCP started their first trial [8].

Chemotherapy studies, involving cooperative or individual centers, in advanced prostate cancer were slow to be undertaken not only because of the perception that many cases were successfully managed with hormones or irradiation, but also because of the lack of good response criteria [9,10]. One of the first tasks of the NPCP clinical trials program was to develop response criteria for evaluating chemotherapy [9]. These have remained largely unchanged in practice, but have been continually refined in statements or reports [5]. Since patients entered these NPCP trials in demonstrated clinical progression, a stabilization of their disease was considered evidence of treatment effect. This category has been criticized by some. However, patients so classified have been shown to significantly outlive those who do not respond ("progression") and do not in fact differ appreciably in survival from those patients judged to experience a "partial regression" [11].

The first trial of the NPCP (July 1973 to April 1975) sought to establish the benefit of chemotherapy (5-FU or Cytoxan) over standard forms of treatment for patients with advanced disease that had failed hormone therapy. This trial entered 125 patients that had not previously been treated with pelvic irradiation. The standard treatment arm included estrogens, anti-androgens, radioisotopes, palliative radiotherapy, and other palliative measures. The results of this study (Table I) clearly demonstrated an advantage for chemotherapy over the standard treatment arm and partial regressions occurred only in the chemotherapy treatment arms [12].

Both agents in the first NPCP trial showed activity, but based on the superiority of that for Cytoxan along with somewhat less toxicity, this agent was selected to serve as the new reference or control for the successor trial (Protocol 300). This trial was conducted from April 1975 to May 1977, and compared Cytoxan with procarbazine and DTIC [5].

TABLE I. Objective response for previously nonirradiated patients randomized to 5-FU, Cytoxan, or standard therapy

| | Treatment | | | | | | | |
| | 5-FU | | Cytoxan | | Standard | | Total | |
Response	No.	%	No.	%	No.	%	No.	%
Partial regression	4	12	3	7	0		7	6
Stable	8	24	16	39	7	19	31	28
Progression	21	64	22	54	29	81	72	65
Total	33		41[a]		36		110	

[a]Response significantly different from the standard arm.

A second NPCP trial (Protocol 200) was developed for patients with bone marrow reserves compromised by previous pelvic irradiation ($\geq 2,000$ rads). For this trial, conducted from July 1974 to March 1976, agents were selected for their low myelosuppressive side effects and consisted of estramustine phosphate (Estracyt) and streptozotocin, each to be contrasted with a standard arm as in the first trial [5]. The results of this trial (Table II) were not as pronounced as those in the first trial, but the chemotherapy arms continued to show better results than did the standard arm. Estracyt was selected as the reference agent in such subsequent trials based on the presence of the only partial regressions, longer responses, and proportion with weight gain. Except for nausea and vomiting the side effects were minimal [13].

At this time the NPCP has completed six protocols for patients (796) with advanced hormone refractory disease; three for nonirradiated and three for irradiated patients. Two more such studies are well underway. Estracyt appears to show some potential in nonirradiated patients, and in irradiated patients the combination of Estracyt and DDP shows promise.

For the nonirradiated patients, Cytoxan remains a drug of choice at this time with acceptable activity (circ 25% + response rate) observed for 5-FU and DTIC [12,14]. Two other agents, procarbazine and methylCCNU, showed similar activity, but this was offset by excessive toxic side effects [12,14]. Minimal activity was observed for hydroxyurea [16].

For irradiated patients, Estracyt remains a drug of choice at this time, followed by streptozotocin [13]. Other agents tested in this group with minimal activity include prednimustine alone or in combination with Estracyt or vincristine [15,17]. Vincristine in combination with Estracyt was no better than Estracyt alone [17].

Other clinical trials in the NPCP program include a trial for newly diagnosed, previously untreated patients with stage D_2 disease, of which one trial (Protocol

TABLE II. Objective response for previously irradiated patients randomized to Estracyt, streptozotocin, or standard therapy

| | Treatment | | | | | | | |
| | Estracyt | | Strepto-zotocin | | Standard | | Total | |
Response	No.	%	No.	%	No.	%	No.	%
Partial regression	3	6	0		0		3	3
Stable	11	24	12	32	4	19	27	26
Progression	32	70	26	68	17	81	75	71
Total	46		38		21		105	

500) has been closed to entry with 301 patients and a successor (Protocol 1300) is underway. In this type of trial, hormone treatment, DES, or orchiectomy in both of these trials were compared with a combination of hormones and antineoplastic chemotherapy.

Another type of trial conducted by the NPCP is for patients with stage D_2 disease that has been stabilized by hormones (Protocol 600). These patients are either continued on hormones (DES) or given a combination of hormones and antineoplastic chemotherapy (DES + Cytoxan or Estracyt). Preliminary results in both Protocols 500 and 600 are beginning to suggest that giving chemotherapy earlier and in combination with hormones may have an advantage over waiting until the disease no longer is clinically responsive to hormones.

The possibility that even earlier administration of chemotherapy as adjuvant to definitive surgery or radiotherapy for localized stages B_2 thru D_1 would prevent recurrence of the disease altogether, is under test by the NPCP in Protocols 900 and 1000, respectively. Estracyt or Cytoxan are being administered on a long-term basis for up to two years and possibly more and are being compared with a third treatment arm that receives only the definitive treatment. Recurring disease is an end point for response. Both recurrence rates and disease-free intervals will be used to evaluate the benefits of these treatments.

This extensive program of clinical trials by the NPCP maintains six active protocols that encompass most types of patients with disease staged B_2 through D_2. Only the very early disease, stages A_1–B_1 are not being treated. To date seven studies have been completed and over 1,700 patients have been entered, making this by far the largest group dealing with prostatic cancer.

The ECOG clinical trial, comparing adriamycin and 5-FU, was terminated in February, 1978, and concluded that adriamycin was a superior agent. One third of the entries at the end of the study were assigned to adriamycin because of the low response experience with 5-FU [8]. This does not agree with the relatively favorable experience with 5-FU in the first NPCP trial. Moreover, the patient population in the two studies appears to vary considerably, with the ECOG study including patients with extensive prior radiotherapy and non-osseous metastases of a critical organ, eg, liver [8,12]. These patients, in our experience, are in a much later phase of their disease than those seen and treated by the NPCP [10].

Several other cooperative groups have relatively large clinical trials in operation. Chemotherapy trials of a smaller nature have been conducted by a number of individual institutions, but these are both too numerous to mention here and are better covered under a general discussion of chemotherapy, for which reference may be made to recent reviews by Torti and Carter [18] and by Schmidt [19].

A cooperative trial of relatively small size (27 patients) was conducted by the Western Cancer Study Group (WCSG) to compare Cytoxan with this agent in combination with 5-FU and adriamycin and found the single agent to be as effective as the combination [20]. This group apparently using the NPCP response criteria observed stable patients to have significantly longer survival than patients with progressing disease, but only in the single agent group [20].

CONCLUSION

The history of cooperative clinical trials in prostate cancer has been reviewed and the current work underway in these programs is also reported. Whereas these cooperative programs are not inexpensive or short-term endeavors, they are able to obtain data that is more reliable than that obtained from individual studies and can do it in a shorter time period. Because most cooperative studies are prospective and randomized as opposed to the usually nonrandomized and often retrospective studies of individual centers, their findings are more readily accepted by the practicing physicians, the general medical profession, and government regulatory agencies.

By nature of the size and organization of a cooperative clinical trial it is possible to conduct ancillary studies that can include pathology, tumor markers, and factors influencing disease history and etiology, prognosis, and response, all to the eventual benefit of the patient. We feel the National Prostatic Cancer Project is currently fulfilling these goals.

REFERENCES

1. Brendler H, Prout G Jr: A cooperative group study of prostatic cancer: Stilbestrol versus placebo in advanced progressive disease. Cancer Chemother Rep 16:323–328, 1962.
2. Byar DP: The Veterans Administration Cooperative Urological Research Group's studies of cancer of the prostate. Cancer 32:1126–1130, 1973.
3. Byar DP: Review of the Veterans Administration studies of cancer of the prostate and new results concerning treatment of stage I and II tumors. In Pavone-Macaluso M, Smith PH, Edsymr F (eds): "Bladder Tumors and Other Topics in Urological Oncology." New York: Plenum Publishing, pp 471–492, 1980.
4. Byar DP, Simon RM, Friedwald WT, Schlesselman JJ, DeMets DL, Ellenberg JH, Gail MH, Ware JH: Randomized clinical trials: Perspectives on some recent ideas. N Engl J Med 295:74–80, 1976.
5. Schmidt JD, Scott WW, Gibbons RP, Johnson DE, Prout GR Jr, Loening SA, Soloway MS, deKernion JB, Pontes JE, Slack NH, Murphy GP: Chemotherapy programs of the National Prostatic Cancer Project (NPCP). Cancer 45:1937–1946, 1980.
6. Berger M, Buu-Hoi NP: Treatment of prostatic cancer with α-bromo-α.B.B-triphenylethylene (Y59). Lancet 2:172, 1947.
7. Schmidt JD: Chemotherapy of hormone-resistant stage-D prostate cancer. J Urol 123:797–805, 1980.
8. DeWys WD, Begg CB: Comparison of adriamycin (ADRIA) and 5-Fluorouracil (5-FU) in advanced prostatic cancer. Proc Am Assoc Cancer Res 19:331, 1978.
9. Schmidt JD, Johnson DE, Scott WW, Gibbons RP, Prout GR Jr, Murphy GP: Chemotherapy of advanced prostatic cancer, evaluation of response parameters. Urology 7:602–610, 1976.
10. Schmidt JD: Chemotherapy of prostatic cancer. Urol Clin N Am 2:185–196, 1975.

11. Slack NH, Mittelman A, Brady MF, Murphy GP, Investigators in the National Prostatic Cancer Project: The importance of the stable category for chemotherapy treated patients with advanced and relapsing prostate cancer. Cancer 46:2393–2402, 1980.
12. Scott WW, Gibbons RP, Johnson DE, Prout GR Jr, Schmidt JD, Saroff J, Murphy GP: The continued evaluation of the effects of chemotherapy in patients with advanced carcinoma of the prostate. J Urol 116:211–213, 1976.
13. Murphy GP, Gibbons RP, Johnson DE, Loening SA, Prout GR Jr, Schmidt JD, Bross DS, Chu TM, Gaeta JF, Saroff J, Scott WW: A comparison of estramustine phosphate and streptozotocin in patients with advanced prostatic carcinoma who have had extensive irradiation. J Urol 118:288–291, 1977.
14. Schmidt JD, Scott WW, Gibbons RP, Johnson DE, Prout GR Jr, Loening SA, Soloway MS, Chu TM, Gaeta JF, Slack NH, Saroff J, Murphy GP: Comparison of procarbazine, imidazol-carboxamide and cyclophosphamide in relapsing patients with advanced carcinoma of the prostate. J Urol 125:185–189, 1979.
15. Murphy GP, Gibbons RP, Johnson DE, Prout GR Jr, Schmidt JD, Soloway MS, Loening SA, Chu TM, Gaeta JF, Saroff J, Wajsman Z, Slack NH, Scott WW: The use of estramustine and prednimustine versus prednimustine alone in advanced metastatic prostatic cancer patients who have received prior irradiation. J Urol 121:763–765, 1979.
16. Loening SA, Scott WW, deKernion J, Gibbons RP, Johnson DE, Pontes JE, Prout GR Jr, Schmidt JD, Soloway MS, Chu TM, Gaeta JF, Slack NH, Murphy GP: A comparison of hydroxyurea, methylCCNU and cyclophosphamide in patients with advanced carcinoma of the prostate. J Urol 1981 (in press).
17. Soloway MS, deKernion JB, Gibbons RP, Johnson DE, Pontes JE, Prout GR Jr, Schmidt JD, Scott WW, Chu TM, Gaeta JF, Slack NH, Murphy GP: Comparison of estracyt and vincristine alone or in combination for patients with advanced, hormone refractory, previously irradiated carcinoma of the prostate. J Urol 125:664–667, 1981.
18. Torti FM, Carter SK: The chemotherapy of prostatic adenocarcinoma. Ann Intern Med 92:681–689, 1980.
19. Schmidt JD: Chemotherapy of hormone-resistant Stage D prostatic cancer. J Urol 123:797–805, 1980.
20. Chlebowski RT, Hestorff R, Sardoff L, Weiner J, Bateman JR: Cyclophosphamide (NSC 26271) versus the combination of adriamycin (NSC 123127), 5-Fluorouracil (NSC 19893), and cyclophosphamide in the treatment of metastatic prostatic cancer. Cancer 42:2546–2552, 1978.

Index

Acid phosphatase, 232, 235, 241,
    244–45, 246–47, 336
Adrenal gland, 33, 58
Ames' test, 200, 203
Androgen receptor, 299–310, 323–24
Androgens and
    canine prostatic epithelium, 235–41,
        245–47
    prolactin, 75–76, 115
    prostatic disease, 33
    prostatic growth, 63
Anti-androgen, 245–46
Aryl hydrocarbon hydroxylase, 183–89,
    191, 193, 202

Benign prostatic hyperplasia, 64, 70,
    98–99, 116, 299, 301–2, 304–5, 308
    and growth hormone, 126–27
    and immunocytochemical techniques,
        122, 125
    and prolactin, 118–20, 127
    and prostatic epithelium, 184, 188
Biopsy, needle, 300, 304–10
B nodule, 336
Bombesin, 27
Breast tumor, 313–15, 321–22, 325

Cancer. *See* Prostate cancer; Tumors
Carcinogens
    chemical, 131–62
    and prostate, 183–89
Castration, 210, 222, 245
Cell
    damage, 329–34
    multiplication, 78–79
    surface markers, 216
Chemical(s)
    carcinogenic, 131–62
    insecticides, 165–79
    and prostate, 131–62

Chemotherapy, 251–53, 341–45
Chlorinated insecticides, 165–79
Concanavalin A-horseradish peroxidase,
    209–10, 219, 221
Cytochrome P-450, 191–204

DDT, 165, 176–79
Dieldrin, 166, 170–79
Diethylstilboestrol, 35, 37–40
Dihydrotestosterone, 279
    and dieldrin, 170–79
    in dog prostate, 247
    and prolactin, 72, 79
    and prostatic cancer, 283
    receptors, 11–12, 14–16
Dimethylbenz(a)anthracene, 183–89
Disease, localized, 335–38
DNA, 279
    binding, 183–89
    and prostate gland growth, 11–12,
        14–16
    synthesis, and insulin, 67–68
    synthesis, and prolactin, 72, 79
Dog
    cystopreputiosomies, 167–70
    prostate, 133, 135–36, 139–42,
        144–46, 148–52, 158–59, 162
    prostatic epithelium, 231–47
Dopamine, 20–27

Endocrine therapy, 299–300, 304
Endocrinology, 31–32
Enzyme
    induction, 192, 202–4
    irreversible inhibitors, 284–85, 290–95
    lysosomal, 208
    and metastasis, 253–55
    see also Specific enzymes
Epithelium
    canine prostatic, 231–47

347

PROGRESS IN CLINICAL AND BIOLOGICAL RESEARCH

Series Editors   Vincent P. Eijsvoogel   Seymour S. Kety
Nathan Back   Robert Grover   Sidney Udenfriend
George J. Brewer   Kurt Hirschhorn   Jonathan W. Uhr

Published in 3 Volumes:
Part A: Psychology and Methodology
Part B: Biology and Epidemiology
Part C: Clinical Studies